OVERTREATED

OVERTREATED

Why Too Much Medicine Is Making Us
Sicker and Poorer

Shannon Brownlee

BLOOMSBURY

Published by Bloomsbury USA, New York
Distributed to the trade by Holtzbrinck Publishers

All papers used by Bloomsbury USA are natural, recyclable products made from wood grown in well-managed forests. The manufacturing processes conform to the environmental regulations of the country of origin.

LIBRARY OF CONGRESS CATALOGING-IN-PUBLICATION DATA

Brownlee, Shannon.
    Overtreated : why too much medicine is making us sicker and poorer / Shannon Brownlee.—1st U.S. ed.
        p. cm.
    ISBN-13: 978-1-58234-580-2
    ISBN-10: 1-58234-580-5
    1. Medical care—United States.   2. Medical care—Utilization—United States.
I. Title.

    RA395.A3B785 2007
    362.10973—dc22

                                                                    2007021968

First U.S. Edition 2007

1 3 5 7 9 10 8 6 4 2

Typeset by Westchester Book Group
Printed in the United States of America by Quebecor World Fairfield

For my parents:

Joan Carroll
Mick Brownlee
Phyllis Brownlee

CONTENTS

INTRODUCTION

WHY CAN'T THE United States seem to fix its health care system? Today, forty-seven million Americans, or one in six under age sixty-five, have no health insurance. Two million of them are veterans who have been denied access to VA hospitals either because they earn more than twenty-five thousand dollars a year or because their condition is not service related. Huge and unpayable medical bills have become the leading cause of personal bankruptcy. Uninsured cancer patients receive half as much care as the insured and may be more likely to die, depending upon the type of cancer. Uninsured car crash victims receive less care in the hospital and have a higher mortality rate than the insured. Women who lack insurance don't get regular Pap smears to check for cervical cancer. Children who are uninsured go without routine vaccinations; those with asthma don't get preventive treatment. In early 2007, a twelve-year-old boy named Deamonte Driver died in a hospital in Washington, D.C., from a brain infection that began as a rotten tooth. His single mother had been trying for weeks to find a dentist willing to take Medicaid payments to care for her two sons. Then the family lost its Medicaid coverage and Deamonte died, because his mother couldn't afford to pay for an $80 extraction. His brain infection cost the District of Columbia $250,000. The Institute of Medicine recently estimated that about eighteen thousand Americans die prematurely each year, simply because they lack health insurance.

It's not as if we haven't tried to fix the system—several times, in fact, over the past century, first in World War I, then again during the Great Depression

1

and the Truman and Eisenhower administrations. Attempt number five was in the 1960s, when Medicare passed—despite vehement opposition from the American Medical Association. Doctors viewed Medicare as the first step on the path toward socialized medicine, which they feared would lead to a loss of income. The most recent effort to reform health care came during the Clinton administration, and foundered in part because of Harry and Louise, characters who appeared in television ads paid for by the insurance industry. The ads scared Americans into thinking that covering the uninsured would mean the rest of us would lose some of our coverage, in order to pay for all those new bodies coming into the system. Most of us feel sorry for the uninsured, but we want no part of a plan that involves rationing.

Instead, we've decided to put up with an unfair, dysfunctional, and spectacularly expensive system. In 2006, we spent an estimated $2.1 trillion on health care. That's almost as much as the worldwide market for petroleum, and more than the United States spends on food. We spend more per capita on health care than the Chinese spend, per capita, on everything. Looking to the future, the Centers for Medicare and Medicaid Services predicts annual health care costs will hit $4.1 trillion by 2016, eating up nearly 20 percent of our gross domestic product. We currently spend nearly $6,000 apiece on health care, two and a half times the median for the rest of the industrialized world.

What do we get for our money? Politicians are constantly telling us we have the best health care in the world, but that's simply not the case. By every conceivable measure, the health of Americans lags behind the health of citizens in other developed countries, starting with life expectancy. In 2001, U.S. life expectancy at birth was seventy-seven years, which put us a few months ahead of Cyprus, Costa Rica, and Chile but years behind Canada, Japan, and Western Europe. We rank twenty-eighth in the world on infant mortality rates, behind Cuba, the Czech Republic, and the United Kingdom, countries that ought to be beating us at soccer, not health. We are no less disabled by disease than citizens of most developed nations, and our medical care is, with few exceptions, no better at helping us survive specific diseases. A recent study of heart attack patients found that Canadians did just as well as American patients—though many Americans consider Canadian health care, which provides fewer expensive, invasive procedures, to be an inferior system.

Why, then, is our health care so astronomically expensive? Conventional wisdom says our system is expensive precisely because we don't ration care. Unlike the citizens of Canada and the United Kingdom, we don't have to wait months for elective surgery or an MRI. But when economists from the Johns Hopkins Bloomberg School of Public Health looked at the fifteen procedures and tests that account for the majority of waiting lists in other countries, they found that those procedures and tests amounted to just 3 percent of costs in the United States, not nearly enough to explain the huge difference in spending.

Many doctors believe malpractice is the culprit, that their worries about lawsuits drive them to practice defensive medicine. Other physicians place the blame on greedy insurance executives and the wasteful bureaucracy they have created with their multiple plans, each of which covers a different set of treatments and pays a different amount for the same treatment. We devote nearly a third of our health care spending to administrative costs—paper pushing, in effect. In 1999, that amounted to $1,000 per capita. Canada's single-payer system, by contrast, was a model of efficiency, spending only about 16 percent of its health care dollars on administrative overhead, which means our system wasted nearly $160 billion. Then there's the $30 billion in after-tax profits earned by health insurance companies. As economist Henry J. Aaron puts it, "I look at the U.S. health care system and see an administrative monstrosity, a truly bizarre mélange of thousands of different payers with payment systems that differ for no socially beneficial reason."

Other health care economists point to "moral hazard," the term they use to suggest that being insured changes the behavior of patients. The moral hazard argument says that because people don't pay out of pocket, they use more health care than they really need. If employers offered their employees vouchers for sports cars, goes the argument, or the government provided universal sports car coverage, we'd all have a little roadster sitting in the garage. Moral hazard says we go to the doctor when we don't really need to; we insist on getting CT scanned for a twisted ankle when ice and an Ace bandage will do; and we demand prescriptions for expensive brand-name drugs we see advertised on TV when a cheap, over-the-counter remedy is more than enough—all because somebody else is paying for it. The concept of moral hazard lies behind the recent enthusiasm for the latest "cure" being prescribed for American health care: health savings accounts. These are low-cost, high-deductible plans that ask patients to pay for the first few thousand dollars of health care out of their pockets before the plan begins picking up the tab. Books like Harvard Business School professor Regina Herzlinger's *Market-Driven Health Care* and a recent presidential report emphasize the need for Americans to have some "skin in the game" in order to become more-prudent consumers of health care.

Some policy analysts argue that American health care costs a lot because prices are higher here than they are in other countries. We pay dearly for innovation, for new technology like cardiac stents and surgical robots and faster CT scanners. We also pay more than other countries for everything from malpractice to drugs to doctors. In a famous paper titled "It's the Price, Stupid," three health care policy analysts and an economist point out that the number of doctors per capita is lower in the United States than the median number in the rest of the developed world, but our doctors have much higher incomes. The average American specialist earns $274,000 a year, and the average general practitioner makes $173,000, amounts that are, respectively, 6.6 and 4.2 times the income of the average patient. The rates in other countries average out to 4 and 3.2. U.S. doctors make so much more than physicians in the rest of the world not so much because they charge more, but because of the volume of services they deliver, the large number of colonoscopies, for example, hip replacements, and office visits. When it comes to hospital and drug costs, on the other hand, the culprit is higher prices. The average cost per day in a U.S. hospital is $1,666, four times the average in the rest of the developed world.

However, while all of these factors—wasteful bureaucratic overhead, malpractice, moral hazard, and high prices—contribute to the high cost of American medicine, throughout the political debate over our health care mess, the most important piece of the puzzle has been consistently overlooked. There's one more factor that contributes to our medical bills, and that's unnecessary care. We spend between one fifth and one third of our health care dollars, an exorbitant amount of money, between five hundred and seven hundred billion dollars (that's billion, with a b), on care that does nothing to improve our health. And while overhead and high prices hurt our pocketbooks, the vast amount of unnecessary care in the system also makes our health care worse than it ought to be. Unnecessary treatment and tests aren't just expensive; they also can harm patients. And unnecessary care is exacerbating in myriad ways the poor quality of American health care—and American health.

The idea that a third of the medicine we receive is unnecessary is undoubtedly hard for many people to believe. Practically everything in our personal interactions with the health care system tells us that far from getting too much care, we're getting too little. If you're like most Americans, everybody from your primary care physician to your insurance company seems bent on denying you the care you think you really need. When you go to the doctor's office feeling sick, you spend time cooling your heels first in the waiting room and then again, sitting in a flimsy paper gown, on an examining table. Finally the doctor rushes in, pausing only long enough to ask a series of questions on a checklist before dashing out again to see the next patient. If the doctor refers you to a specialist, getting an appointment takes weeks. If the doctor prescribes a drug, your insurer refuses to pay for it. Where's the unnecessary care in all of this? There wasn't any unnecessary care when Deamonte Driver's mother tried to find a dentist who would pull out her son's abscessed tooth.

The notion that we are getting too much treatment is made all the more difficult to grasp by the soaring achievements of twentieth-century medicine. The eradication of smallpox, the polio vaccine, organ transplantation, penicillin, the ability to control asthma and surgically correct defects in an infant's plum-sized heart, and all the other milestones in medical science gave us a sense of medicine's power and beauty; they imbued the century with a feeling of hope. Medicine seemed to lift us from the sordid, bloody brutishness of injury and disease that was an inescapable part of life for most of human history. It made us imagine that as medical science progressed, everything was becoming possible—long life, no suffering, no crippling disease—eventually creating the fantasy that we could thwart even death. Today, Americans believe devoutly in the power of medicine not only to heal but to cure. In surveys conducted by a group of Harvard researchers, 34 percent of respondents said they believed that modern medicine "can cure almost any illness for people who have access to the most advanced technologies and treatments." "We are the new priesthood," says Stephen Baker, one of the doctors you'll meet in this book. "The myth we are peddling is not everlasting life in heaven, but everlasting life here on earth."

Against this backdrop, it's hard to imagine unnecessary care, and it is also often difficult to measure it, but it happens in big and small ways. Each year, Americans undergo millions of tests—MRIs, CT scans, blood tests—that do little to help doctors diagnose disease, and that sometimes lead them to find and treat conditions that would never have bothered their patients had they never been found. We undergo back surgery for pain in the absence of evidence that the surgery works, and while some patients improve, others are left in far worse shape—making surgery a crapshoot. Patients contract lethal infections while in the hospital for elective procedures. They suffer strokes when they undergo a surgery that, ironically, is intended to prevent stroke. Unnecessary treatment, or "overtreatment" in medical parlance, increases the chaos level in hospitals. It leads to unnecessary suffering. And it is killing people. One estimate puts the number of deaths due to unnecessary care at thirty thousand Americans a year. That's the equivalent of a 747 airliner crashing and killing everyone aboard at least once a week. It's hard to imagine the airline industry being permitted to kill thirty thousand people a year. If overtreatment were a disease, there would be a patient advocacy group out there raising money for a cure.

Unnecessary care also makes medical errors more likely, because the higher the volume of care you receive, the greater the odds are that somebody, somewhere, will make a mistake. In its 1999 report *To Err Is Human*, the Institute of Medicine estimated that as many as ninety-eight thousand Americans are killed each year by medical error. Another ninety thousand to four hundred thousand patients are harmed or killed by the incorrect use of a drug—they received the wrong drug, or the wrong dose of the right drug, or two drugs that interacted in the wrong way. A friend of mine was hospitalized recently with a condition that caused her to be partially paralyzed temporarily from the chest down. She also suffers from another disorder that prevents her blood from clotting, a condition that was clearly noted in her chart. Yet one day she had to stop a nurse from giving her an injection of a drug intended to prevent clotting in patients who are immobilized in bed for long periods of time. Not only would giving my friend the drug have been useless, but it could have caused her to bleed internally had she fallen out of bed or while trying to get to the bathroom.

Hospitals are rife with such confusion. In the introduction to his book *Best Care Anywhere: Why VA Health Care Is Better than Yours*, my friend and colleague Phillip Longman tells the story of his wife Robin's treatment after being diagnosed for breast cancer, and how the problems of American health care suddenly became more than an abstraction to them. Robin was treated at the prestigious Lombardi Comprehensive Cancer Center, which is part of Georgetown University Hospital, in Washington, D.C. The couple, writes Phillip, "felt blessed that our gold-plated health insurance allowed us unfettered access to all the doctors and specialists we would care to see." But during the ten months that elapsed between the time Robin was diagnosed and her death, the couple saw firsthand how poorly even one of the most respected hospitals could handle care, beginning with the fact that Phillip found himself having to explain to his distraught wife why he hadn't been in the post-op recovery room to comfort her after her lumpectomy. The reason was that nobody in the hospital could tell him where his wife was located.

The Longmans' experience is far from unique. In most hospitals, patient records are routinely kept in multiple places, with CT scans and X-rays in one department and medical records in another. During handoffs of patients between one shift of nurses and the next, or when patients move between floors, critical information is regularly lost. Sometimes it seems, as in my friend's case, as if nurses and doctors don't even read a patient's chart before deciding how to treat them. Home Depot does a better job of tracking a box of nails than your local hospital does in tracking you, the patient.

Later, the Longmans discovered how little the various specialists involved in Robin's case seemed to consult with one another. In one emotionally devastating meeting, Phillip writes,

The discussion began with various members of Robin's "team" optimistically discussing her prospects for reconstructive surgery. Robin and I were both thrilled that the lumpectomy was an apparent success and that her chemotherapy seemed to be working to contain the cancer. But well into the meeting, one doctor began to fidget, finally asking if anyone had looked at the results of a recent liver scan. The team quickly departed, leaving Robin and me in an empty examining room for 30 or 40 minutes. Eventually, a grim faced oncologist returned. The cancer had metastasized to her liver. It looked as if she was terminal.

Robin's doctors would subsequently press her to try a bone marrow transplant, an expensive last-ditch treatment for breast cancer that was popular throughout the 1980s and '90s, despite the fact that it put the patient through a ghastly, monthlong ordeal that proved more deadly than the cancer for many women. The Longmans instinctively resisted her doctors. Later, after she died, clinical trials would finally show that bone marrow transplants are no more effective than standard treatment for breast cancer.

Why do doctors and hospitals deliver so much unnecessary care? There are many reasons. Doctors lack the evidence they need to know which treatments are most effective and which drugs and devices really work. They also lack the training to interpret the quality of evidence that's available. They overtreat patients out of a desire to help even when they don't know the right thing to do. Malpractice fears drive defensive medicine, and then there is medical custom, which varies from region to region of the United States. But the most powerful reason doctors and hospitals overtreat is that most of them are paid for how much care they deliver, not how well they care for their patients. They get paid more for doing more. This simple fact has led not only to overtreatment but also to the profound disorder of the American health care system. Modern medicine is a team sport, requiring coordination between primary care doctors, specialists, and hospitals. This is especially true when it comes to caring for patients with chronic diseases, like asthma, heart failure, and diabetes. But in this country, medicine is still practiced much as it was fifty years ago—a time of fewer specialists and less technology. We've never structured the delivery system to ensure that patients get all of the treatments and procedures they need and aren't subjected to care they don't. One doctor often doesn't know that another physician has already ordered a battery of tests, or that they have both prescribed two different drugs that do the same thing. They often don't know how drugs will interact. The simplest treatments often fall through the cracks—making sure a patient knows how to use an asthma inhaler, for instance. And when doctors and hospitals try to deliver the right kind of care, such as keeping track of a heart failure patient's weight gain to make sure he or she doesn't land right back in the hospital, they lose money.

Overtreated is an exploration of three simple questions. What drives unnecessary care? Why should we worry about it? And once we understand how pervasive it is in American medicine, how can we use that knowledge to create a better system? I became interested in this topic while on staff at U.S. News & World Report, where I wrote about the latest medical breakthroughs and cutting-edge research. Like most Americans, and most medical journalists, I viewed medicine as an "epic of progress," as sociologist Paul Starr puts it, an unbroken string of discoveries, each of which improved medical care. That is, until 1999, when I began researching the breast cancer treatment known as high-dose chemotherapy with bone marrow transplant, the treatment Robin Longman's doctors wanted her to try. Brutal, dangerous, and extravagantly expensive, the treatment was nonetheless touted by oncologists—and by my colleagues in the press—as a cure for advanced breast cancer. More than forty thousand women would receive it over the years, and nine thousand of them would die from it, before a series of clinical trials finally showed in 1999 that it was no better than standard treatment. As I dug more deeply into the history of high-dose chemotherapy, I learned that medicine was often driven more by money than by science, and that many of the "cures" that we in the press wrote about over the years didn't pan out when—and if—they were actually put to a test. I also began to wonder about the connections between the lack of good science behind a lot of medicine and our health care system. Why was American health care so much more expensive per capita than health care in other industrialized countries, and getting pricier by the year? And why were our health statistics so much worse?

In running down these questions, it became clear to me that the lack of rigorous science and evidence was just one of many factors that lead physicians and hospitals to deliver care that doesn't improve health. I also discovered along the way that most of the solutions to our various health care crises—consumer-driven care, malpractice reform, universal coverage, pay for performance, electronic medical records—only nibble around the edges of fixing the system. None of them can remedy the poor quality of American health care unless we simultaneously address the issue of overtreatment.

Yet in politics, overtreatment is routinely left out of any discussion of health care reform. That's partly because getting rid of it smacks of rationing. But rationing is when you deny patients care that could potentially help them. Rationing is when you say to a patient with kidney failure that he can't have dialysis because dialysis is expensive and he's too old. Rationing is when you limit the number of MRI machines in order to discourage doctors from ordering an MRI test for a patient. But getting rid of overtreatment, care that's useless and potentially harmful? That isn't rationing; that's improving the quality of medicine.

The issue of overtreatment also gets short shrift in political discussions about health care because it's difficult to point to individual patients whom it has harmed. We tend to reform systems in this country in response to highly publicized tragedies, stories about real people. Amendments strengthening the Food, Drug, and Cosmetics Act were passed in 1962 in the wake of thalidomide, the drug that caused devastating birth defects when it was given to pregnant women. A series of midair collisions prompted the passage of the Federal Aviation Act twenty years later. Today, heart-wrenching stories like that of Deamonte Driver are helping focus the nation's attention once again on the plight of the uninsured. One state, Massachusetts, has already passed legislation aimed at insuring all residents. Others are considering similar proposals. As the 2008 presidential campaign began heating up in early 2007, there were signs that the richest country in the world was preparing, maybe once and for all, to find the eighty billion dollars a year that's needed to cover every last one of its citizens.

Thus far, however, the candidates have been notably vague about the other major problem in health care—soaring costs. Maybe that's because talking about costs means talking about overtreatment, and bringing up overtreatment means facing the fact that reducing unnecessary, wasteful care would lead inevitably to a smaller health care industry. The seven hundred billion dollars we currently spend on unnecessary care doesn't just go down the drain—it goes toward paying for drugs and medical devices, which are manufactured by American workers. It helps pay the salaries of doctors, hospital administrators, nurses, orderlies, and pharmacists. It covers part of the cost of hospital beds and the construction of new hospital wings, which are built by American construction workers. It helps support the insurance industry and the salaries of all the clerks who shuffle those mountains of paperwork. Think for a moment what it would mean to eliminate this wasteful, unnecessary care. Getting rid of seven hundred billion dollars' worth of useless medical care is roughly the equivalent of wiping out the entire U.S. high-tech industry, including all the jobs it provides and the money it makes for shareholders.

Hospitals, nurses, specialists, and all of the industries that produce medical goods have a vested interest in maintaining the status quo; they don't want to see health care shrink. Drug companies don't want doctors to write fewer prescriptions, and latex glove manufacturers don't want cardiologists to perform fewer angioplasties. And nobody would want to put thousands of people who are currently employed by the health care industry out of a job, unless it was absolutely necessary. But it is necessary, because the alternative to rightsizing health care is worse. Some economists, notably Harvard's David Cutler, claim that we should stop worrying so much about rising costs, that we can afford to spend 20 percent of the gross domestic product on health care, because there's so much "good stuff," as he puts it, to be gained from medicine. Besides, says Cutler, it's too hard to get rid of the bad stuff. But American businesses are already staggering under the burden of paying for health insurance. They will become increasingly less competitive in a world market as they pay more and more for care that does less and less to improve the health of their workers. For the economy as a whole, wasting seven hundred billion dollars on useless care represents an enormous opportunity cost.

Solving the problem of the uninsured requires a solution to our mounting national medical bill, and we can only get a grip on costs by facing overtreatment head-on. Doing so will lead to improvements in health care that go beyond the ability to provide access to everyone. It will guarantee that all Americans, including those of us who are already insured, won't simply get more medicine; we'll get better medicine.

ONE Too Much Medicine

JOHN E. WENNBERG is one of the heroes of modern medicine, but not because he discovered a new treatment or invented a lifesaving medical device. His career spans American medicine's shift from a collection of solo practitioners at midcentury to one of the largest single industries in the world, and his life is a parable for both the power of individual doctors to heal the sick and the capacity of medicine to cause harm. At the heart of the story is New England, where he has spent the better part of his adult life, and where doctors in small towns in Vermont, New Hampshire, and Maine showed him that more medicine is not necessarily the best way to improve America's health.

Wennberg, who goes by Jack, lives in Hanover, New Hampshire, just a few miles down the road from Dartmouth Medical School, where he has been a professor for thirty years. He is both a physician and a Ph.D. in public health. Above the fireplace in his living room hangs a photograph of him as a small boy, bundled in a heavy jacket, with short wooden skis strapped with leather bindings to his feet. Peeking out from under a woolen cap with flaps over his ears, Wennberg smiles shyly for the camera—his head enormous on his little boy's body. The photo was taken in 1937, on the slopes near his hometown of Bellows Falls, Vermont, where his father managed the paper mill. A Norwegian immigrant, the elder Wennberg made his son read the plays of the great Norwegian writer Henrik Ibsen. The family snowshoed and skied in the long New England winters; Wennberg fished in the summers. When he was ten years old, the family moved to Vancouver,

Washington, a raw Western mill town in the shadow of Mount Saint Helens. Wennberg spent his summers at Spirit Lake, on the flanks of the volcano, fishing and working at a YMCA camp. In the winters, as a teenager, he served on the ski patrol on Mount Hood. Although Wennberg excelled in science and math, he graduated from Stanford in 1956 with a degree in literature, intending to get his Ph.D. in German literature and teach. But when it came time to read the Bible in Gothic, Wennberg realized he was more interested in science than words. By the time he graduated from McGill University Faculty of Medicine in Montreal, in 1961, he had grown into a handsome man of middling height, with wavy dark hair covering his large head, broad shoulders, and a heavy jaw. He had also met his first wife, Emma Ottolenghi, who was also a medical student at McGill, and they had their first child, David, the year Wennberg graduated.

In 1962, the family moved to Baltimore, where Wennberg had won a prestigious residency at Johns Hopkins, long one of the premier academic medical centers in the country. He thought he wanted to study the kidney, with its microscopic tubules that maintain a perfect balance of fluids and salts in the blood, but he was a terrible experimentalist. "I wasn't good at pipetteing and the careful work and the clean desks," he would later say. At Hopkins, he split his time between the dialysis ward and classes in epidemiology. The Wennbergs' third child, Diana, was born at Johns Hopkins with what at first appeared to be pyloric stenosis, a defect in the muscular valve that sits at the bottom of the stomach. Because they can't pass food from the stomach to the small intestine, babies with pyloric stenosis vomit everything they eat. Surgery introduced in the early twentieth century had transformed pyloric stenosis from an almost invariably fatal condition into a curable disorder. But when Diana's surgeon, Jacob Handelsman, known as "Jake the Snake" for reasons that have been lost over time, cut open the Wennberg baby's tiny abdomen, he found her pyloric valve was normal; her vomiting was completely inexplicable. Handelsman refused to give up. Over the course of two more operations, he realized her small intestine was missing a layer of muscle, and he invented a way to bypass the defective section of her gut, giving her the ability to pass food in the right direction. When she needed a transfusion during the third surgery, one of Wennberg's fellow residents whose blood type matched Diana's gave her a transfusion directly from his own vein. Wennberg never forgot the kindness of the doctors at Johns Hopkins, or the miracle of his daughter's cure.

The heroic surgery was also tangible evidence for Wennberg of the transformation that had taken place in modern medicine over the previous four decades. The discovery of penicillin meant that by the 1940s patients no longer had to die from infected wounds or a burst appendix, and that abdominal surgery no longer had to be a life-threatening ordeal. The discovery of high-blood-pressure medication prevented strokes, while cortisone transformed the treatment of several illnesses, including Addison's disease, the disorder that afflicted President John F. Kennedy. Without regular cortisone shots, Kennedy would never have been able to serve as president. Routine vaccination for polio, smallpox, and whooping cough meant that losing a child to infectious disease was no longer the norm but a rarity. Hospitals were no longer simply warehouses for the sick and dying, where little more than comfort could be offered; they had become factories whose product was miracles—"gleaming palaces of medical science," as sociologist Paul Starr puts it, where doctors were in the midst of pioneering work that would soon allow them to mend damaged hearts with open-heart surgery, transplant organs, and routinely postpone death with kidney dialysis.

After America's victory in World War II, which was won in part by the invention of such technologies as radar, sonar, and, of course, the atomic bomb, all of science assumed a symbolic as well as practical role in helping shape America's destiny as leader of the free world. Supporting scientific research became a responsibility of government, while American technological know-how—along with the destruction of Europe's economies during World War II—allowed American factories to produce more than half the world's goods, and 80 percent of its automobiles. Medical research held a special place in the scientific pantheon. Americans literally rejoiced in the streets at the news that Jonas Salk had created a vaccine for polio. By 1960, the insecticide DDT had eradicated malaria from the United States, along with yellow fever. Dysentery, typhus, and tetanus were now preventable with vaccines; pneumonia and meningitis could be cured with antibiotics. Newsmagazines ran weekly reports on medicine under hopeful headlines:

"Machine of Life," a story about dialysis, and "Hunt for Cancer Vaccine Closes In." Newsweek quoted U.S. Surgeon General Luther L. Terry, who predicted that by 1985 nine out of ten diseases would be eradicated and "spare parts for the human body . . . may seem almost commonplace." Television aired shows about heroic doctors, including Dr. Kildare, Ben Casey, and Marcus Welby, M.D., which in 1969 was the nation's favorite program. Americans thought they had the best health care in the world, and doctors were convinced they had the best job in the country.

And yet, patients still died unnecessarily. Wennberg learned this in 1963, midway through his residency, when a middle-aged woman slipped into a coma in the dialysis unit at Johns Hopkins with him attending. In her forties, the woman had undergone surgery for gallstones a few days before and was recovering normally, when her kidneys suddenly began to fail. At that time, dialysis had only been around for a few years and it took a machine the size of a bathtub to accomplish what two little fist-sized organs do in the human body. The woman was lucky to be at Johns Hopkins, which had one of the few dialysis units in the country.

She was on Wennberg's watch for only a short time—he can no longer recall exactly how long. He could find no reason for her to go into acute kidney failure, save one: Before her surgery, the woman had received a dose of the drug Orabilex, which was used to visualize her gallstones on an X-ray. Other drugs in the same class were known to have potentially harmful effects on the kidneys, yet the manufacturer, E. Fougera, neglected to warn doctors that Orabilex shared this drawback. In fact, the drug's label claimed it had "spectacularly low" toxicity and "notable absence of side-effects." To find out if his instinct about Orabilex was right, Wennberg set up a series of experiments in which he injected cats with escalating doses of the drug. After all the cats died of kidney failure, Wennberg went to the Johns Hopkins administrators, persuading them to take Orabilex off the formulary, the hospital's list of approved drugs. But they ignored his suggestion that they put pressure on the FDA to withdraw the drug, saying it was not their responsibility.

The administrators' refusal to protect patients beyond the walls of Johns Hopkins was an "epiphany" Wennberg would recall, a moment that seemed connected both to his future as a doctor and to the political and social up-heaval that was occurring in the outside world. Within the gleaming palace of medicine that was Hopkins, Wennberg was still an underling, only twenty-nine years old—hardly in a position to challenge the authority of his employer. On the outside, the Vietnam War was escalating, and the power of authority in American culture was breaking down; students were taking over university buildings and forcing administrators to make changes in curricula; protesters were disrupting political conventions. Wennberg decided it was his duty to ignore his superiors and act. He began canvassing physicians at other hospitals: the University of Maryland; Georgetown University; Sibley Memorial Hospital; George Washington University. Every hospital had seen patients suffer kidney failure after being given Orabilex, including more than twenty-five patients in the Washington, D.C., area alone.

Wennberg wrote to the company, notifying it of his findings. He never received a reply. He later learned that the company had already received several reports of kidney failure and deaths associated with its drug, but had brushed them aside with the argument that physicians had administered too high a dose. The company never passed the reports on to the FDA. Wennberg then wrote to the FDA himself, detailing the cases he had uncovered and citing several papers in medical journals about the drug's potentially deadly side effect. He urged the agency to remove Orabilex from the market. Again, Wennberg got no reply and the agency did nothing.

Wennberg continued to collect cases involving the drug, uncertain what to do next. Then, in November 1963, President Kennedy was assassinated, an event that left Wennberg shaken yet more determined than ever to do what he believed was right, to stop other physicians from killing patients with Orabilex. In May 1964, he sent a letter to Senator Hubert H. Humphrey, urging him to go to the FDA about the drug. Writing that he was "embarrassed [a letter] was necessary," Wennberg told the senator that neither the company nor the FDA seemed willing to take the drug off the market in order to protect patients. Extrapolating from his data for the Washington, D.C., area, he estimated that at least one hundred people had died around the country from a drug that was still being touted by its manufacturer as entirely safe. Humphrey took Wennberg's letter to the White House. When managers at E. Fougera learned that the Johnson administration was preparing to call a meeting with FDA officials over Orabilex, the company voluntarily withdrew the drug.

The Orabilex episode set Wennberg on a new course. He realized that there was more to being a doctor than simply treating one patient at a time; that doing the right thing, asking what he could do for his country, meant working to improve the health of communities.

Growth industry

Medicine itself was also setting out on a new course, one that would lead to the dramatic expansion of the health care industry, to more cases like Orabilex, and to many of the problems that would reach crisis proportions by the turn of the next century. In 1965, Congress passed the Medicare Act, which for the first time provided the elderly with free hospital insurance and coverage for physicians' fees. The act's passage was the culmination of one of the most bitter, divisive, drawn-out fights in congressional history, during which the American Medical Association spent fifty million dollars campaigning against what it called at various times, a "dangerous device, invented in Germany," a "communist plot," and "socialized medicine."

The AMA's opposition dated back to the time of the Progressive Party and President Teddy Roosevelt, who supported many forms of social insurance, including universal health insurance, on the grounds that no nation could be strong if its citizens were impoverished and sick. At that time, opposition to universal coverage came largely from private life insurance companies, which had begun to market health insurance too. Many physicians supported government-provided insurance at first, until they realized that the Progressives didn't want simply to insure citizens; they intended to encourage doctors to form prepaid, group practices, modeled after early HMOs like the Mayo Clinic. Doctors at Mayo, and later Kaiser Permanente, in California, and Group Health Cooperative of Puget Sound, in Seattle, worked in multispecialty groups and accepted salaries rather than fees for their services. Several European countries, notably Germany, had already successfully adopted a government health system modeled on group practices, making affordable, modern medical care available to all citizens, many for the first time in their lives. Despite the success in other countries, by the late 1930s the AMA was arguing that the government should never intrude on the "sacred doctor-patient relationship." The AMA maintained that salaried doctors would lose their "professionalism," the code of conduct embodied in the Hippocratic oath.

The most pressing reason for the AMA's opposition to universal health insurance boiled down to money. As medicine's star was rising during the twentieth century, so were physician incomes, so that by the mid-1960s, doctors were among the highest-paid professionals, earning an average of $22,000 a year, or about $141,000 in today's dollars. The AMA leadership persuaded the rank and file that one of the effects of "socialized medicine" would be to lower their incomes. As the chairman of a California commission set up to look into a statewide health insurance program wrote in 1938, "My own experience in speaking to physicians is that the only questions they ask are . . . how much money they would get, whether they would have to get up nights at the demand of whoever called them . . ."

Only a few decades before, doctors were paid little more than the laborers they took care of. Like blacksmiths, pharmacists, and later auto- and dockworkers, they depended upon collective action to raise their status and their income. The AMA was in effect a labor union, and its message to the public was, and still is, that patients do best when doctors are paid fairly (according to their own definition of fair) and left alone, to practice as they were trained to do. Like most Americans, doctors wanted to be free to earn a good income; to work where, when, and with whom they liked. By the 1950s, the AMA, as the profession's political mouthpiece, had beaten back universal health insurance proposals in several states, including California and New York, along with a string of bills in Congress, including one that was heavily favored by President Harry Truman.

But the AMA's efforts to quash national health insurance accomplished something the group never intended: They stirred a national debate among Americans about the right to health care. Most workers had health insurance through their employers by the 1960s, largely as a result of collective bargaining by unions, but there were two groups of Americans who were still "going bare": children and the elderly. Two thirds of the more than thirteen million Americans who were over age sixty-five had incomes of less than one thousand dollars a year—a third less than the rest of the population—yet their medical needs were roughly three times higher. Only half of the elderly had any form of health insurance, and many of them were living and dying without benefit of any medical care at all. Social Security, which was enacted in the 1940s, was a hugely popular program, inspiring proponents of universal health insurance to narrow their sights shrewdly on getting coverage for the aged poor; they would worry about children and the rest of the population later. When Kennedy made the medical plight of the elderly a pivotal issue in his 1960 presidential campaign, Medicare became, in the words of an editorial in Life magazine, "the hottest political potato" of the year.

The AMA responded by stepping up its attacks. In 1962, it demanded equal time opposite a televised speech by the president. When the networks turned the AMA down, it simply bought an hour of prime time. The AMA formed the American Medical Association Political Action Committee, or AMPAC, which drummed up donations from physicians with these words: "The dollars you use for political purposes may well mean more to your children and your family's future than any other investment you will ever make." AMPAC took out ads, warning citizens that proponents of "socialized medicine" viewed Medicare as just the first step toward universal health insurance—which was true. It exerted constant pressure on its friends in Congress, most of them Republicans, but also many powerful "Dixiecrats," Southern Democrats like Tennessee's Albert Gore Sr. The group arranged for incessant phone calls from influential constituents and organized letter-writing campaigns by physicians back home. It launched "Operation Coffee Cup," a campaign to get thousands of physician's wives to hold afternoon letter-writing parties. As the ladies sipped their coffee, they listened to a recording of an actor named Ronald Reagan, who warned: "One of the traditional methods of imposing Stalinism or socialism on a people has been by way of medicine."

By 1964, Lyndon Johnson had won the presidency by a landslide, the

Democrats dominated Congress, and no amount of AMA-sponsored coffee klatches and lobbying could stop Medicare. Yet the politics of Medicare's passage set the stage for many of the ills that would beset American health care over the coming decades, including its skyrocketing cost, the poor quality of care, and, ironically, the rising number of younger Americans who lacked health insurance. The bill's passage was shepherded by Representative Wilbur Mills, a Democrat from Arkansas, chair of the House Committee on Ways and Means, and a wily politician who had long opposed the government getting involved in health insurance. Mills changed his mind about Medicare when polls showed that two thirds of Americans supported it, but he intended to protect the financial solvency of the Social Security Administration, which would manage Medicare once it passed, by becoming the bill's sponsor. His defection, Michael J. O'Neill wrote in the *New York Daily News*, stunned the AMA: "They considered [it] the ultimate perfidy . . . And Mills was furious with them for their blind refusal to accept reality."

Unable to stop the bill, Mills figured he might as well use it to further his own ambition, to be elected president of the United States. The majority of voters supported Medicare, but they also believed it offered more medical coverage than it actually did. Mills worried that many citizens would be disappointed in the program—and angry at the party that gave it to them— once they discovered how little it really covered, a possibility the AMA and several Republicans were already exploiting by telling the public that Medicare would reimburse only a tiny fraction of their medical bills. In reality, it covered more than a tiny fraction—80 percent of sixty-five days a year in the hospital—but still, less than the public thought. It did not cover physician fees at all. The Republicans and the AMA were pushing a competing bill, dubbed "Bettercare," that did cover physician fees. But there was another difference between the two pieces of legislation: Bettercare would allow recipients to have a small deduction taken from their Social Security checks. Those deductions, which were entirely voluntary, were to be used, along with funds from the general treasury, to purchase private health insurance policies only for the senior citizens who wanted them. Bettercare was entirely voluntary, and it would give private insurers a piece of the action.

Members of the Ways and Means Committee were still bickering over which bill to support when Mills launched a preemptive strike on March 2, 1965, calling Wilbur Cohen, an assistant secretary for the Department of Health, Education, and Welfare, to a meeting of the committee. At the meeting, Mills told the Republicans he liked their Bettercare idea so much that he intended to fold it into the Medicare legislation, creating a three-tiered program. The bottom layer would become Medicaid, which would cover the indigent; the middle layer would be Medicare, which would cover the costs of hospital, nursing home, and home health care for the elderly; and the top layer he borrowed from Bettercare, a voluntary supplemental insurance to cover doctor's fees, in and out of hospitals. Cohen said later, "Like everyone else in the room, I was stunned by Mills' strategy. It was the most brilliant legislative move I'd seen in thirty years. The doctors couldn't complain because they'd been carping about Medicare's shortcomings and about its being compulsory. And the Republicans couldn't complain because it was their own idea. In effect, Mills had taken the AMA's ammunition, put it in the Republicans' gun, and blown both of them off the map."

The restructured bill moved swiftly through Congress. On July 30, 1965, President Johnson flew to Independence, Missouri, to sign Public Law 89-97 at the Truman Presidential Museum and Library. In attendance was President Truman himself, the first chief executive to publicly support government health insurance.

Mills was hailed by senior citizens' groups as one of the fathers of Medicare, which was a good sign for his presidential hopes. Physicians, on the other hand, threatened to boycott the program. They would go to jail, said many doctors, before they would fill out a government reimbursement form. But as Richard Harris wrote in the New Yorker a year after Medicare passed, "There was no way for them to carry out this threat short of forcing their way into jail, for the law provided that if a doctor refused to fill out a Medicare form, the patient could collect from the government by simply sending in the doctor's bill and a record of it having been paid."

For all their worries about socialized medicine imperiling their livelihoods, doctors would in the end reap a bonanza from Medicare, a windfall that would last until 1992, when a new payment system would lead to cuts in reimbursements. One of the great social programs of the twentieth century, Medicare made health care available to millions of elderly citizens, but it also spurred the desegregation of hospitals in the South—and brought down infant mortality rates among blacks as a result. Though they didn't know it at the time of passage, Medicare would prove to be a cash cow for both physicians and hospitals, and it would help fully capitalize the health care sector, thus transforming American medicine from a cottage industry of solo practitioners at the beginning of one century into the medical-industrial complex by the turn of the next.

Meanwhile, Mills's presidential aspirations ended in 1974 in the shallow water of the tidal basin in Washington, D.C. Mills staggered, drunk, from his car one night when the police stopped him. His passenger, Fanne Foxe, a stripper known as the "Argentine Firecracker," ran from the vehicle and jumped into the tidal basin.

Gaping holes

In 1967, Jack Wennberg left Johns Hopkins for a position at the University of Vermont as director of one of several newly established Medicare programs for regional planning. The National Institutes of Health was handing out block grants of several hundred thousand dollars to medical schools around the country, with the intention of creating new regional programs to improve the treatment of cancer, stroke, and heart disease. Much of the money, Wennberg would say later, "was going down the drain," because deans of medical schools were using it not to improve the delivery of health care to the population around them but rather to fund whatever departments they happened to favor. Wennberg intended to use his federal grant to find out what the citizens of Vermont actually needed, so the federal government could build new medical facilities that would really make a difference in the health of the population. He installed his family on a farm just outside of Stowe, Vermont, and set out to uncover pockets of medical need in the state.

Like most doctors, Wennberg assumed that the most serious problem in American health care was that many citizens were not getting enough of it. He and Alan Gittelsohn, a statistician from Johns Hopkins who spent several summers in Vermont working with Wennberg, expected their research would show that many small towns, "mostly in the hinterland," as Wennberg put it, were hurting for good medicine, filled with sick people and not enough doctors, or too far away from a hospital to provide all the care citizens needed. Medicare could remedy that, by putting money into local clinics.

To get a clear picture of the medical state of the state, the pair went from hospital to hospital, offering them small grants to computerize their patient data. Wennberg and Gittelsohn then gathered the data to look at rates of illness in the population and the medical care patients received. At that time, most health care researchers approached the question of whether or not the sick were being provided for by looking at whether or not hospitals were working at capacity. If all the hospitals in a region were full most of the time, the assumption was that there weren't enough beds to go around and another hospital was needed. Wennberg turned that question on its head, deciding to ask how sick people in a particular area were and whether that corresponded with how much care they were getting. He and Gittelsohn combed through computerized data that had been collected by the state from 251 towns—stacks and stacks of folded computer printouts, which covered every spare surface of Wennberg's office at the university. They mined the printouts for a wealth of information, including the rates of diseases ranging from measles to heart attacks; the number and type of doctors in each town; the number of hospital beds; every surgery performed in every hospital; nursing home admissions; deaths; and medical costs.

Vermont's small size allowed Wennberg and Gittelsohn to organize their information according to which hospital people went to when they were sick. With a population of 444,000, the state had only sixteen hospitals, most of them scattered fairly evenly. They divided the state into regions, each of which contained a hospital that served the majority of the citizens in that region. Three regions had two hospitals, while another ten had just one. The population in each ranged from about 8,000 to 110,000 people.

But when the researchers looked at the amount of medical care people were receiving in different regions, nothing made sense. In Middlebury, a small town south of Stowe, 7 percent of children under the age of sixteen had their tonsils removed. In Morrisville, just a two-hour drive away, nearly 70 percent of children had the procedure. Soon they noticed other strange patterns. Hernia operations and hospitalizations for heart attacks and strokes seemed to occur at a constant rate across regions, while other procedures, like back surgery for pain, varied wildly. In one region, there were twenty hysterectomies performed for every 10,000 people; in another, there were sixty. Hemorrhoid removal went from a rate of two per 10,000 to ten per 10,000; there were threefold differences in the rates of appendectomies and mastectomies and a fourfold difference in the rate of surgery for varicose veins.

Baffled by their results, Wennberg and Gittelsohn came up with various hypotheses to explain the "small area variations." Maybe it was patient demand—people in some parts of Vermont were choosing to have more surgeries than people in other parts of the state. Another possibility was that people in one region were simply healthier, on average, while the people in a neighboring region, for whatever reason, had more tonsillitis, varicose veins, appendicitis, or breast cancer.

But neither explanation sat well with Wennberg and Gittelsohn. For one thing, the idea that patient demand could account for such huge variation, that parents in Morrisville, for instance, were insisting that their children undergo surgery to remove their tonsils ten times more often than parents in Middlebury, didn't make much sense. Tonsillectomies were not a major operation, but they were painful, and they did pose a small risk of death from anesthesia and bleeding. And the researchers simply couldn't believe that the children in Morrisville were suffering ten times the number of swollen tonsils and ear infections as the kids in Middlebury. They also knew that people living in different regions of Vermont were strikingly similar in terms of their education and income, which predict how often people get sick. (The poor, not surprisingly, suffer more illness than the rich.) Different levels of illness simply couldn't account for the huge variation in tonsillectomies and other surgeries that Wennberg and Gittelsohn were seeing in different parts of the state.

Other physicians did not share their skepticism. When Wennberg went to his colleagues at the University of Vermont and showed them the data, they dismissed it as self-evident: Of course differences between patients were driving the differences in the amount of surgery. Patients in areas where surgery rates were higher obviously needed more surgery. Either that or patients in areas where rates were low simply weren't getting *enough* surgery. When he and Gittelsohn tried to publish their results, they were turned down curtly by the editors of every major medical journal, all of whom were convinced that the variations in the small state were entirely due to variations among patients in different regions—or to a shortage of physicians. Their results would not be published until 1973, in *Science*, a prestigious publication for basic scientists, but a journal of last resort for medical researchers. The paper was almost entirely ignored by their fellow physicians.

Gittelsohn returned to Johns Hopkins in 1972, while Wennberg set out to determine once and for all what was causing the small area variations: Was it patients, or something else? He teamed up with Floyd "Jack" Fowler, a sociologist from the Massachusetts Institute of Technology, to craft a survey designed to determine how sick people were in different regions of the state and whether they were going to the doctor and demanding care more or less often. Wennberg, Fowler, and a team of researchers completed more than four thousand interviews among Vermont citizens selected at random in each of six areas of the state.

Just as Wennberg had suspected, the people living in different parts of Vermont were remarkably homogeneous in their health, their socioeconomic status, their level of education, and how well-insured they were. Practically everybody was white; nearly everybody had a personal physician, whom they visited on average about as often from one region to the next. Practically nobody was going to the emergency room for routine care. It was absolutely clear. The high rates of surgery were not being driven by patients but rather by doctors. In the case of tonsillectomies, it turned out that the huge numbers of surgeries in Morrisville, which had the highest rate in the state, were being performed by just five physicians, a mix of family practitioners and surgeons. Little consensus existed in the early seventies about when a child really needed to have his tonsils removed. When

Wennberg went to Morrisville and sat down with each doctor he learned that they were simply very quick to use the scalpel compared with their colleagues in other parts of the state. Morrisville physicians were yanking out tonsils when more-conservative doctors might have waited to see if their young patients outgrew their susceptibility to sore throats and ear infections—as most children do.

When Wennberg set out his results for the doctors in Morrisville, they were astounded. They had no idea how different their practices were from their colleagues, that they were subjecting children to unnecessary tonsillectomies. They decided to adopt a system of seeking a second opinion when they thought a child needed his tonsils removed. This simple change led the doctors of Morrisville to perform two-thirds fewer tonsillectomies over the next five years.

Slowly, Wennberg came to an unsettling conclusion. Medicine had wrapped itself in the mantle of science, yet much of what doctors were doing was based more on hunches than good research. There were gaping holes in medical knowledge even when it came to something as seemingly mundane as a tonsillectomy. Maybe medicine wasn't an unbroken string of increasingly sophisticated scientific discoveries about the nature of disease and the human body.

In fact, as research would show over the coming decades, stunningly little of what physicians do has ever been examined scientifically, and when many treatments and procedures have been put to the test, they have turned out to cause more harm than good. In the latter part of the twentieth century, dozens of common treatments, including the tonsillectomy, the hysterectomy, the frontal lobotomy, the radical mastectomy, arthroscopic knee surgery for arthritis, X-ray screening for lung cancer, proton pump inhibitors for ulcers, hormone replacement therapy for menopause, and high-dose chemotherapy for breast cancer, to name just a few, have ultimately been shown to be unnecessary, ineffective, more dangerous than imagined, or sometimes more deadly than the diseases they were intended to treat. By the 1990s, progressive doctors were talking about a new movement called "evidence-based medicine," but well into the twenty-first century, much of what doctors do remains evidence-free. Medicine is both an art and a science, they say, the art being the intuition and informed guesswork they apply in the absence of clear symptoms or good data for what treatments work best. Deans of medical schools often tell graduating doctors that half of what they have learned in the past four years is wrong—but nobody knows which half. Still, many doctors did not appreciate having Wennberg point out to them that the medicine they were practicing fell in the category of the wrong half.

In the early 1970s, when Wennberg and Gittelsohn conducted a study in Maine similar to what they had done in Vermont, they saw just as much variation in the rates of surgeries in different areas of that state. Two procedures in particular stood out: the hysterectomy, in which a surgeon removes a woman's uterus and sometimes her ovaries and cervix, and the prostatectomy, or removal of a man's prostate gland, which sits at the base of the penis and helps produce seminal fluid. Hysterectomies were performed for a variety of reasons: to get rid of fibroid tumors, a noncancerous type of growth on the uterus that can cause bleeding and cramps; to reduce premenstrual symptoms; to cure the pain from another abnormal growth called endometriosis; and sometimes as an expensive form of birth control. Even young women in their late teens and early twenties were being given hysterectomies, which left them unable to have children. Doctors were excising prostates mostly in older men who had developed benign prostatic hyperplasia, a condition in which the gland swells and can press on the urethra enough to make urination slow and difficult.

The two procedures clearly helped some patients, just as tonsillectomies are necessary for a few kids, but there was, and still is, little agreement among physicians about when patients really needed to have their reproductive parts removed. In the case of prostatectomies, some doctors performed them to prevent their patients from having urine sit in the bladder, where, it was believed, it could lead to infection. Others viewed prostatectomies and hysterectomies as an effective way to protect patients from developing prostate cancer and uterine cancer later in life, a view that happened to be aligned with their financial incentives. More-conservative doctors felt they should take up the knife only when the patient complained of symptoms, and debilitating symptoms at that. Once again, there wasn't a lot of evidence either way, and once again, Wennberg and Gittelsohn knew that the variations they were seeing were not being driven by differences in how sick patients were, or how often they were coming to their doctors and asking to be relieved of their organs.

Wennberg also noted that what patients wanted was often being left out of the decision. The side effects of both surgeries could be huge, even life-altering: The hysterectomy was major surgery, and some women died. Others suffered a sudden and complete loss of interest in sex. For men, a prostatectomy might make urinating easier, but it could also leave them so incontinent they needed adult diapers, or impotent, or both. Wennberg wondered how many men and women would actually submit to the surgery if they were made aware of the potential consequences and the uncertainty about its supposed benefits. Such questions weren't welcomed by surgeons. When Wennberg went to speak in Lewiston, Maine, where the rate of hysterectomies was the highest in the state, the physicians in the audience were incensed. They argued that women in other parts of the state, where fewer hysterectomies were being performed, were being deprived of surgery they needed. "They were mad as hell," Wennberg recalled.

He was making a lot of doctors mad as hell. He alienated several powerful members of the department of obstetrics and gynecology at the University of Vermont when he pointed out that practically every woman over the age of fifty in the area around the university's hospital had been relieved of her uterus. There were two possible implications to what he was telling them: Either the physicians and residents at the medical school were not using good science to decide whether or not to operate—which they weren't, of course, since there wasn't much good evidence to justify the surgery—or they were performing unnecessary operations in order to train young obstetrics residents. By then, Wennberg had worn out his welcome at the university. The dean of the medical school wanted to use the grant from the NIH as he saw fit, rather than leaving it to Wennberg for gathering his data on small area variation—data that hardly anybody, the dean included, deemed significant. As Wennberg put it later, "Exposing the scientific weaknesses of medicine was not something academic medicine particularly relished." He found himself assigned to a smaller and smaller office each year, with a less prestigious title. In time, Wennberg would be recognized as the Christopher Columbus of health services research, an entirely new branch of medical science; his work would be considered "groundbreaking," "remarkable," and "revolutionary." Yet he was run out of town on a rail, as one colleague from Dartmouth puts it. He left the University of Vermont in 1973, the same year his landmark paper was published in *Science*, for an unpaid position at the school of public health at Harvard. He commuted to Cambridge, Massachusetts, from his home near Stowe, bunking in Cambridge with his colleague Jack Fowler during the week.

Too much medicine
While Wennberg continued gathering his data on variations in how doctors cared for their patients, the nation's medical bill was rising far faster than the Social Security Administration had anticipated, or budgeted. There were several reasons for the dramatic increase, one of them being more doctors, and in particular more specialists, than ever before. By the 1970s, several reports recommended increasing the number of physicians in order to care for a growing population, to redress the shortage of doctors in rural areas and the inner cities, and to meet the increased demands for care that would result from the passage of Medicare and Medicaid. The federal and state governments approved funds to support the building of more medical schools and opened the doors to more foreign-trained physicians. Medicare, and in some states Medicaid, began subsidizing hospitals for the cost of training residents. At the peak of federal funding, in 1973, more than two billion dollars a year was going toward subsidizing medical school education. Between 1960 and 1980, the number of medical school graduates doubled to sixteen thousand a year, and over the following two decades, the number of physicians would increase four times faster than the population, doubling to more than 600,000.

In passing the legislation that led to the dramatic increase in the number of doctors, politicians and policy makers imagined that they were expanding the old version of medicine and graduating more Marcus Welbys: physicians who knew their patients well; who kept fees low for their poorer patients; and who carried their black bags on house calls. They also believed that increasing the number of physicians would lead doctors to hold down fees as they competed for patients. But as Dr. George Lundberg, former editor of the *Journal of the American Medical Association*, writes in his book *Severed Trust*, the politicians "completely misunderstood what was happening in medicine." Boosting the number of doctors in a community did not lead to lower fees, because medicine does not function like other economic markets. If doctors found they weren't getting enough business, they didn't have to slash their fees in order to attract new patients; they could simply give more medical care to patients they already had, especially those who were now insured by Medicare and thus insulated from the price of their care. This was especially true for proceduralists—surgeons, orthopedists, gastroenterologists. General practitioners, now called primary care physicians, were the diagnosticians—thinkers—of medicine. They had more trouble maintaining their incomes by doing more, but even they could always tell patients to come back for a follow-up visit to keep their appointment books filled. Patients complied, because now most of them were buffered by insurance from the price of their care—and because they trusted their doctors. The subsidies for medical education also helped drive all those new physicians toward specialization. "No one seemed to notice that patients and physicians were both attracted to more specialized care," writes Lundberg. "Instead of producing more general practitioners, the new federal dollars dramatically increased the number of specialists."

All those new specialists would be kept gainfully employed by private insurance and Medicare. Far from reining in medical fees, as the AMA had feared throughout the Medicare battles of the 1950s and '60s, the federal program's enactment helped drive the steep and unprecedented escalation in the incomes of both hospitals and doctors that had already begun a decade earlier. Hoping to ensure a "smooth take-off " for the program, one that would avoid rekindling virulent opposition from physicians and the AMA, Congress and Medicare administrators bent over backward to reimburse doctors well for their services. They were paid on the basis of "usual, customary, and reasonable" fees. That meant that Medicare tracked what the doctors in a given area were charging and set reimbursement at the

seventy-fifth percentile, or a rate equal to just over whatever three quarters of
the doctors in that area were charging. If most physicians in a town charged,
say, between seven and fifteen dollars for an office visit, then Medicare reimbursement would be set at about twelve dollars, which was a little low for
the highest-priced doctors but a hefty increase for everybody else.

Before Medicare, many physicians had sliding fee scales, depending on
their elderly patients' ability to pay. Others simply kept their charges low in
areas where most of their patients were poor and paying out of pocket. This
was partly out of a sense of duty, but also because doctors were well aware
of how they were perceived by their communities, and this awareness had
generally disciplined the prices they charged the poor and elderly. Writer
Phillip Longman tells the story of his grandfather, a physician in the Midwest, agonizing over what sort of car to buy. Longman's grandfather still
made house calls, and he did not want to arrive in a Cadillac for fear of
looking ostentatious; but he also didn't want to drive a Chevy for fear his
patients would think he was not a very good doctor and therefore wasn't
making any money. (He settled on a Ford Galaxy.) Medicare effectively removed the social controls on the fees physicians charged the elderly. With
the disembodied government now footing the bill, the doctor was no
longer charging his elderly patients directly, and it no longer mattered as
much whether he drove a Cadillac or a Chevy.

Medicare also made it possible for physicians to discover how much
their competitors were charging. Physicians were barred by law from fixing
fees, but they could now find out what prevailing rates were simply by going to their local medical societies, which had the Medicare data on what
usual, customary, and reasonable rates were in their region. Many doctors,
particularly specialists, then adjusted their own fees accordingly. Young surgeons, just moving in to a community, would often charge higher prices
than older, more-established doctors, who had felt constrained by their
long-standing relationships with patients. With the advent of Medicare, surgeons whose fees were at the low end discovered they weren't charging
nearly as much as their peers, while physicians charging in the middle found
they could raise their rates a little bit too. Since the federal government—
and many private insurers—set fees on the basis of the distribution of what

physicians were charging in the previous year, rates began going up, and fast. Every time individual physicians raised their fees, Medicare and private insurers were forced to raise reimbursements, and soon physician payments were in an inflationary spiral.

The government's payment system helped physicians' incomes grow at a far faster rate than that of general inflation. In the first year after Medicare's enactment, average physician income rose by 11 percent, although some were bigger winners than others. Primary care doctors did not play the usual, customary, and reasonable game as effectively as specialists did, so their incomes rose more slowly. The earnings of some specialists, by contrast, were soon rivaling those of small-business owners. A cardiac surgeon writing in the *New England Journal of Medicine* estimated that in 1980 members of his specialty were earning an average of $350,000 a year on bypass surgeries alone. When the other surgeries they performed were included, their incomes could easily top $500,000, the equivalent of more than $1 million in 2005. Between 1950 and 1978, physician fees rose 43 percent faster than other wages, and within a little more than a decade of Medicare's enactment, total spending on health care exceeded 10 percent of the gross national product.

In the spring of 1979, Wennberg arrived at Dartmouth Medical School. He had been recruited by the new chair of the department of community and family medicine, an economist by training, who had been following Wennberg's work and recognized its importance. Wennberg kept to himself at Dartmouth, working alone out of a tiny office in Strasenburgh Hall, a converted dormitory near the medical school, with noisy pipes and narrow halls lined with painted cinder block. As he published more papers, a few researchers and physicians around the country began to take note. Elliott Fisher, an internist who had a master's degree in public health, wrote to Wennberg in 1989, asking if he could work with him. Wennberg said he didn't really want a colleague, but if Fisher wanted to come to Dartmouth, that was his business. Fisher came. So did H. Gilbert Welch, a young doctor who had worked in Alaska and on Indian reservations. Eventually they would be joined by Jonathan Skinner, an up-and-coming young economist.

The rest of the medical school remained either uninterested in Wennberg's message or distrustful. Megan McAndrew came from the Office of Public Affairs at Dartmouth-Hitchcock, the medical school's hospital, in 1993 to help the team create reports for the Clinton health care plan. When colleagues asked her whom she was working for, she would tell them, "the Black Prince," with no further explanation needed. Even so, a team of researchers, statisticians, public health experts, and economists had flocked to Wennberg. Together, they expanded their investigations far beyond New England, looking at variations in how much medical care was being delivered in different regions of the entire country.

What they found was that medicine was all over the map, literally. If Wennberg had been using a microscope to look at medical care in New England, his team was now standing on a mountaintop looking at the entire nation, yet they were seeing precisely the same patterns he had found in Vermont and Maine. Only now they could tell it wasn't just tonsillectomies, hysterectomies, and prostatectomies that were being used far more in one region than in another. It was CT scans, office visits, cardiac catheterizations. It was blood tests and hospitalizations, back surgery, chest X-rays, and knee replacements. In one part of the country, practically every woman with breast cancer was still getting a mastectomy long after clinical trials had shown that a breast-sparing lumpectomy with radiation was just as effective. In another, babies were being put in neonatal intensive care units when they didn't need it. They found that patients with back pain were 300 percent more likely to get surgery in Boise, Idaho, than in Manhattan. Doctors in hospitals affiliated with Harvard Medical School admitted patients to the intensive care unit four times more often than their colleagues at Yale University School of Medicine. Arthroscopic knee surgery—which would later be shown to be entirely ineffective at treating knee pain due to arthritis—was performed five times more often on arthritic patients in Miami than in Iowa City.

Soon, Wennberg's group began mining Medicare records, a vast database that allowed them to look at not just the medical care received by every citizen over age sixty-five but also the cost. By 1995, Medicare's bills had hit a staggering $181 billion, an increase of 6,000 percent in the thirty years since the program's inception. Medicare costs per recipient rose from under

$500 per person in 1965 to $5,000 in 1995—a rate of increase more than
double the rate of inflation. Not all parts of the country were getting an
equal share of Medicare dollars. Wennberg's team spent three years sifting
through Medicare records to replicate for the nation what Wennberg and
Gittelsohn had done for Vermont. They figured out which hospitals Medicare
patients were most likely to be admitted to and then divided the country into
306 "hospital referral regions," each of which was a little bigger than the average county. Once the group had determined where Medicare patients were
getting their care, they looked at how much Medicare spent, on average, on
recipients in each region. The numbers were amazing. In 1996, for example, the average recipient living in Miami cost Medicare $8,414; the average
recipient in Minneapolis, $3,341—a little more than a third as much.

The differences in cost weren't due to variations in how much doctors
and hospitals were charging in different parts of the country. Charges varied, of course. A hip replacement in Miami was a little more expensive than
a hip replacement in Minneapolis, but not by much. Price alone couldn't
account for the variation in how much Medicare was spending in different
regions. Nor was it due to differences in how sick people were. Wennberg's
group looked at rates of heart attacks, strokes, hip fractures, cancer, and
bleeding in the stomach in order to measure whether level of illness could
account for how much care people got. There were differences, but they
were slight. The elderly in Birmingham, Alabama, for instance, were less
healthy on average than those living in Palm Springs, California, largely because the residents of Birmingham were poorer. But rates of illness had little to do with rates of medical care in Palm Springs and Birmingham, or
with how much Medicare spent. The conclusion was inescapable: Americans were being subjected to unnecessary medicine in many parts of the
country—and paying for it in more ways than one.

Moose hunting
Wennberg's office is still located in Strasenburgh Hall, the same building
he has occupied since arriving at Dartmouth three decades ago, and
which now houses the Center for the Evaluative Clinical Sciences, the team

of nearly sixty researchers and staff who have gathered at Dartmouth. Wennberg's work has gained worldwide respect, yet Strasenburgh still feels like an academic gulag. Dingy gray carpets cover the floors; the radiators snap and gurgle. A cardboard box filled with at least a dozen framed awards and certificates of appreciation sits in one corner of Wennberg's office. A dilapidated couch that looks as if it was new sometime back when Medicare was enacted is shoved against a wall. Wennberg likes it that way, because the medical school forgets he's there when it comes time to look for faculty to serve on committees.

In 1993, the group began compiling data from around the country in order to help the Clinton administration plan health care reform. When reform fell through, the group started publishing their data in The Dartmouth Atlas of Health Care, selling it to hospitals and health plans to try to cover publication costs. By 1994, the Robert Wood Johnson Foundation, a private organization with an interest in improving the quality of health care, began supporting the group with one million dollars annually. Year after year, on map after map, the atlas served to reinforce the message that patients living in some parts of the country were being subjected to unnecessary care—huge amounts, in some places. There were obvious hot spots, in Boise, Idaho, and Redding, California, where hospitals and doctors were doing absurd numbers of certain surgeries and procedures.

In 2000, Wennberg's colleague Elliott Fisher launched a study that would finally persuade many of the skeptics that the variations the Dartmouth group were seeing were real and were causing patients harm. He showed that Medicare recipients living in high-cost regions were no healthier and no less disabled than those living in regions where recipients got less care. Nor were they living any longer. In fact, their chances of dying were slightly higher. More medicine not only meant higher costs; it also meant more deaths, not fewer. Fisher later estimated that at least thirty thousand elderly Americans were being killed each year by too much medicine. That's four times the death rate from skin cancer; twice the number of deaths from brain cancer; two times the number of murders committed annually in the United States. More and more medicine wasn't necessarily helping the elderly; sometimes it was killing them. Fisher eventually showed that Medicare recipients were dying in high-cost regions largely because they were spending far more time in the hospital than people in lower-cost regions. For all the miracles that hospitals deliver, they are also dangerous places, where patients risk suffering a medical error, a life-threatening infection, complications from surgery, or getting a diagnostic test that leads to unnecessary and life-threatening treatment.

Beyond the excess deaths that excess health care causes, it is also costing us all an enormous amount of money. Wennberg, Fisher, and their colleague Jonathan Skinner estimate that as much as 30 percent of the medical care that is paid for by Medicare as well as private insurers is useless, unneeded, a waste—a figure that has been arrived at independently by other researchers. As of 2006, when the total health care budget reached two trillion dollars, Americans were spending as much as seven hundred billion dollars a year on health care that not only did them no good but caused unnecessary harm. With the most sophisticated medical care in the world, the most skilled doctors, and more technology per square foot of hospital real estate than at any other time in history, more health care in America, as Wennberg's team was discovering, doesn't always mean better health.

Just how useless too much medicine could be came home to Megan McAndrew in 1998, when her frail, elderly mother mentioned she had had a mammogram. By then, McAndrew had been working with Wennberg for more than five years, editing The Dartmouth Atlas. Sitting with me in her cramped office in Strasenburgh Hall, she tells me the story of how her husband was dying of colon cancer while her mother, Jean, was suffering from pulmonary hypertension, a condition that most likely had been caused by a cancer treatment Jean had received thirty years before. In 1962, Jean underwent a radical mastectomy and "cobalt bomb therapy," intense radiation treatment that her doctors hoped would prevent the cancer from returning. Eventually, clinical trials would show that cobalt bomb therapy was no better than standard, less-damaging radiation treatment. The immediate result of the therapy was that her mother's chest, says McAndrew, "looked like she'd been sunbathing topless at Hiroshima." The long-term result for Jean was that by the early 1990s she was having chest pains and finding it increasingly difficult to breathe. The radiation treatment had scarred her right lung, and this subsequently overtaxed her heart as it tried to pump blood to her stiffening lung. By 1995, Jean was tethered to an oxygen tank and declining steadily. It was clear she was going to die of either sudden heart failure or her lungs simply giving out.

In March 1998, nine months before her death, Jean told her daughter she'd had a mammogram on the remaining breast. McAndrew questioned her mother about what the referring physician had said they would do if she were diagnosed with cancer, since she was obviously so weak she could never have withstood general anesthesia to remove a tumor, much less the pain and trauma of surgery with only local anesthesia. "My mother was telling me about getting a mammogram in the context of saying how great Medicare is, that it would pay for everything. But this is somebody who has the life expectancy of a fruit fly," says McAndrew. "Neither the doctor who referred her, the technician who did the exam, nor the radiologist who read it had discussed with her what they would do."

A few months later, an ophthalmologist performed surgery on Jean in his office for what he told her were "incipient" cataracts. "I've never looked into what incipient cataracts might be, but it sounds to me like my husband's dermatologist's recommendation, a year before his death from colon cancer, that he come back annually because cells taken from his ear were 'potentially precancerous,' " McAndrew says. "Also that year, my mother had what she thought was blood in her stool and was referred for a colonoscopy. The person who was going to do that fortunately panicked at the last moment and decided that it would not be a good idea to put her through it, and diagnosed hemorrhoids. Again, I asked her what she had been told they would do if she was diagnosed with colon cancer. Again, nobody had considered that. Since I was intimately familiar with surgery for colon cancer, it was apparent to me that there would be absolutely no chance of treating it in her case.

"In the end, she was driven home from Vermont after Thanksgiving weekend at my sister's, probably having cardiac symptoms but not reporting them, and went into the bathroom when she got home. She was in there for about fifteen minutes before the people who'd driven her home got concerned, found her, and called 9 1 1. The ambulance arrived, and seeing a basically dead person who was hooked up to oxygen and who probably hadn't been breathing for at least fifteen minutes, they intubated her and must have done cardiac resuscitation and took her off to the emergency room." Being intubated meant that one end of a slender tube had been slipped past her vocal cords into her trachea so that the other end could be hooked up to a ventilator, the last thing Jean would have wanted. "She had spent more time on advance directives than anyone I've ever known," says McAndrew. "She discussed it at length with her pulmonologist, who served as her primary care physician, asking not to be intubated if there was no prospect of ever coming off the ventilator, which was clearly the case with her lungs. All those records were at the hospital where she was taken. In spite of all of that, she was sent from the emergency room to the ICU, and when her pulmonologist arrived at the hospital several hours later, he insisted that all five of us children explicitly agree to withdraw life support." Jean was pronounced dead in the ICU.

Wennberg's home is a ten-minute drive from Strasenburgh Hall, down a narrow lane, where he lives in a converted farmhouse with his second wife, Corky. The rooms are airy and open. Big windows look out over the once-polluted Connecticut River, and the walls are hung with Corky's oil paintings, landscapes and nudes that possess some of the unsettling beauty of Andrew Wyeth's work. It is late March. Snow still blankets the ground; ice grips the river with no sign of a spring melt in sight. Wennberg, Corky, their black lab, Mattie (short for Matisse), and I climb into their car so we can drive to their favorite hiking spot. We pull off near an abandoned road, where Corky and I fit our boots with gizmos called Yaktrax, which look like miniature tire chains. Wennberg straps on a pair of snowshoes and takes up his ski poles, and the three of us strike off into a mixed stand of conifers and deciduous hardwood. Mattie zigzags across the path, darting from splashes of shadow into dazzling sun. Nearly seventy, Wennberg has no trouble making the steady climb over the snow. His face is craggy, with bristling brows and gray hair curling around his ears. With big, beefy hands, he looks more like a gentleman rancher than a maverick medical researcher.

At the top of a ridge we stop, our breath coming fast, to look out over the rolling hills and compact houses of Lyme, New Hampshire, which is not unlike one of the dozens of small towns Wennberg visited during his research in Vermont. I ask him why doctors deliver so much medical care that is useless and even harmful.

"Most doctors don't know they are doing it," he says. "The general attitude is more medicine is better. I went to Vermont believing in the paradigm that science was being translated into effective care, and that the doctor was competent to decide what was best for the patient." What he found, instead, was that whenever there is uncertainty about when to use a particular test or surgery, when there is incomplete or conflicting evidence about whether a procedure is effective, some doctors will be more aggressive about using it than others, especially if money is a motivation. Fee-for-service reimbursement, still the dominant form of payment in the United States, makes most physicians pieceworkers; they are paid for how much they do, not how well they care for patients. If orthopedic surgeons earn more when they perform more back surgeries, and the decision about whether a particular patient's pain will be relieved by the procedure depends upon the physician's clinical judgment, then some orthopedists will be doing lots of questionable surgeries, perhaps unconsciously deciding that patients will be helped by the procedures even when they won't.

"Doctors find ways to maintain their incomes," says Wennberg. "Look, a medical license is like a hunting license. They go out and find enough patients to bag their limit, and their limit is set by some income target."

"You mean like hunting for moose?" I ask.

"Yeah, like hunting for moose, only they are hunting for a certain type of patient. Orthopedic surgeons have a number of procedures they can become familiar with—knee replacements, hip repair, back surgery. They subspecialize in certain procedures that they become comfortable with, and then they hunt for opportunities to do those procedures."

"They hunt for patients?"

"They look for patients who fit the paradigm, the kind of case they spe-

cialize in," he says. "They get known for a particular procedure: this orthopedist is a knee guy; this one does backs. If a patient comes in who doesn't
fit what they do, they refer them to another doctor. Or because they are orthopedists, they ignore other possible remedies." Such remedies include
telling a patient with back pain to go home and take some pain medication
and wait, or to try moderate exercise and stretching, which may work as
well or better than surgery for most patients. When your only tool is a hammer, everything looks like a nail.

Wennberg's discovery of huge variations in the rates of different surgeries was partly a reflection of the uneven distribution of doctors around the
country. When several doctors with a particular subspecialty live in a particular region, he says, and they happen to be aggressive, then a lot of unnecessary surgery will be performed, as in Lewiston, Maine, where there were
unneeded hysterectomies, and Morrisville, Vermont, where doctors were
doing countless tonsillectomies. In other words, he says, the supply of
physicians can determine how much surgery is performed, rather than how
much surgery patients actually need.

"The really fascinating thing to me is to think that what predicts your
risk of surgery today in a particular region is what it was ten years ago in
the same region. That is just incredible," he says. This pattern of practice, or
"surgical signature," as Wennberg puts it, persists over time; there's a kind
of cultural transmission of when and how to treat patients that gets shared
among doctors in a particular area and passed down to the next generation
through teaching hospitals in the region, or when doctors form group
practices. For patients, then, geography is destiny. If you move from Tampa
to Fort Myers, Florida, your chances of getting back surgery go up 60 percent. If you happen to live in a region where there are lots of aggressive gy-
necologists and obstetricians who are performing too many hysterectomies
and C-sections, or where physicians are admitting patients to the intensive
care unit unnecessarily or sending them for unneeded CT scans, you risk
being subjected to the dangers of too much medicine.

"Nothing has changed since our *Science* paper in 1973," says Wennberg.
Nothing, of course, except the fact that American medicine has swelled into
a behemoth industry equal in size to the entire economy of Italy. Today,

there are more technologies and drugs available to doctors and patients than ever before, and they are more expensive. For many patients, of course, the medical progress of the past several decades has meant the difference between life and a premature death or a disability. But for others, it has simply meant more opportunities to receive even more costly unnecessary care. For some it has meant premature disability and death.

"The resistance to change is structural," says Wennberg. "It relates to the fact that doctors don't want to think they aren't doing the right thing. You can understand why doctors would feel that way; they've done it all their lives. But we don't need professionals who are trained with licenses to hunt for fifty years with no requirements of accountability."

I ask Wennberg if he gets discouraged.

"No," he answers. "But we'll probably keep doing it this way for a few years more."

TWO The Most Dangerous Place

ON A CHILLY TUESDAY evening in February 2001, eighteen-month-old Josie King arrived at the pediatric intensive care unit of Johns Hopkins Medicine with second-degree burns covering 60 percent of her small body. The accident had happened in a flash. Earlier that evening, the King family was gathered around the fire after dinner, when Josie crept upstairs behind one of her three older siblings, toddled to a bathroom, and turned on the scalding hot water. Josie had already scrambled out of the bath by the time her mother, Sorrel, heard her screams and raced up the stairs after her. The child's rubber duck and a washcloth were floating in the tub.

Though Josie was seriously burned, Sorrel and Tony King had no doubts their daughter would fully recover at Johns Hopkins, which they knew by reputation was one of the best hospitals in the country, if not the world. Even before moving to Baltimore a year earlier—when Tony, a trader for Wachovia Securities, was transferred there from Richmond, Virginia—they had heard of Johns Hopkins. A wry, no-nonsense thirty-four-year-old, Sorrel King found comfort in the calm competence of the team of doctors caring for Josie. There was Milissa McKee, a pediatric surgical fellow, who provided much of Josie's day-to-day doctoring, always under the supervision of Charles Paidas, the director of pediatric trauma at the hospital and a world-renowned pediatric trauma surgeon. An entire team of pain specialists, anesthesiologists, and nurses kept Josie comfortable with methadone, a powerful narcotic, and other painkillers. Half a dozen intensive care nurses rotated through the unit over the course of a day. Amal Murarka was Josie's

43

pediatric intensive care specialist. A warm, handsome thirty-two-year-old who was just at the beginning of his career, Murarka stopped in to check on Josie regularly and became one of her mother's favorites.

The gravest dangers facing Josie, like any patient with extensive burns, were infection and dehydration. Without the first two protective layers of skin, burn victims are acutely vulnerable to bacteria trying to get in and the water in their bodies leaking out. Infants and toddlers lose water through their damaged skin more quickly than older children and adults, because the surface of their bodies is larger in comparison to their bodies' volume. To keep her hydrated, Josie's doctors needed to give her intravenous fluids, but with so much of her skin burned, they had trouble finding a place to put an IV line. Two days after she arrived at the hospital, she was sent to the operating room, where she was given a "central line," a tube inserted just under the collarbone into the large central vein leading directly to her heart. She underwent repeated skin grafts, and her caregivers took pains to keep her wounds as sterile as possible.

Within two weeks, the toddler was well enough to be moved from intensive care to a "step-down unit," a sort of halfway house for patients who are ready to leave the ICU but not quite well enough for the regular wards. Sorrel King, who had spent much of the time at her daughter's side, confided to Paidas that she was worried about the move. None of the nurses were familiar, she told him. Was Josie really ready? Paidas reassured King that her daughter was practically healed. Yet within a day of the move to the step-down unit, Josie began vomiting and having bouts of diarrhea. She spiked intermittent fevers, a signal to her doctors that she had a systemic infection. Paidas suspected the source was her central line, a common portal for bacteria unless it is kept scrupulously clean. Tests came back negative, but he decided to remove the central line anyway and treat Josie with oral antibiotics.

As Josie's vomiting and diarrhea tapered off over the next two days, King noticed that her daughter seemed perpetually thirsty. The child whimpered or screamed as she reached for a cup or soda can if anyone nearby was drinking. The nurses instructed King not to give Josie anything by mouth; they were carefully monitoring her intake of fluids and did not want her to drink anything that went unrecorded. On February 18, the night before her discharge, Josie seemed listless to her mother, who noticed she sucked furiously on her washcloth while she was being bathed. By the time King tucked her daughter into bed, the child was unable to raise her head. King summoned a nurse, asking her to page a doctor.

The nurse checked Josie's vital signs—her temperature, blood pressure, and heart rate—and reassured King her daughter was fine. King said again that her daughter seemed thirsty and asked that another nurse be called. When the second nurse confirmed that all was well, King went home, reluctantly, to see Tony before he left the next morning on a business trip to California. She woke twice in the middle of the night and called the hospital, only to be told not to worry.

King arrived at the hospital at five thirty the next morning. After one look at Josie, she ran into the hall. "Get in here now," she said to McKee, the surgical fellow who performed many of Josie's skin grafts. "I need a team in here now, now, now."

McKee found a lethargic and pale child, her eyes dilated and sunken in their sockets. The doctor and nurses gathered around the bed, wondering aloud if perhaps Josie was reacting to the methadone. This theory seemed to be confirmed when she perked up after an injection of Narcan, a drug that reverses the effects of narcotics. King told McKee her daughter was thirsty and asked a nurse to bring her something to drink. Josie gulped down a liter of juice, the equivalent of more than four cups.

McKee paged Paidas. After consulting with McKee about Josie's response to the Narcan, he wrote in the girl's chart that she was not to be given any more pain medication unless he was consulted. Then he left for surgery. About an hour later, Josie got another shot of Narcan. She seemed more alert to King, looking around the room and watching a Scooby-Doo cartoon on television. Still worried, King asked McKee to be ready to return at a moment's notice.

Just before lunch, a pediatric anesthesiologist from the pain team stopped in. Worried that Josie might suffer withdrawal symptoms without another dose of methadone, the doctor paged Paidas to get his permission to reinstate the drug. He was still in surgery, so the pain doctor consulted with another member of the pediatric surgical team before ordering a lower dose of methadone. At one in the afternoon, a nurse on duty entered Josie's room with a syringe of the drug.

Knowing only that Paidas had ordered a halt to the methadone, King questioned the nurse, who told her there was a new order in Josie's record. King asked her to double-check. After confirming the change, the nurse gave Josie the medicine. Within minutes, Josie's eyes rolled back in her head, and her body went slack.

Murarka, the young intensive care specialist who had watched closely over Josie's recovery in the pediatric ICU, heard the code for cardiac arrest over the loudspeaker. When he rushed into her room, he did not recognize the patient at first, or her mother, standing horrified in a corner. Nurses and doctors crowded around the little girl, pumping her chest, trying to find a vein for an IV needle, slipping a breathing tube down her trachea. Murarka drew close enough to realize it was Josie. Later he would recall thinking to himself, "This is not happening. I can't believe this child is going to die right here."

A million patients

A string of errors—oversights and a crucial miscommunication—led to Josie King's death in what may seem the least likely place for such a thing to occur. In a prestigious medical center, under the care of rigorously trained specialists and experienced, caring nurses, the toddler became profoundly dehydrated, so dehydrated that a small dose of methadone pushed her over the edge into cardiac arrest. There was no overt or gross negligence, no disregard for a little girl's well-being. Josie might have survived her burns without being hospitalized and treated, but she probably would have been disabled by the scars. Certainly her parents never once considered the possibility that her life was in jeopardy either from her burns or from being hospitalized. Yet she died as a result of treatment intended to prevent her from being scarred for life.

Although nobody likes to think about it, hospitals are filled with such contradictions. We go to the hospital expecting to be cared for, hoping we will benefit from the miracles that happen there every day. At the same time, hospitals are rife with opportunities for harm. Unlike many industries, the medical field rarely faces the problem of an indifferent workforce. For the most part, patients are cared for by people who are competent and dedicated—who want nothing more than to do their very best to heal. Yet in a hospital, the most innocent of mistakes can, and with astonishing frequency does, result in dire peril. Every patient admitted to a hospital risks being hurt or even killed by the very people who wish to help her. In addition to human error, patients risk hospital-borne infection and complications from treatment—even when the treatment is correctly administered. The more often a patient is hospitalized and the longer the stay, the greater the chance of something going wrong. More invasive procedures—injections, IVs, central lines, surgeries—equal more potential dangers.

This is not to say that hospitals must or should be avoided, or treatment refused. Overall, the benefits of modern medicine far outweigh the risks. The Kings did precisely the right thing when they rushed to get the best medical help for their injured daughter. Yet that care, the most advanced care available, failed because of the opportunities it presented for something—or a cascade of somethings—to go wrong.

Such opportunities for disaster become even more worrisome when considered in light of the research compiled by the Dartmouth group and others. Unlike little Josie, many patients enter the hospital not because they need to be there, and are given tests and treatments not because they are necessary, but because of other factors—reasons that stem from the culture and economics of medicine as it is practiced in the United States. What is customary, preferred, or expected among peers at a particular hospital or within a geographic region has great influence over a doctor's decisions. Those customs, in turn, trace at least in part to factors such as how many specialists and subspecialists are locally available and what equipment is at hand for conducting tests. Underlying any consideration of what drugs to prescribe, what referrals to make, and what tests and procedures to order is the widely held belief that more medicine is better medicine—the more doctors and money applied to a medical problem, the more positive the outcome. Yet that maxim gives little weight to the fact that more care also brings with it more risks.

In 2003, the *Annals of Internal Medicine* published a landmark pair of papers, the results of the study led by Dartmouth's Elliott Fisher that showed for the first time the potential for harm inherent in unnecessary medical care. An internist and one of the first researchers to join Jack Wennberg at Dartmouth back in the 1980s, Fisher and his colleagues had a seemingly simple objective for their massive study, which analyzed the medical care received by nearly one million Medicare beneficiaries. They wanted to determine whether or not regions of the country that spend more on health care provide better care.

This is the general assumption among many physicians and the public: that health care is like other goods and services. If you could afford the luxury of the Four Seasons, where the staff cater to your every need, you wouldn't set foot in a Motel 6, where they don't do much more than change the sheets and make sure there's soap in the bathroom. In the same way, we assume that more health care is better, and better care naturally costs more.

But is more care better? Are hospitals that use the most Medicare dollars producing better outcomes? And are they any better at delivering the treatments that are considered the most effective—a prescription for heart attack patients to take an aspirin a day, for instance, and flu shots? Are they making sure their female patients get regular Pap smears, and do they take steps to ensure that surgical patients don't contract infections? Physicians and hospitals are so wedded to the notion that more dollars buy better care that despite thirty years of data, the Dartmouth group's findings had gained only grudging acceptance. Fisher was looking to produce a study that would persuade his medical peers.

If you wanted to create the perfect study that would show how spending affects patient outcomes, you would first find lots and lots of people with the same diagnosis and roughly the same risk of dying from their disease. You would then tell several hospitals how much each could spend on its patients with that particular diagnosis. Then you would randomly assign your patients to the various hospitals. Finally, you would look at how the patients fared over time.

Of course, researchers can't very well go around telling patients where to get their medical care and hospitals how much they get to spend, so Fisher and his team did the next best thing. First, they categorized the nation's 306 hospital referral regions into five groups, or quintiles, according to how much the regions had spent in the past, on average, on Medicare recipients in the last six months of life. (Just to give an idea of the huge range of spending, the highest-spending regions devoted $14,644 worth of care to the average Medicare patient compared with $9,074 on average for patients in the lowest-spending regions.)

Next, the team combed through millions of Medicare records in order to find three groups, or cohorts, of patients who were equally sick at the time of diagnosis. The patients they chose all had one of three conditions: 159,393 patients had had an acute myocardial infarction, or heart attack; 195,429 had colorectal cancer; and 614,503 had a fractured hip. The researchers had to dig deep into the medical records of their Medicare patients to extract information not only about how much was spent on their care but also about any "comorbidities," other conditions they had that might influence their outcomes. The team looked at what procedures and tests patients underwent; which drugs they took; and whether or not their health was improved by any of it. They even looked at socioeconomic status, which can independently affect health outcomes.

The research team then followed the patients, through their medical records, over the course of several years. They could see if the members of their cohorts in high-spending regions were more likely to receive high-quality care than those in low-spending regions—and were more likely to recover from their illnesses as a result. Two years—and hundreds of hours of number crunching—later, the study's findings surprised even Fisher.

The son of a professor at Harvard Business School, Fisher grew up in Cambridge, Massachusetts, and got both his undergraduate and medical degrees at Harvard before heading west to the University of Washington's school of public health. It was there that Fisher began studying Wennberg's early research and resolved to work with him. On a winter day in his office at Dartmouth, Fisher tells me he came there "motivated in part by a sense that if we could get our hands around the unnecessary, wasteful stuff in medicine, we might be able to help the poor and the uninsured."

A blunt, cerebral man in his early fifties, Fisher is tall and craggy. He looks like a more-handsome version of the actor and playwright Sam Shepard. Today, he is holding a chart from his *Annals of Internal Medicine* article, which Dr. Donald Berwick, a leading health care reformer, considers "possibly the most important paper of the decade." The chart shows how much care each cohort in Fisher's study received and how the amount of care varied wildly, depending upon which hospital the patients went to. Fisher and his team looked at several dozen different things that could be done for patients, from office visits to brain CTs to having a feeding tube inserted. They looked at how many days patients spent in an ICU; how often they were given a pulmonary function test, a measure of lung capacity and strength; and how many times they underwent an intubation.

True to form, hospitals that historically spent the most money on Medicare recipients in the last six months of life also spent the most on Fisher's cohorts over the course of several years—and gave them lots of tests and procedures. Remember, all of these patients were basically identical in terms of how sick they were and what they needed to get better. Yet patients received 60 percent more care in the highest-spending regions than in the lowest-spending regions. This result reinforced what the Dartmouth group had been saying for years. Just as groups of doctors in Vermont and Maine had surgical signatures, hospitals and regions have spending signatures, if you will, that reflect the pattern of care that the physicians and hospitals in each region tend to deliver.

But it was the outcomes of the researchers' three cohorts that proved to be the most startling finding. Fisher and his colleagues discovered that patients who went to hospitals that spent the most—and did the most—were 2 to 6 percent more likely to die than patients who went to hospitals that spent the least.

The upshot of this finding is inescapable. More care may not only be useless (and expensive), it may also be downright dangerous. "The most reasonable explanation for the higher mortality rate," says Fisher, "is that the additional medicine patients are getting in the high-cost regions is leading to harm." When doctors give unnecessary treatment, patients are exposed to all the risks—but not the benefits—of medicine, risks that include hospital-borne infections, the complications and side effects that can come with any treatment, and medical errors like the ones that led to Josie King's death. Hospitals, says Fisher, "can be dangerous places."

Bad doctors

Just how dangerous? Consider some typical medical disasters. A thirty-seven-year-old man was admitted to Allegheny General Hospital, in Pittsburgh, with pancreatitis, an inflammation of his pancreas. Treatment seemed to be going well until four days into his hospital stay, when the staff discovered that an intravenous line delivering fluids and medicine into his groin was infected. The man developed a massive, systemic infection that couldn't be stopped, even with intravenous antibiotics. Abscesses in his abdomen required repeated surgeries to drain the infection. The man finally went home, after eighty-seven days in the hospital.

A medical student in an emergency room was asked by the attending physician to check the blood pressure on both arms of a patient racked with chest pains. The student couldn't get a proper reading from one arm because the man was thrashing about. When the student didn't report the second reading, the attending assumed the patient's blood pressure was the same in both arms, which suggested he was in the throes of a heart attack. In fact, the man was suffering from a dissecting aortic aneurysm—a rupturing blood vessel—not a heart attack, and he bled to death internally before anybody figured it out.

Betsy Lehman, a reporter for the *Boston Globe* who had breast cancer, was killed at the prestigious Dana-Farber Cancer Institute, in Boston, after receiving massive, repeated overdoses of a chemotherapy drug. A doctor mistakenly ordered a dose nearly four times higher than it should have been, and not a single person who looked at the order noticed her error—neither the pharmacists who filled it nor the nurses and physicians who administered the incorrect dose repeatedly to Lehman over the course of four days.

In 1999, the prestigious Institute of Medicine published *To Err Is Human*, a report that documented the scope and outcome of medical error in American hospitals. The report stunned even health care professionals. The institute estimated that medical errors kill between forty-four thousand and ninety-eight thousand Americans each year. Some 4 percent of the thirty-three million people who are hospitalized annually, about 1.3 million patients, suffer from a complication—or in medical argot, an "adverse event"—that leads to a longer stay in the hospital, disability, or death. One in seven adverse events tallied in the study involved an infection acquired in the hospital. More than half of the adverse events were due to mistakes the reviewers deemed were preventable. In one out of three of these errors, there was actual negligence—a surgeon cut off the wrong limb or left a retractor inside a patient's abdomen by mistake, for instance, a pharmacist provided an incorrect dose, or an emergency room doctor misdiagnosed a serious condition. Some critics of the two large studies that formed the basis for the Institute of Medicine's report argue that the number of adverse events may be inflated. Yet even using the institute's lower, more-conservative estimate makes preventable hospital error the eighth leading cause of death annually, ahead of motor vehicle accidents (43,458), breast cancer (42,297), and AIDS (16,516).

Drug errors are the most common mistakes of all, and on average at least one occurs for every patient admitted to the hospital. No lasting harm is done most of the time, yet even so, according to a 1995 study, two out of every one hundred patients admitted to hospitals were hurt when they received the wrong drug, the wrong dose of the right drug, or two drugs that interacted badly. Estimates for the number of patients injured or killed by adverse events involving a drug range between ninety thousand and four hundred thousand. The Institute of Medicine calculated that drug errors alone add on average nearly $5,000 to the cost of every hospital admission, or about $2.8 million annually for a seven hundred-bed teaching hospital.

Why are so many errors committed? To much of the public, medical error seems to be a problem primarily of bad doctoring. We think physicians and nurses who make mistakes are either incompetent or uncaring, or some lethal combination of both. A San Diego surgeon who had no license botched several sex-change operations and cut off the wrong leg of a man who subsequently developed gangrene and died. An orthopedic surgeon became fixated on doing more surgeries than any other physician in his group, sometimes working eighty hours a week to keep up his productivity. The more surgeries he did, the sloppier he got, until he was routinely committing errors and getting sued for malpractice. In one case, he put in the wrong size screw to repair a patient's bone and refused to correct it when the head of the screw poked through the patient's skin.

It's tempting to lay all medical error at the feet of bad doctors, but that can't be the whole story, as Harvard surgeon Atul Gawande points out, for the simple reason that good doctors make mistakes too. Studies of specific types of medical error suggest that it is not just a small subset of doctors who commit them, a rotten few who are responsible for all the problems. Rather, every physician is destined to make at least one horrible mistake in the course of a career—and most will carry the memory and shame of it for the rest of their lives.

It isn't just doctors who err. Virtually every person who has direct responsibility for the care of sick people falls down on the job sometimes, and the more people involved in an individual patient's care—and the more procedures the patient undergoes—the more likely it is that somebody in the medical supply chain is going to blow it.

Just think for a moment about the sheer number of people who have a hand in whether a patient lives or dies. There are the orderlies who must deliver blood samples to the lab on time and the pathologists who must correctly identify infectious agents so doctors can prescribe the right antibiotic. Pharmacists have to provide the right drug at the right dose to the right patient. Somebody has to scrub down every bacteria-harboring nook of an operating room, thoroughly sterilize equipment and linens, stock supply closets, fill soap dispensers, and maintain heart monitors and ventilators. Every single person must do his or her job right every single time or risk the well-being of patients.

When you think about how many people touch a patient, either directly or indirectly, and how many tasks they must perform with precision in order to keep patients safe, it's hard not to wonder how patients ever leave a hospital intact. The sense that hospitals are dangerous places is only intensified by studies of near misses. This research suggests that the errors that get recorded represent only a fraction of the number that actually occur. One ICU that tracked near misses reported 1.7 errors per day per *patient*, about 30 percent of which could have been serious or fatal.

A doctor I know relates the story of a near miss involving his own daughter in his own hospital, which is one of the most respected academic medical centers in the country. His daughter had developed a DVT—deep vein thrombosis—or blood clot in her leg. DVTs are not uncommon among women in their twenties, and they can occasionally be fatal if they break free and move up to the lungs, where they can block a major blood vessel. The usual treatment is to dissolve the clot with anticoagulants, drugs that also prevent more clots from forming. The young woman flew home from overseas, where she was pursuing her Ph.D., so she could be admitted to the hospital where her father practiced.

One night, the young woman's brother arrived at the hospital after visiting hours and sneaked into his sister's room—only to find her lying unconscious in her bed. He called his father, who paged a doctor from the ICU. The father suspected a clot had broken free and gone to her lungs, depriving her of oxygen. He was wrong. The intensive care specialist ordered all of the woman's intravenous bags taken down and replaced with new ones. He then gave her a dose of dextrose, a kind of sugar, which revived her. It turned out one of her IV bags had contained insulin, not heparin, the anticoagulant she was supposed to be getting. The insulin had caused her blood sugar to crash to such a low level that she was on the verge of suffering brain damage. She recovered fully, but her father says he will never view a hospitalization in quite the same way again.

In his book *Human Error*, British psychologist James Reason argues that complex systems that depend upon everybody doing everything right all the time are inevitably filled with what he calls "latent errors," accidents just waiting to happen. Not surprisingly, latent errors abound in medicine. Workloads for doctors and nurses can be staggering; communication between multiple caregivers can be hit or miss; and in teaching hospitals, young, inexperienced doctors provide the lion's share of the day-to-day care of patients, and they do it on minimal sleep. (Doctors have a saying: Never get admitted to a teaching hospital in July, because that's when all the new interns arrive fresh from medical school.)

Yet despite the abundance of latent errors in complex systems, a single misstep rarely results in disaster. Rather, adverse medical events generally evolve over time, according to Reason's logic, largely because human beings possess the capacity to change course when they realize things are going terribly wrong. The ICU specialist who took down the IV bags of the doctor's daughter was able to think through the most likely possibilities fast enough to prevent the young woman from suffering irreparable harm.

It's when multiple, often small, errors are missed that catastrophes blossom. In his remarkably candid book *Complications*, Atul Gawande tells the story of botching an emergency tracheotomy, a surgical procedure that involves cutting a hole in a patient's neck just below the larynx in order to insert a breathing tube when the patient's trachea is obstructed. As a young surgical resident, Gawande was ill prepared in every possible way for the procedure. He had previously performed only one emergency "trach" (pronounced "trake") in his life—on a goat. He failed to get out the equipment he needed—the lighting, suction tubing, sterile instruments—the moment he first suspected the patient's airway was shutting down. He waited too long to call a more-experienced doctor. Finally, as panic threatened to take hold, he cut into her neck in the wrong direction, causing so much bleeding that he could not see well enough to complete the job. Luckily, the patient survived, because another doctor was finally able to slip a breathing tube past her vocal cords. Gawande describes his feelings after the event as a "burning ulcer." He writes, "This was not guilt: guilt is what you feel when you have done something wrong. What I felt was shame: I was what was wrong."

Things just happen in hospitals

The chances that multiple errors will snowball into full-blown disasters have grown in recent decades, for the simple reason that medical treatment has grown more complex. Just think about the sheer number of things doctors can do for patients today that they couldn't do a generation ago. Here's an example. Thirty-five years ago, a sixty-year-old man who was carried into an emergency room in the midst of a heart attack might have gotten morphine, to ease his pain, and lidocaine (a drug that has recently been shown to cause more harm than good in stable heart attack patients). Physicians could have administered an electrical shock to his heart if it had stopped, or if he had gone into fibrillation, an abnormal rhythm of the heart. Beyond that, there was little else his doctors could have done but hope he survived. Today, that same patient would be treated according to a complex algorithm, depending upon what kind of myocardial infarction, or MI, he was having and how serious it was. He would probably get clot-busting thrombolytics. He might receive drugs called glycoprotein inhibitors, nicknamed "super-aspirins," to help prevent further clots from forming; beta-blockers to restore an even heartbeat; and maybe angioplasty and a stent to hold open the blocked artery.

All that new technology has helped cut the death rate from heart attacks by nearly two thirds for men in their fifties and sixties—a spectacular medical achievement. But it has also created a paradox: The same new drugs and treatments that have decreased a man's chances of dying from his acute MI have also increased the number of latent errors that are possible and the potential for complications. A physician gives an injection of heparin without first performing a rectal exam, to make sure the patient isn't bleeding in his gut, and the blood thinner causes the patient to hemorrhage. Thrombolytics, the very drugs that can bust the clot in his coronary arteries, can also cause catastrophic bleeding in the brain. The man could suffer an allergic reaction to a drug. Maybe the beta-blocker causes his blood pressure to drop precipitously and he "bottoms out," a side effect of the drug that can aggravate the damage to his heart and even cause sudden cardiac arrest. The cardiologist could accidentally perforate an artery while she's threading a catheter into the man's heart.

On balance, of course, the new treatments are obviously well worth such risks. Far more heart attack patients' lives are saved than lost by new technology, and nobody in his right mind would want to go back to the days when all doctors could do was give a heart attack patient a painkiller and hope for the best. Yet physicians and nurses know that a certain number of their patients are going to be killed not by their heart attacks but by the treatment that is supposed to save them.

Doctors and nurses are acutely aware that the treatments they provide carry inherent risks. In medicine, writes Gawande, "the stakes are high, the liberties taken tremendous." Physicians tinker with body chemistry, slice patients open, remove parts, add synthetic bits, and send patients into a coma and then revive them, knowing all the while that everything they do represents a balancing act. Every treatment, no matter how commonplace or seemingly safe, offers the hope of improving health while simultaneously posing the very real possibility of a complication—a term that embraces medicine's uncertainties and dilemmas as well as the known risks. Some percentage of patients will suffer a deadly allergic reaction to the dye that physicians inject into the bloodstream in order to detect an aortic aneurysm on a CT scan. Nobody has figured out how to predict who will react badly, and no doctor or nurse who has watched a patient go into shock after receiving an injection of the dye ever forgets it. One surgeon performing abdominal surgery lost control of the bleeding while removing what turned out to be a benign tumor; the patient died. A simple blood draw, the most common and seemingly innocuous invasive procedure in all of medicine, occasionally causes debilitating nerve damage.

Even aspirin can be lethal. If you've already had an acute MI, taking an aspirin a day can reduce the odds of dying from a second one by more than 15 percent, a bigger risk reduction than any single treatment or surgery a doctor can prescribe for heart disease. But taking aspirin daily when you aren't likely to have a heart attack might not be such a good idea, since aspirin can trigger hemorrhaging in the brain, stomach, and intestines.

At least the trade-offs for aspirin are well defined. Given clear information about the risks and potential benefits of this drug, patients and their doctors can choose whether they are willing to trade short-term safety for possible long-term gain. Most of the time, however, the scales of medicine aren't so easy to read. The benefits of many treatments have never been demonstrated with any certainty, so doctors are flying at least partially blind when it comes to weighing the odds that a particular patient will be healed or hurt. Often, patients and doctors don't have the luxury of being able to mull over a complex cost-benefit analysis before embarking on a course of treatment. If doctors paused to fret about the possibility of a massive brain bleed every time they were about to administer a clot-busting drug, more patients would die of their heart attacks. When a little girl is burned over 60 percent of her body and needs fluids, fast, nobody stops to ponder the risk of infection while putting in a central line.

This unhappy fact is epitomized in a story told by Dr. Stephen Grund about a patient he encountered during his second year of residency at Massachusetts General Hospital, one of the institutions affiliated with Harvard Medical School. Early one morning, near the end of his overnight shift in the cardiac ICU, Grund found himself headed for the surgical recovery room in response to a page. His new patient, a homeless, alcoholic man in his forties whom we'll call Richard Black, had walked into the emergency department the night before, holding up a grossly infected pinkie finger. Swollen and pus-filled, the finger needed to be cleaned thoroughly and debrided—meaning the dead tissue had to be removed surgically—in order to drain the infection. Black was wheeled into the operating room for the procedure.

Once in the post-op recovery room, Black became dangerously belligerent, threatening the nurses and pulling at his intravenous line. He was given a small dose of Haldol, an antipsychotic drug used routinely to calm agitated patients, along with Ativan, a drug similar to Valium. Black quieted down for about fifteen minutes, only to become agitated once again. He was given another dose of Haldol and Ativan, which calmed him. When Black grew agitated a third time, a psychiatrist was paged. The psychiatrist directed the post-op team to continue administering Haldol and Ativan, as needed.

After several more doses, an alarm bell sounded. Black's heart had gone into a rare arrhythmia known as torsades and then arrested. After the team was able to get his heart started again, Grund was summoned to take the patient to the cardiac ICU. Grund asked how much Haldol and Ativan the man had received. The answer was a lot, perhaps ten doses of each drug, which in itself wasn't surprising, given how dangerously agitated Black had been.

But when administering Haldol, doctors always run the risk of triggering torsades, a complication that is rare but often fatal. In this case, Black's alcoholism may have made matters worse.

Grund rushed his patient to the cardiac unit, where an attending cardiologist assured him that the Haldol would be out of the man's system within a day or two, and his torsades would resolve. In the meantime, Grund would have to monitor him closely. But the patient didn't get better. By the time the young doctor went off rotation, a few days later, Black was still unconscious and hooked up to a ventilator. Grund forgot about his patient until several years later, when he learned that the man had never regained consciousness. After some weeks in the hospital, Black was sent to a "vent farm," a nursing facility for people on permanent life support.

The case of the man with the pinkie still haunts Grund, a thoughtful, intense physician who now heads the oncology department at the Hospital of Central Connecticut, in New Britain. Recalling those few days when he cared for Black, Grund says, "There was no mistake here. Nobody in that whole line, from the orthopedist who operated on his finger to the post-op team to the psychiatrist to the cardiac unit, nobody made a mistake. Everybody did everything right. Things just happen in hospitals."

Controlled chaos

Here, then, is an explanation for Fisher's discovery that Medicare patients with the same well-defined medical conditions, the same chances of survival, and even the same socioeconomic status are more likely to die in parts of the country where Medicare spends the most. Spending more means doing more, and doing more increases the chances of errors being committed and of patients being hit with a complication. The corollary to this stark fact is that the more days a patient spends in the hospital, and the more complex treatment he receives, the greater the odds he'll suffer an adverse event.

In his office in the rabbit warren of Dartmouth's Strasenburgh Hall, Fisher pulls out yet another chart, one that illustrates just how much more care patients with a given diagnosis can receive at certain hospitals. Fisher still sees patients as an internist at the Veterans Health Administration hospital in

White River Junction, just over the border from Dartmouth in Vermont. He is intimately familiar with each of the nearly three dozen tests and procedures he and his team combed through during their study.

"Look at the extra stuff that's done more often in the high-cost regions," Fisher says. "Most of it is relatively minor procedures and imaging and diagnostic tests." Most major surgeries, on the other hand, hardly vary at all between regions. Surgery for colon cancer, for instance, is relatively constant, as is hernia repair. For cataract removal, the rate is only slightly higher in hospitals in high-spending regions compared with low-spending ones.

For many other procedures, however, the differences are striking. Fisher runs a finger down the list and stops at a procedure called a laryngoscopy. "That's for looking down your throat to see why you're hoarse," he says. "It's done three and a half times more often in high-cost regions. Here's another. The pulmonary function test tells you how good the lungs are. Two and a half times more often in a high-cost region. Look at vena cava filter; you put in a thing to catch clots before they can get to your lungs. It means very sick people are getting treated with an aggressive device, and this is in the last six months of life. You are three and a half times more likely to get that at a high-cost region. Days in the ICU: one and a half times more likely. The thing that's really startling is that the differences we see are all explained by these decisions around discretionary treatment, things that don't fall into the category of absolutely necessary, important medicine."

This is a central point. Patients in high-spending regions are not getting more big-ticket surgeries; rather, they're being given more of the small stuff of medicine—tests, procedures, and drugs—some of which may be prescribed defensively to avert lawsuits. What all of these treatments and tests have in common is that there are no hard-and-fast rules about when to use them.

"Discretionary" means these procedures and tests are employed at the doctor's discretion. The question is, why are physicians at high-spending hospitals using discretionary procedures so much more often than doctors in low-spending hospitals? Even when their patients are equally ill and equally likely to survive—as Fisher showed of the three cohorts in his gigantic study—the doctors at one hospital are far more likely to decide to perform a laryngoscopy or a pulmonary function test than the doctors at another.

Dr. Diane Meier, a palliative care specialist at Mount Sinai Hospital, in Manhattan, makes the point that physicians who throw lots of procedures and tests at their patients are merely doing what they've been taught. Beginning in their first year of school, young medical students learn that they will "see one, do one, teach one," an expression that conveys the importance of apprenticeship in medicine. One day, a first-year resident watches a third-year resident slip a three-inch needle into a patient's chest, just under the collarbone, to insert a central line. The next day, he's putting in a central line himself, with some coaching. A year later, he's teaching another first-year resident.

Young physicians don't just learn to perform procedures by example; they also absorb lessons about when it's appropriate to use a particular test or treatment. Residents learn from attending physicians, who learned when they themselves were residents, when to put in a vena cava filter, which patients need a central line, and how to treat postsurgical abdominal pain. "It's called the hidden curriculum," says Meier. "Most of what's taught is not in the medical school curriculum."

A telling little study by Fisher seems to support that view. Fisher looked at the results for several hundred internists who took their initial qualifying exam, a test that's required for certification by the American Board of Internal Medicine. The test consists of approximately three hundred questions about several hypothetical cases. The doctors need to know when to order a lumbar puncture in diagnosing meningitis, for instance, and how to tell the difference between a viral sore throat and one caused by a *Streptococcus* bacterium. Out of those three hundred questions, the right answer for thirty-two of them is that the doctor should either do nothing or withdraw therapy. For example, a patient presents with acute bronchitis, accompanied by fever and coughing up of blood. After two weeks, the fever is gone, the patient is no longer coughing, and a chest X-ray shows the lungs are clear. Should the doctor (a) do a chest CT; (b) perform a bronchoscopy, which involves putting a flexible scope down the bronchial tubes to take a look at them; or (c) do nothing? The right answer is c—do nothing. The patient is cured. What Fisher found was that doctors who trained at hospitals where the pattern of care was most intense and aggressive were significantly more likely to get many if not all of the thirty-two "do nothing" questions wrong.

Young doctors learn to be more or less aggressive in their treatment during their internships and residencies, but they don't stop absorbing the cultural messages around them the minute they finish their training and enter practice. Physicians who work in the same hospital share knowledge and opinions whenever they are thrown together, discussing cases over coffee or standing in front of the nurses' station—and shaping, in the process, a kind of groupthink about how best to handle different conditions. One surgeon wants all of his patients to receive a vena cava filter. Another physician disagrees, arguing the device should only be used in patients who can't be given heparin to prevent clots. Since there's often little evidence to support one approach over another, this give-and-take can drive the collective clinical decisions made by doctors at a particular hospital.

But while cultural transmission of practice styles certainly plays a central role, it isn't the whole explanation for why the care in high-spending regions is more intense—and expensive—than in low-spending regions. Another key factor, says Fisher, is the high number of specialists in the highest-spending regions. "These are specialist-oriented systems," he says. "The pattern of practice is one of having lots of different specialists involved. Most of the doctors in high-intensity hospital regions are doing more; they're more likely to test, they're more likely to hospitalize, but most of all, they have a lower threshold for referring to other specialists."

What Fisher is saying is that the care that patients are likely to get results from the interplay between culturally transmitted practice styles, which evolve at individual hospitals, and the availability of different kinds of doctors. The more specialists around for any given physician to call in for a consult, the more likely it is that a specialist will be called in. If your patient has a fever, and there's an infectious disease specialist around, you call her. If your patient is having trouble breathing, you call the pulmonologist. And if this is happening in a teaching hospital, the residents and interns are learning the lesson that calling in another specialist is the right thing to do. Yet as Fisher's research suggests, involving another specialist leads to more procedures and tests—and the more procedures and tests, along with more days in the hospital, the greater the opportunity for complications and for latent errors to pile up into catastrophic adverse events.

At first, the idea that more specialists can make for worse medical care seems thoroughly wrongheaded. After all, isn't the specialist the doctor with the most knowledge about a given condition and therefore the one person most able to help us get better? Well, yes and no. Specialists have detailed knowledge that at times can be critical in making a correct diagnosis, and they acquire skills, by dint of years of practice, that make them far more qualified to perform certain procedures. You wouldn't want a gastroenterologist operating on your knee.

At the same time, anyone who has witnessed the whir of activity in a busy hospital can see how more specialists can lead to more confusion. Here's an example of how the confusion starts. A physician sees a patient, prescribes a drug, and then records the order in the patient's chart—sometimes illegibly. The next specialist comes along, misreads the previous doctor's hieroglyphics, and proceeds to give the patient another drug that causes a bad reaction with the first. (Electronic medical records can greatly reduce if not virtually eliminate instances of this type of error, along with many other mishaps, but most hospitals have yet to invest in the technology.) Busy specialists don't always consult one another directly, even by phone, and it's almost unheard of for all the doctors involved in a single patient's care to gather together in one room and actually discuss how best to treat him.

And so each specialist focuses on the part of the body he or she knows best. The pulmonologist doesn't concern himself with the surgery patient's infected abdominal wound site; he's got the lungs to worry about. The surgeon is not focused on the patient's failing kidneys; she's calling in the infectious disease guy for a consult about the patient's infection. The nephrologist is too busy treating kidney failure to think about the patient's growing despondency over her worsening condition. Very sick patients may be seen by several dozen doctors, each of whom may order a separate set of the same blood tests and images—relating his or her findings and orders to the others through notes scribbled in the patient's chart.

That leaves only two people in the entire hospital who may know what's happening to the whole patient. If you come in for surgery, one of those two people might be your surgeon, except for the fact that surgeons are often far too busy to keep tabs on what all the other specialists are doing to their patients. If you're lucky, your primary care physician takes time off from his office schedule to make regular visits to the hospital and check up on you. (Some hospitals have begun to hire "hospitalists," primary care physicians who rotate in shifts to watch over the care of specific patients.) If you have a terminal condition or you're in pain, a palliative care specialist, like Meier, may be available. Palliative care specialists make a point of looking at the whole patient and the entirety of her care. But most of the time, the only person in a position to be aware of everything that is happening during a hospital stay is you, the patient—and often you're too sick to pay attention. Even family members can't be expected to stand watch twenty-four hours a day, much less keep track of the complexities of modern medical treatment.

All of which points to one of several weaknesses in the new health care reform movement called "consumer-driven health care." Backed largely by political conservatives and free marketeers, consumer-driven health care is aimed at improving quality and bringing down health care costs by putting more decisions in the hands of patients. In consumer-driven plans, insurers offer lower health insurance premiums in return for high deductibles, on the order of four thousand dollars a year. The idea here is that if patients have more "skin in the game," or more of a financial stake in their care, they will pay more attention to cost and quality.

In his slim and eloquent volume *Escape Fire: Lessons for the Future of Health Care*, Donald Berwick illustrates just how absurd it is to expect patients or their families to monitor their own care when they're in a hospital—even when a family member is a physician. A Massachusetts pediatrician, Berwick is now president and CEO of the Institute for Healthcare Improvement, a group that advises hospitals on how to reduce error and improve quality. Berwick was radicalized, as he puts it, in 1999, when his wife, Ann, was hospitalized six separate times for a mysterious and debilitating spinal cord disorder.

Over the course of several months, Ann Berwick spent a total of sixty days at three different hospitals, including one of the most prestigious hospitals in the country. Most of the people who cared for her, writes her husband, showed extraordinary kindness, goodwill, compassion, and commitment, but Berwick was stunned nonetheless by the lack of coordination he witnessed. During one admission, he writes, "The neurologist told us in the morning, 'By no means should you be getting anticholinergic agents'; and a medication with profound anticholinergic activity was given that afternoon. The attending neurologist during another admission told us by phone that a crucial and potentially toxic drug should be started immediately. He said, 'Time is of the essence.' That was on Thursday morning at 10:00 am. The first dose was given 60 hours later—Saturday night, at 10:00 pm. Nothing I could do, nothing I did, nothing I could think of made any difference. It nearly drove me mad."

Each time Ann Berwick was discharged from a hospital, there was little follow-up care. Out of the fifty different doctors who treated her over several months, only three, writes Berwick, made any effort to follow her course outside the doors of their hospital: "Continuity of care was based on acts of near heroism. Ann's primary neurologist travels frequently for speaking engagements. When he was away during crucial times, he phoned Ann every day, whether from Amsterdam, London, Geneva, or San Francisco."

The whole patient

What Berwick saw firsthand is sometimes called the "network effect," the barely controlled chaos of multiple caretakers in an environment where there is little coordination of care. A former head of Kaiser Permanente dubbed it the "adhoc-cracy" of medicine. Whatever you call it, health care doesn't work well when there is no single individual, in particular no generalist, who's in charge of coordinating a patient's care. This persistent and widespread lack of coordination may help explain the "undertreatment"— the failure to deliver needed care—that Fisher and his colleagues recorded in the highest-spending regions. The group found that high-spending regions weren't delivering better care, or even needed care, just more of it.

This may be Fisher's most stunning finding of all. If you are a patient who happens to live in a region where hospitals have lots of resources and lots of specialists, you are more likely to be undertreated—that is, your hospital may fail to deliver care that's known to be effective for your particular condition. In the highest-spending regions, for instance, about 75 percent of heart attack patients were sent home from the hospital with orders to take a baby aspirin a day—the single most effective drug for reducing a patient's risk of suffering a second event. In the lowest-spending regions, by contrast, more than 83 percent of heart attack patients went home with their baby aspirin. Only 48 percent of patients in high-spending regions were given a flu vaccination, compared with 60 percent in the low-spending regions. Major teaching hospitals, which are considered the crème de la crème of American medicine, were only a little better than most, and on only a few quality measures. Hospitals that spent more and were overtreating patients with certain kinds of care were simultaneously undertreating them.

This astonishing finding, that many hospitals are failing to deliver the simplest—yet often most effective—care, has been corroborated by another massive study, which was published in 2003 in the *New England Journal of Medicine*. Led by Elizabeth McGlynn, a researcher with the RAND Corporation, the study involved combing through thousands of medical records for information about 439 indicators of the quality of health care. Did migraine sufferers get the right drugs? Did people who came to the hospital with a broken hip receive heparin to prevent a stroke or heart attack? Did elderly patients get a pneumonia vaccine when they were admitted to the hospital? Did diabetics receive counseling to improve their diets and get more exercise?

McGlynn's results were so arresting that the article has been cited in the medical literature hundreds of times by other researchers since it was published. Her team reported that on average, patients were given recommended care a little less than 55 percent of the time. People with certain conditions were more likely to get what they needed. Cataracts, for example, were treated correctly nearly 80 percent of the time. On the other hand, only 24 percent of participants in the study who had diabetes consistently received an important test over a two-year period. Only one in five patients with chronic pulmonary disease was advised to quit smoking; one in ten alcoholics received counseling. While counseling smokers and drinkers may hardly seem like advanced medicine, it can persuade a certain percentage of patients to change their habits—and dramatically improve their health. The bottom line is this: Whether you are rushed to the hospital or you walk in the door, your chances of getting all the treatment that is recommended for any given condition are about the same as flipping a coin.

Nobody can quite explain why so much necessary treatment simply falls through the cracks—and why it happens more often, as Fisher found, at hospitals that are delivering the most intensive treatment. It may be the result of the network effect, a case of confusion that leads health care providers to repeatedly drop the ball. Or maybe physicians and hospitals don't make sure their patients get what they really need because they aren't specifically paid for it.

That's the idea behind Medicare's new reimbursement system, called "pay for performance," which offers small bonuses to hospitals for sweating the small stuff, like ensuring that heart attack patients get their aspirin and giving every Medicare recipient who walks through their doors a flu vaccine. This approach assumes that hospitals (and the physicians and nurses who work in them) fail to do what's right because there's no money in it, and that paying them will get them to focus on reducing undertreatment. This assumption could well be true, though the pay-for-performance initiative is too new to produce results that would tell us one way or another.

What is known is that regions that have fewer specialists in relation to the population—and more primary care physicians—have better overall health, a result that has turned up time and time again in various studies. In his big study, Fisher noted both less undertreatment and lower mortality rates in hospital regions where there are more primary care physicians and fewer specialists. While Americans worship the specialist for his knowledge and technical expertise, the most important doctor for ensuring good health may be the underappreciated primary care physician.

What all of this says is that somebody needs to keep watch over the whole patient, not just his various parts. Consider the following case of a woman who was misdiagnosed for more than half her adult life. The woman, whom we'll call Rebecca Dawes, presented herself to Jeanne Lenzer, who is now an investigative journalist but was working as a physician's assistant in family practice at an academic medical center in 1997. Dawes had come to the clinic that day so dizzy she could hardly sit, much less stand. She didn't want Lenzer to treat her, however; all she wanted was a referral to an ear, nose, and throat specialist or a neurologist. Referrals were the only reason she went to a primary care practice. Like many patients, Dawes had never seen the need for a primary care physician. Specialists were so much more highly trained. Why waste time with a generalist? When Lenzer asked Dawes if she could do a thorough physical exam and get a complete history before making any referrals, Dawes was taken aback. Nonetheless, she agreed to allow Lenzer to take her history and examine her.

Thirty-seven years old at the time, Dawes had begun having complaints twenty-four years earlier, when she fainted for the first time at the age of thirteen. Since then, she had passed out more times than she could count. Most days, she could hardly stand up without feeling woozy. She was hospitalized at twenty-five for a "nervous breakdown," as she put it. At thirty-one, she underwent a total hysterectomy for symptoms of endometriosis. Besides the fainting spells, Dawes suffered from nausea, vomiting, exhaustion, dizziness, blinding headaches, depression, and anxiety. Her symptoms left her unable to work, and she spent most of her time in bed or on the sofa. With no primary care physician, Dawes had made more than two hundred visits to emergency departments over the years and had referred herself to a string of specialists whenever one symptom or another grew intolerable. Each visit to a specialist led to a different set of tests—and a different diagnosis. Suspecting that colitis or a peptic ulcer might be causing her vomiting and nausea, a gastroenterologist did an upper GI series, a set of X-rays taken to look for abnormalities in the stomach and small intestine. A psychiatrist suspected an eating disorder or depression. A neurologist gave her a head CT scan to rule out a tumor. She was diagnosed at various times with gastroenteritis, dehydration, depression, and "functional disorder," a term physicians use when they can find no organic or physical explanation for a patient's symptoms and conclude the patient's complaints are all in her head. Dawes had been prescribed everything from antacids to sedatives. Nothing relieved her symptoms.

As a physician's assistant, Lenzer was trained to think like a generalist. Noting the woman's emaciated appearance, slightly darkened skin, and history of fainting, she asked Dawes to get off the examining table. As the woman stood there, swaying, Lenzer performed the most basic of tests: She took Dawes's pulse and her blood pressure. Dawes's heart rate went up when she went from sitting to standing, while her blood pressure dropped. Next, Lenzer drew blood and sent it to the lab. The results came back showing Dawes had low levels of salt in her blood and high levels of potassium. Lenzer immediately suspected Addison's disease.

A relatively rare condition that is found in about one in one hundred thousand people, Addison's is nonetheless one of the first diagnoses a young doctor commits to memory. It occurs when the adrenal glands don't produce cortisol, a hormone that's critical for the body's ability to maintain everything from blood pressure and salt-potassium balance to appetite and a sense of well-being. Lenzer ordered a more-complex blood test that showed the woman had dramatically diminished levels of cortisol. A CT scan further confirmed the diagnosis when it revealed that Dawes's adrenal glands were shrunk to mere nubbins. Lenzer referred the woman to an endocrinologist, who treated her with synthetic cortisol. Over the next five months, Dawes gained twenty-nine pounds, regained a sense of well-being, and stopped fainting. For the first time in her adult life, she was no longer confined to her bed and the sofa.

There is something deeply and disturbingly counterintuitive about the picture of American medicine that emerges from these examples. Elliott Fisher's study showed that more medical care doesn't necessarily help patients; sometimes it harms them. Because modern medicine, for all the hope it can offer, always carries some risk, Richard Black could walk into an emergency room holding up his infected pinkie finger only to be wheeled out of the hospital brain-dead. No matter what Donald Berwick did, the lack of coordination between his wife's caregivers made it impossible for him to make sure that she got the drugs she needed—and didn't get drugs that might harm her. Rebecca Dawes had lived with untreated Addison's disease for nearly two thirds of her life, even though the clue to her condition was there in her blood the whole time. Numerous emergency room doctors had drawn her blood, seen the imbalance of sodium and potassium, and undoubtedly thought at least in passing of the possibility that she was suffering from Addison's. But by then, she was already on her way to another specialist. She was everybody's patient, and nobody's.

These stories reflect the structural flaws inherent not only in the way hospitals are run but also in the way health care is reimbursed. Hospitals and physicians are not rewarded for keeping patients safe or coordinating their care. Doctors aren't paid to keep decent records and hospitals aren't reimbursed for retaining the right mix of specialists and primary care physicians. Both physicians and hospitals are paid, by and large, to do more, and distortions in what gets reimbursed most richly have ensured that the simplest, most effective care often falls through the cracks in favor of more-invasive, complicated treatment—care that involves more doctors than necessary and that may put patients at unnecessary risk.

In Josie King's case, it's difficult to pinpoint exactly what went wrong and when. First there was the infection that her doctor initially suspected had entered through her central line. Central line infections are so common in hospitals that they are not even considered to be errors in the strictest sense, or the result of negligence—though they should be—but simply a complication of care, a potentially lethal adverse event. About 250,000 patients a year suffer a central line infection, and as many as 60,000 die from it. (This hazard declines dramatically when hospitals institute well-defined protocols for keeping the insertion of central lines fastidiously clean.) Josie's infection did not kill her directly; it led to vomiting and diarrhea, which dehydrated her little body so severely that her weight dropped 15 percent in the twenty-four hours that preceded her cardiac arrest. That's like a two-hundred-pound man losing thirty pounds in a single day. Nobody knows how such a clear warning sign of dehydration could possibly have been overlooked, but one way or another it was missed by every person who scanned Josie's chart that day; or if it was noted by anyone, he or she failed to act. Perhaps it rang an alarm bell in the mind of a nurse, but in the fiercely hierarchical social order of hospitals, a person near the bottom may sometimes hesitate to speak up. Allowing Josie to drink a liter of juice in one sitting also may have contributed to her death, by suddenly diluting the electrolytes in her blood. Even if her sudden intake of fluid played no role in her death, it was a sure sign she was extremely dehydrated.

The final straw was when the pain specialist ordered another dose of methadone, unaware that the child's body was already so weakened that even a low dose of the drug might be enough to stop her small heart. By the time Josie was revived, she had already suffered massive brain damage. She spent two days on life support, and then, as her parents held their daughter tenderly in their arms, she died.

Josie King was killed by a third-world condition, dehydration, in a first-world—indeed a first-class—American hospital. Yet it's impossible to fix blame on any single person or event in the string of tiny missteps that led to her death. Perhaps the most devastating error of all was that nobody paid sufficient attention to Sorrel King's observation that her daughter was desperately thirsty.

THREE Your Local Hospital

To reach Shasta Regional Medical Center, just drive north from San Francisco on Interstate 5 for four hours, until you see Mount Shasta, floating over Siskiyou County in its permanent cloak of snow. The hospital sits in the middle of downtown Redding, near a bend in the winding Sacramento River. Known as Poverty Flats in the early nineteenth century, Redding was first settled by miners and loggers, who stayed until the mines were tapped out and the redwoods and pines were all cut down. The town revived in the mid-twentieth century, when it became a mecca for fishermen, hikers, and skiers headed for nearby Shasta and Trinity lakes, Lassen Volcanic National Park, and snowcapped Mount Shasta. Tourism is now one of two main businesses in this town of ninety thousand residents and more than four hundred hotels. The other main business is medicine. Between them, Shasta Regional Medical Center and Mercy Medical Center employ more than two thousand people, and generate nearly one hundred million dollars a year in revenue.

Dr. Patrick Campbell arrived in Redding with his wife and two children in 1993, less than two years out from his internship and residency at the University of California, Davis. Campbell had been working in an urgent-care facility in Sacramento when he was recruited by Redding Medical Center (which would be renamed Shasta Regional Medical Center in 2003). Redding offered a two-year salary guarantee, which would give Campbell time to build a practice and pay off medical school debts. From the hospital's perspective, good relationships with primary care physicians like

Campbell were a matter of branding, well worth the recruitment costs; primary care doctors who were loyal to Redding Medical would admit patients to the hospital and refer them to the hospital's specialists, especially those in its busy cardiac program. To Campbell, Redding seemed to offer a good life. The crime rate was low, the schools were good, and the area was beautiful. He could have a small-town practice that would let him get to know his patients over the years, while still having access to a modern, high-tech hospital.

Campbell's high hopes and idealism at the outset of his career made the events that would unfold in Redding over the next decade—the lawsuit he would file in 2002, the evidence of malpractice and fraud committed by several heart specialists at Redding Medical that he would uncover, and the town's anger at him for exposing two of its most prominent physicians—seem all the more surreal. After blowing the whistle on the hospital and its specialists, he would lose practically everything he valued, his medical practice, his family, and his home. The tale of Campbell and Redding Medical Center tells a larger story about the forces that drive all hospitals to deliver unnecessary care—and how difficult it is to rein them in.

Campbell grew up in Portland, Oregon, the son of a secretary and a customs inspector, the first person in his family to go to college. An accomplished violist in high school, he entered Lewis and Clark College with a full music performance scholarship. But after two years of college and a move to California, the early dream of an orchestral music career faded. He enrolled at the University of California, Santa Cruz, and switched to natural sciences. After an undergraduate degree in chemistry and three years as a graduate student, he finally settled on medicine, enrolling in medical school at the University of California, Irvine, where he met his wife. Both Campbell and his wife went into primary care, an idealistic decision at a time when more and more of their classmates were choosing to enter specialties, where the money was much better.

One of the first doctors Campbell met in Redding was a cardiologist, Chae Hyun Moon. The son of a Korean physician, Moon was a more ambitious breed of doctor. According to the New York Times, he graduated in 1972 from the College of Medicine at Yonsei University in Seoul and completed an internship and residency at Metropolitan Hospital Center in New York.

His forceful personality and constant availability allowed him to quickly build a thriving practice in Redding. When Moon arrived in northern California in the early 1980s, all invasive cardiac services—cardiac catheterization, angioplasty, and open-heart surgery—were being done in bigger cities like Sacramento, two hundred miles away. Moon pushed for a cardiac catheterization laboratory—a special room containing the equipment needed to perform such procedures as balloon angioplasty—and open-heart-surgery capability in Redding. First Mercy Medical Center and then Redding Medical opened labs, followed by an open-heart-surgery program, in 1987. Five years later, Moon and Fidel Realyvasquez Jr., a Stanford-trained cardiothoracic surgeon, were the dominant figures in their respective specialties. Together, the men built the California Heart Institute within the once-sleepy Redding Medical Center. Primary care physicians sent their patients from all over northern California, from tiny towns like Weed and Paradise, and from as far away as southern Oregon. Moon was always willing to accommodate another patient. As he would later tell the *Sacramento Bee*, "When these guys call me up day or night or holidays, it doesn't matter. I am in a health profession to save lives."

Both heart specialists were workhorses, but Moon especially so. He focused his practice on catheterization, an invasive procedure that involves snaking a thin catheter, or tube, up through a major blood vessel in the groin into the coronary arteries, the blood vessels that supply the heart muscle with oxygen. Moon also performed balloon angioplasties, threading a tiny balloon up a wire inside the catheter. When the balloon was inflated, it could smash a clot against the arterial wall, allowing blood to flow freely once again. By the 1990s, cardiologists were also employing stents, tiny mesh tubes that could prop open a blockage inside a coronary artery. Moon sometimes performed as many as a dozen cardiac catheterizations in a single day—four to five times the number his peers in northern California were performing. In one year, he performed more than eight hundred invasive cardiac procedures. Between June 2001 and 2002, he billed Medicare for four million dollars. At its peak, Redding Medical Center was performing nearly eight hundred open-heart surgeries per year—many of them done by Realyvasquez.

With the enormous volume of procedures came high incomes and lavish lifestyles. Moon owned a rambling hilltop estate on the west side of Redding, with a view of Mount Shasta and No Trespassing signs posted at the bottom of the driveway. Realyvasquez lived on the east side, at the end of a tree-lined street behind an electronic gate. The doctors were popular figures in town. Realyvasquez donated his collection of fifty original Ansel Adams prints to a local museum. For eight years, Moon donated five thousand dollars annually to a scholarship for Shasta High School graduates interested in science or medicine. In a letter to the editor of the Redding Record Searchlight, the local paper, a resident wrote, "How lucky we have been that Dr. Moon chose this country to practice in."

In the summer of 1993, a new patient, Mary Rosburg, came to Patrick Campbell with a multitude of physical complaints, including mild chest pains and shortness of breath. Rosburg and her husband spent summers living in their trailer in Trinidad, a small resort town on the California coast, just north of Eureka. Because she was having chest pains, Campbell gave Rosburg, who was in her sixties, a stress test, which involved asking her to walk on a treadmill while hooked up to a cardiac monitor. The test was inconclusive, but out of an abundance of caution, he referred his patient to Moon. Campbell assumed that the specialist would "work up" Rosberg—that is, give her a series of mildly invasive tests, including another kind of treadmill test, that would help determine whether her complaints indicated heart disease. Instead, Moon went straight to a coronary artery catheterization and promptly declared that she needed immediate bypass surgery and a heart valve replaced. Campbell was surprised both by the speed with which Moon used catheterization and by the diagnosis, but he assumed the cardiologist knew best.

Later that same day, however, Campbell got another call, from a young cardiovascular surgeon who was a newly arrived partner of Realyvasquez's. In that doctor's opinion, Rosburg did not need surgery. Campbell was startled, but as a primary care physician just starting out in the community, he didn't feel he was in any position to question Moon's judgment. He suggested the surgeon talk to Moon directly. The next morning, Campbell's patient underwent the operation. Her recovery was uneventful, but several weeks later, while in Trinidad with her husband, Rosburg abruptly developed severe chest pain and shortness of breath. Flown back by helicopter to Redding, she was found to have a large blood clot on her new heart valve and underwent emergency surgery that night to replace it. Rosburg went into acute kidney failure and died within a week.

Shaken by the death of a patient who had been essentially healthy just three months earlier, Campbell wondered if perhaps the surgeon who had called him had been right—that Moon's diagnosis had been incorrect. He concluded that he was in no position to review the records independently, and the surgeon in question left the area after one year. But after witnessing further examples of Moon's quickness to send patients to the cath lab and recommend open-heart surgery, Campbell began to worry in earnest that Moon and his group were being far too aggressive in their management of cardiac patients. Two years later, Campbell would have hard evidence that patients were being given unnecessary care by the cardiologists in Moon's practice. During a routine office visit, Emma Jean Montgomery complained to Campbell about chest pain. Campbell reports that he sent her to one of Moon's partners. The cardiologist performed a stress test, then catheterization, and told Campbell by phone that the patient had severe, three-vessel coronary artery disease and needed immediate bypass surgery. The surgery was done the next day. When Campbell received the written report from her catheterization, two months after her surgery, he was shocked to see that the cardiologist had indicated that the patient had only mild to moderate coronary artery disease and that her chest pain was not caused by her heart. Not knowing which version to believe, Campbell obtained the images of her heart that were taken during her procedure and looked at them with Dr. Roy Ditchey, a local, board-certified cardiologist who had just relocated to Redding. Campbell says that Ditchey agreed: The woman's coronary arteries were not severely blocked, and she had not needed surgery.

More than once, Campbell and other physicians who were concerned about the hospital's cardiology program and its doctors would complain to Redding Medical Center administrators. At least once, a review was promised, but over the years, as far as Campbell could tell, one was never actually undertaken. In the end, Redding Medical Center would be forced to shut down its cardiac program, after Campbell finally succeeded in alerting the Federal Bureau of Investigation and the Department of Justice. Medical records seized from the hospital were given to several outside heart specialists, who found that in twenty-seven years at Redding, Moon had catheterized some 35,000 patients, a huge number for just one physician working in a lightly populated, largely rural area. In the opinion of the outside specialists, between one quarter and one half of the patients who underwent catheterization or surgery at Redding Medical Center had been operated on inappropriately. Justice Department documents stated that at least 167 patients had died during cardiac surgery, or shortly after, as a direct result of the Redding doctors' aggressive treatment. Either the patients had been too weak to withstand the surgery, or the doctors had been negligent, or they had committed errors, sometimes in haste to go from one patient to the next.

In May 2006, the California State Medical Board moved to revoke Moon and Realyvasquez's licenses. By then Redding Medical's parent company, Tenet Healthcare Corporation, had agree to pay $59.5 million to the federal government to settle charges of Medicare fraud, at the time the largest settlement made by a health care company. A flurry of news reports appeared across the country, tracking the spectacular fall of Redding Medical Center. Most of the articles interpreted the events as an exceptional example of doctors run amok, or an isolated case of Medicare fraud, or an especially egregious episode in the ongoing saga of for-profit health care. But the story of a small hospital in northern California symbolizes a flaw in American medicine that goes far deeper—and is shared by nearly every single medical institution in the country.

No margin, no mission

The one concept that the media missed in covering the events at Redding Medical Center was that most hospitals deliver unnecessary care. As patients, we want to believe that places like Redding and doctors like Moon and Realyvasquez represent the rare case, and that a for-profit hospital so busy making money that its administrators did not want to acknowledge what was going on in their cardiac center is the exception, not the norm. Unfortunately, Redding Medical and its doctors were simply outliers at the far end of the spectrum of useless, unnecessary, and potentially dangerous care that hospitals provide (even as they simultaneously fail to deliver other kinds of care that patients need). Unnecessary care, it turns out, is inevitable in a health care system like ours, partly because of the way hospitals are paid. All hospitals need to make money, and for the most part, as we've seen, hospitals and the physicians who work in them get reimbursed for how much care they deliver, rather than how well they care for patients—let alone how efficiently they deliver that care.

When hospitals and doctors give patients medical procedures and tests they don't need, or when they fail to give patients care they do need, they are responding to the perverse incentives built into the byzantine and often-precarious reimbursement system that keeps them all afloat. In the days before health insurance and Medicare, most hospitals were run by religious charities, which operated under the motto "No margin, no mission." Their mission, of course, was tending to the sick, regardless of the patient's ability to pay; they tried to earn a small margin on the patients who could pay in order to cover the cost of their mission.

Today, hospitals still need to run a profit to stay open, even nonprofits, which make up more than three quarters of the more than five thousand hospitals in the United States—and most still turn to paying (or insured) patients in order to do so. From the humblest rural clinic to the most prestigious academic center, nonprofit hospitals generally earn at most between 2 and 6 percent profit on annual revenues, in part because forty-seven million Americans under sixty-five, or about one in six of us, have no health insurance. At most nonprofits, about 3 to 5 percent of patients are uninsured; at public teaching hospitals, it's a whopping 15 to 20 percent. In 2003, hospitals reported losing twenty-five billion dollars providing care for which they received no compensation. (Outside researchers suggest hospitals may be inflating their losses, which may be closer to sixteen billion dollars.)

In their search for margin, hospitals are constantly looking for ways to attract affluent customers—or at least, patients with well-paying insurance. One sign of that search began appearing in the 1990s, when the entrances to hospitals started to resemble hotel lobbies. Even nonprofits with religious affiliations began sporting soaring atria, booths offering fancy coffee, and valet parking. Hospital boards began hiring vice presidents for marketing and branding, and approving the construction of "VIP suites," where cash-carrying patients, many of them from foreign countries, can enjoy such special treatment as fluffy white bathrobes, daily newspaper delivery, and gourmet meals. One hospital arranged for a dinner of freshly slaughtered goat for a Muslim patient. These days, billboards can be seen along freeways and in airports touting hospital amenities and procedures, with headlines like "We Do Botox!" and "The More You Know About Uterine Fibroids, the Better You'll Feel." The tagline on a series of ads in the *New York Times Magazine* extolling the healing powers of Mount Sinai Hospital, in Manhattan, was "Another Day, Another Breakthrough." And while hospitals publicly deplore the competitive atmosphere fueled by rankings in *U.S. News & World Report*, those that top the list are happy to advertise their position. When Massachusetts General was deemed "America's Best Hospital" by *U.S. News* in 2003, the venerable institution hung a two-story-tall banner outside its front door.

Billboard ads and lattes in the lobby are only the most obvious signs that hospitals have become more-commercial enterprises. To get a clearer idea of how hospital finances work, take a stroll around the main campus of Johns Hopkins Medicine, probably the most prestigious academic medical center in the world. Founded in 1889 by Johns Hopkins, a Quaker and successful businessman who made his money investing in the Baltimore and Ohio Railroad, the hospital is now the second-largest private employer in the state of Maryland, after Wal-Mart. The original building at Hopkins, a somber gray eminence topped with peaks and spires, sits on the top of a hill in the middle of a deeply depressed section of east Baltimore. Hospitals have been called the modern equivalent of Renaissance cathedrals, which were important commercial centers as well as places of solace and hope in the face of death. That would make Johns Hopkins the Vatican of hospitals, the site of some of the most significant milestones in modern medicine, including the development of the radical mastectomy, open-heart surgery on blue babies, and kidney dialysis.

Today, the slate-clad spires of the original building are flanked by a sprawling, forty-four-acre complex of modern structures housing dozens of medical departments, including the emergency room, which can be found in a nondescript brick building on the north side of the old hospital. Designed to handle thirty-seven thousand patients a year, the ER at Johns Hopkins sees sixty thousand, the vast majority of them from the impoverished, largely black neighborhoods that stretch out on all sides from the hospital. One busy Monday, I spend an evening shift shadowing Dr. Gabor Kellen, the chief of the emergency department. The ER is jammed with patients, filling every bed and lying on gurneys in the hallways. Rich or poor, insured or not, patients who come to this emergency room have access to one of the most respected hospitals in the nation, and some of the world's best doctors. Even so, says Kellen, "People have no idea how dangerous it is to be in the emergency room when it is this crowded." Patients can wait for more than an hour before being worked up, and those who need to be admitted upstairs to the hospital may wait a day or more. The two trauma rooms, where the seriously injured are brought, are so cramped that staff members constantly bang their heads against equipment that has no proper place. The linoleum floors are scuffed and discolored; the dark blue Naugahyde covering the beds is fraying at the corners; and there is not enough room for the stacks of patient records that pile up at the nurses' station, waiting for physicians to scribble their notes hastily before moving on to the next patient.

On the other side of the old hospital, a different world awaits at the Sidney Kimmel Comprehensive Cancer Center, a 350,000-square-foot clinical facility devoted exclusively to caring for cancer patients. The lobby soars two stories high, all burnished cherry woodwork setting off the white marble floor, with the sound of piano music floating on the air. Twelve-foot-tall potted fig trees dot the brightly lit space, and tastefully upholstered purple and mauve couches are scattered about the room. The contrast between the cancer center and the emergency room at Johns Hopkins reflects one of the financial realities of running a hospital: It is better to invest capital resources in departments that will attract paying patients, who will contribute to the bottom line, than to put money into departments, like the ER, that run at a loss. The hospital is competing with other hospitals for paying cancer patients—and implicitly discouraging patients from coming to the emergency room.

A glass-and-chrome door leads off the elegant lobby to the cancer center's administrative offices. When I met with her, Terry Langbaum, the center's chief financial officer, looked like she would fit in at any corporate board meeting in her purple suit with black trim, her dark hair cut stylishly short. Treating cancer patients, she explained, is a moneymaker for Johns Hopkins, as it is for many other big hospitals. "If you look service by service, there are things that lose money and things that make money," said Langbaum. The Kimmel Cancer Center runs a tidy margin on gross revenues of about $135 million a year—a margin that Langbaum and Hopkins administrators declined to name. But Langbaum did say that the margin on cancer care is enough to generate some of the cushion needed to protect against losses in departments like the emergency room, which hemorrhages money the way a gunshot victim hemorrhages blood. About 20 to 25 percent of Hopkins emergency room patients are uninsured, and another 15 to 20 percent are "underinsured," which means they are on Medicaid or a private plan that barely covers the hospital's expenses. Caring for the poor is part of the hospital's mission, but it comes at a cost.

The cancer center, by contrast, lures a better-insured clientele, in part because the disease itself is most common among Medicare recipients. Chemotherapy represents a major source of profit for any cancer center, because the hospital buys the drugs wholesale and is permitted by Medicare and the state of Maryland to mark up the price by about 16 percent. Radiation therapy is also profitable. "There's an incentive to say we're not going to do psychiatry because we lose money," said Langbaum. "So we really should refuse to admit psychiatry patients and admit more surgery patients. The problem with that is this is a teaching institution, and we can't pick and choose what we will take care of. So we try and develop programs that do make money to [be able to] run the programs that don't make money."

In other words, Hopkins does what all hospitals must do: It uses the profits it makes on some patients to cross-subsidize the care of others. A hospital's "refuges of profit," as departments that make money are sometimes called, can include cardiology; neurosurgery; orthopedics; high-end imaging, like CT scans and MRIs; and most recently, bariatric surgery, a technique for reducing the size of the stomach to help morbidly obese patients lose weight. Obstetrics departments, which earn razor-thin margins, can be winners in some hospitals and losers in others, depending on whether the hospital delivers enough insured babies in a year to cover such fixed costs as staffing and maintaining birthing rooms and malpractice insurance. (Malpractice insurance is particularly high for obstetricians and obstetrics departments, because parents frequently sue and juries frequently side with them.) The big losers are psychiatric wards, which are magnets for poor, uninsured patients suffering from debilitating mental illness and substance abuse problems that require lengthy, expensive treatment. Medical departments, which care for patients with infectious diseases like pneumonia and chronic diseases like heart failure, are routinely in the red. The emergency departments at many hospitals break even only if they're lucky, in large measure because while their reimbursements are high, so are their costs, and many of the patients they see are uninsured. It's no surprise that between 1993 and 2003, according to a report from the Institute of Medicine, hospitals closed 425 emergency departments. In one study of California ERs, hospitals lost an average of $84 per patient seen on an outpatient basis in the ER and not admitted to the hospital. For trauma centers, where ambulances bring the critically injured, the cost of caring for patients can be mind-blowing. In the 1990s, the trauma center at the UC Davis Medical Center incurred losses of nearly $2.2 million on gunshot victims alone over a three-year period.

Much of the disparity between hospital departments can be laid at the feet of the convoluted reimbursement system that sprouted after Medicare's enactment. Medicare and some private insurers reimburse on the DRG (diagnosis-related groups) system, which pays hospitals a set fee for each diagnosis, regardless of how much the individual patient actually costs the hospital. A Medicare patient with pneumonia earns a hospital one fee, while a patient undergoing an appendectomy earns another. The DRG system came online in 1983, after seventeen years of what can only be called the golden age of government largesse, when Medicare paid hospitals on the basis of a wildly inflationary cost-plus system. In an effort to appease the hospital industry after Medicare's politically rocky start, the Social Security Administration instructed Blue Cross to gather data on how much each hospital had spent in the previous several years; the administration then reimbursed the hospital for its average annual expenses—plus another 2 percent to provide a small profit.

It was a payment plan that rivaled the cushiest of Pentagon deals, and it proved to be a recipe for fiscal disaster. Just a year after enactment, a report to Congress stated that Medicare's system for paying hospitals "contains no incentives whatsoever for good management and almost begs for poor management." Between 1970 and 1975, Medicare reimbursements to hospitals doubled, and then doubled again by 1980, far faster than anybody had anticipated at the start. Total health care spending went up an average of 12.7 percent a year throughout the 1970s, in large measure because hospitals had no reason to be efficient and every reason to run up the bill, which they did by keeping patients around for as long as possible and by buying equipment and expanding the number of beds and staff. Hospital expansion had already been encouraged by the Hill-Burton Act, passed in 1946, which provided funds to states to build new hospitals and expand existing ones. Hospitals that let costs run wild were rewarded by Medicare with even higher reimbursements; those that brought costs down were punished, often for many years to come, because each year's reimbursement was based on the costs they had reported for several previous years.

By the time Ronald Reagan took office, in 1981, Medicare looked like it would be bankrupt within the decade. Private insurers could quietly pass on their rising costs to employers, who covered increasing insurance premiums by cutting back on wage increases that might otherwise have gone to employees. But Medicare's budget was in full view of Congress, taxpayers, and the administration. Even as inflation chilled in the early 1980s, an ominous thing happened: Medical costs, unlike most other prices, kept on rising.

With its ideological preference for market-driven solutions, the Reagan administration was not about to approve price controls on hospital payments. Instead, the president signed a plan to impose the DRG system, an entirely new, draconian payment plan intended to create incentives for efficiency and reduce the number of details over which government and hospitals could quibble. The fee for each diagnosis group is set to reflect the average cost of treating that condition in an efficient hospital. If a patient is sicker than average and requires extra care, the hospital eats the difference. If the patient is healthier than average, or the hospital gets him back on his feet more quickly than average, and he consequently costs less than average, the hospital gets to keep the change. The DRG system succeeded in providing a market incentive for efficient hospitals to make a small profit, while forcing inefficient hospitals to cut expenses. Many hospitals responded by shutting down excess beds and slashing their lengths of stay, which had stretched out during the cushy cost-plus years. The system slowed the rate at which Medicare spending was rising to 8.6 percent between 1983 and 1984, the smallest annual increase since the program began. The following year, the rate of increase dropped to 5.5 percent. (The rate of increase for hospital payments went to zero the year that Redding Medical Center's shenanigans came to light, with hospitals bending over backward to avoid overcharging Medicare.)

But the DRG system also had an unexpected side effect, one that has helped drive the delivery of unneeded care in certain branches of medicine. Even though DRG fees are supposed to reflect actual costs, in reality they overpay for many procedures, especially many surgeries. At the same time, they underpay for other kinds of care. Take cardiac bypass, an exceptionally profitable surgery. In 2002, Medicare paid $24,000 per bypass surgery with cardiac catheterization, while the average cost per case, according to a report put out by the Medicare Payment Advisory Commission (MedPAC), was $14,400, leaving $9,600 profit for every bypassed patient. Other cardiac procedures offer even higher margins: Replacing a heart valve, the surgery Patrick Campbell's patient Mary Rosburg underwent, can yield as much as 60 percent profit. The net profit hospitals make from these procedures drops when Medicare patients are sicker, of course, but even so, the most common cardiac procedures typically performed on a heart attack patient earn about 6 to 16 percent over costs from Medicare reimbursement—and more than one hospital has made its entire margin on invasive cardiac procedures alone. Most private insurers don't use the DRG system, but rather a combination of negotiated payments and per diems that wind up being more generous in some markets than Medicare—and they too overpay on many procedures. From private payers, hospitals can reportedly make around $20,000 for an angioplasty procedure, about 40 percent of which is profit. On the flip side of the profit equation, the DRG payment for treating a heart attack patient with drugs alone and no surgical intervention—which for many patients is just as effective—produces about an 11 percent *loss* for the average hospital.

What all this means is that any hospital administrator with an ounce of good business sense is going to want to maximize the number of patients in profitable service lines, which they have taken to calling "centers of excellence," whether or not they are, in fact, excellent. Even at academic medical centers, administrators exert subtle pressure on the physicians working in profitable departments to keep up their productivity by performing more-profitable procedures. In this sense, a hospital is no different from any other business. In recent years, IBM has shifted its focus from selling hardware to servicing large database systems, where profits are higher. An even better analogy for the hospital industry is a low-margin, high-volume business like personal computers. Dell earns only about 5 percent profit on each computer it sells, but it sells millions and millions of them.

Similarly, hospitals want as many "bed turns," or as much "throughput," as possible in their profitable departments. The best way to accomplish this is to expand the capacity of high-margin departments to increase volume. You can think of it as the Willie Sutton strategy: Willie Sutton robbed banks because that's where the money is; hospitals invest in their moneymaking product lines because that's where the profit is.

Yet, when hospitals focus not on profits, but instead on providing care that helps patients, they often wind up being punished financially. Several hospitals around the country have experimented with integrated, supportive programs for patients with congestive heart failure. When you have congestive heart failure, your heart can't pump blood effectively, and fluid slowly builds up in your lungs. Congestive heart failure is the most common diagnosis leading to hospitalization among the elderly, and it's a miserable condition to have, because when you go into a crisis and your lungs fill with fluid, you feel as if you're drowning. Several hospitals have demonstrated that an integrated approach to care can keep heart failure patients from having a crisis and out of the hospital for long stretches. In 1995 for example, Duke University Medical Center instituted a program that allowed nurses to call heart failure patients regularly at home to check on their breathing, and to make sure they were taking the right medication, and taking it properly. Nutritionists helped patients improve their diets. Doctors shared information about them, and came up with new ways to improve care. The number of hospital admissions for congestive heart failure at Duke declined, and patients who were admitted spent less time in the hospital, bringing down costs for insurers by 37 percent. There was only one problem: Duke lost money. Bringing down costs meant hospital revenue went down, due to a decline in heart failure admissions and the premium hospitals make from Medicare for complicated cases. Other hospitals have run into the same problem when they implemented similar integrated care programs for such conditions as pneumonia, diabetes, and heart failure. That leaves hospitals looking for profit where they can, and providing care that loses money only when they must.

Langbaum offered the example of a program at Hopkins for cochlear implants, a $25,000 device that is implanted in the skull and can restore hearing to some deaf patients. The cochlear implant program is not profitable, because many insurers don't yet reimburse the hospital for the device. Every time a Hopkins surgeon implants one, the hospital must absorb its cost. "Would we want to grow the cochlear implant program? No," said Langbaum. "Are we going to advertise it? No. But we make money taking care of leukemia and lymphoma patients. Are we going to try to grow that program? Yes." Profit centers like Langbaum's helped Johns Hopkins stay open by contributing to its slender 2.5 percent margin, which netted the hospital $25.5 million in 2004 on revenues of $1.06 billion.

Investing in profit, not health

All of this goes a long ways in explaining why, in 1998, Redding Medical Center decided to expand its moneymaking product line—the cardiac procedures being performed by Realyvasquez and Moon. That year, the hospital earned $50 million in pretax profits, most of it from the California Heart Institute. "We were beyond full," one former administrator would later tell the *New York Times*. "We were flying." The hospital constructed a five-story addition, known around town as "the Tower," much of which was devoted to expanded cardiac facilities. The Tower allowed Moon and Realyvasquez to recruit other cardiologists and surgeons to the area—and to bring in more patients.

The cardiology specialists were not actually employed by the hospital; they had private practices and what's known as "admitting privileges," a relationship that is beneficial to both physician and hospital. Once known as the "doctor's workshop," a hospital is a little like a hotel filled with nursing staff, technology, and beds, where physicians are granted the privilege of admitting and treating patients. For hospitals, doctors are the medical equivalent of rainmakers in a law firm, the people who bring in the paying customers, and most hospitals bend over backward to attract and keep physicians who can bring in patients who are insured. "Hospitals need to understand who their customer is—the doctor who admits patients," as one neurosurgeon aptly puts it.

With so much riding on the cardiac team, Redding administrators and the hospital's parent company, Tenet Healthcare, stroked and pampered Moon and Realyvasquez. The hospital appointed Realyvasquez chairman of cardiothoracic surgery and made Moon chairman of the cardiology department. Moon was also a member of the hospital board, and was eventually made head of the committee charged with overseeing the quality of cardiac care. The hospital sponsored golf tournaments to benefit the cardiac unit, sometimes offering Moon the use of its emergency helicopter to fly to the golf course. Moon's success and prestige gave him unusual clout for a physician; at one point, he was instrumental in persuading Tenet to dismiss a hospital executive. "No one would ever want to take [Moon] on," a former Redding administrator told the *New York Times*. "Moon was Redding Medical Center, and he knew it."

By 1999, Campbell had stopped sending patients to Moon if he could avoid it. He left his group practice and moved to another office, preferring to send his patients to Mercy Medical Center, the hospital across town. Still, he felt compelled to call attention to the situation at Redding. He strongly suspected that Moon, Realyvasquez, and their colleagues may have been charging Medicare and Medi-Cal, the state's Medicaid program, for unnecessary procedures, not to mention putting patients at terrible risk. In March, he approached a local Redding attorney, asking his advice about how to get the government to investigate the hospital and its cardiac team. The attorney, Jerrald Pickering, a longtime Redding resident who was a patient of Campbell's at the time, listened to the doctor's story for two hours before promising to look into the matter. Over the next two weeks, Pickering made several confidential inquiries to local Medicare officials, outside physicians, and the local district attorney's office. The lawyer then wrote Campbell a letter, telling him that the public authorities were not interested in pursuing the case. "The Medicare people shuffled around and around . . . and were not really interested unless someone handed them a case fully worked up," he wrote. The district attorney was equally disinclined to pursue the issue, according to Pickering, even after he mentioned the death of one of Campbell's patients. Several of the people Pickering contacted knew about the problems at Redding Medical Center, wished any whistle-blower well, but "would undoubtedly disappear when the first shot was fired. The conclusion is inescapable: Do not blow any whistle! Period. Rationale for this is: (1) you would be very alone, (2) there is too much money involved, (3) except for the victims and/or their families, no one cares, and (4) you would instantly find yourself with a bunch of new vigorous enemies."

Several of those predictions would turn out to be painfully accurate for Campbell, who ignored the lawyer's advice and continued to search for a way to get Medicare to pay attention. Later that year, he came across an article in the magazine *Medical Economics* about a successful physician whistle-blower and the federal False Claims Act, which is intended to encourage employees of companies that do business with the federal government to report fraud and abuse. Campbell called the physician, who referred him to a New York law firm that specialized in whistle-blower cases. The firm told Campbell he needed more cases to persuade the government that there was a serious problem worth investigating. But Campbell was unable to get other Redding physicians to produce any cases, even physicians who in private complained about Moon, Realyvasquez, and Redding Medical Center. By the summer of 2001, Campbell was deeply discouraged. He'd exhausted every option he could think of for alerting the authorities. His wife was fed up with his obsession, and he still had a busy primary care practice to tend to.

A year later, Campbell got word that an FBI agent was nosing around town, asking questions after a few patients or their families had complained to the agency about the cardiac program. Throwing his lawyer's advice to the wind, Campbell called the agent. That was on a Thursday afternoon in August; the next morning he was sitting in the agent's office in Redding. Worried that the FBI agent would not believe him, Campbell arrived with over sixty pages of documents. After showing the agent his material, Campbell steered him to a nurse and two other physicians, who would eventually back up his claims that Redding's cardiac team was performing unnecessary cardiac procedures. On October 30, 2002, the FBI filed a sixty-seven-page search warrant affidavit with a judge, based largely on Campbell's information. That same day, more than forty agents from the FBI and the federal Department of Health and Human Services showed up without notice at Redding Medical Center and the doctors' offices and seized thousands of patient records and other evidence. Two weeks later, the stock price of Tenet Healthcare had tumbled from nearly fifty dollars a share to fifteen dollars.

The Justice Department's outside experts and a cardiologist hired by the state medical board would find a pattern of unnecessary and sometimes negligent care that represented "an extreme departure from standards of medicine," according to one physician who reviewed the records. In one case at Mercy Medical Center in 1996, Moon left a sixty-seven-year-old man who had suffered a massive stroke on the catheterization table, in the care of nurses without adequate instructions, and returned to his office. The man died soon thereafter. Moon would later defend his actions by saying he had done everything he could by picking up the phone and calling in a neurologist and a critical care specialist. When brought before peer review committees at Mercy to explain his actions, Moon fought back, ultimately filing lawsuits in state and federal courts against the hospital. The suits were eventually dismissed.

Other patients of Moon and Realyvasquez survived but suffered long-lasting, debilitating effects from their unnecessary surgeries. A local rancher named Stephen Hunt was only thirty-eight years old when he walked into the emergency room at Redding Medical Center just before Christmas in 2001, complaining of blurry vision in one eye. Hunt knew he had high blood pressure, but he was shocked when Moon told him he needed immediate bypass surgery—that he could suffer a heart attack and die on his way back to his car. Moon also told him there just happened to be an opening in the hospital's operating schedule on Christmas Eve. Hunt went ahead with the surgery. When the Justice Department gave Hunt's medical records to outside cardiologists, they found no evidence that the surgery had been needed. Hunt's blurry vision cleared up once his blood pressure was successfully treated with drugs, but his life would never be the same after his surgery. He suffered a hernia at the incision site, which meant he could no longer do the physical labor of ranching: the fencing, bucking hay, and moving cattle. Five years later, he lost his ranch.

On August 4, 2003, Tenet Healthcare Corporation agreed to pay $54 million to settle fraud charges brought by the federal government. In return, Redding Medical Center and Tenet were granted immunity from criminal prosecution. Ultimately, Tenet paid nearly $60 million to settle federal fraud allegations, and the Department of Health and Human Services permanently banned Redding Medical Center from receiving Medicare, Tricare (which insures members of the military), or Medi-Cal payments, effectively forcing Tenet to sell its former flagship hospital. The company eventually agreed to pay an additional $395 million in restitution to more than 769 patients and their families who sued the company. In all, Tenet would pay the federal government more than $900 million to settle charges of unlawful billing practices at Redding and other hospitals. Shareholder lawsuits amounted to $215 million. In January 2003, Moon voluntarily suspended his practice. The California State Medical Board opened an investigation.

Moon and Realyvasquee agreed to pay $1.4 million each in fines to the federal government, in lieu of criminal prosecution, while their Medicare billing privileges were revoked.

There are many lessons to be drawn from the story of Redding Medical Center, beyond the obvious fact that physicians don't like to point fingers at colleagues, even when their reticence allows patients to be harmed. But perhaps the most important lesson concerns the powerful effect that distortions in the reimbursement system can have on the decisions that hospital administrators make about how to invest capital resources. These distortions, coupled with policies dating back before the beginning of Medicare that built up the number of hospital beds until the early 1980s, have conspired to leave some cities, or parts of cities, with a surplus of certain kinds of beds and facilities—while simultaneously creating a shortage of others. In Los Angeles, for instance, there are two and a half times more intensive care unit beds per Medicare recipient than there are at the renowned Mayo Clinic, in Rochester, Minnesota, where nobody would argue that patients get substandard care. The result of this surplus of ICU beds in Los Angeles has meant that doctors are more likely to put patients in the ICU, whether or not they really need to be there. This kind of overinvestment in profitable service lines can be seen in cities and towns across the country, in New York, Miami, and Los Angeles especially—precisely the cities where Jack Wennberg's group has found the highest rates of unnecessary care. We all wind up paying for it, as this overinvestment drives up costs for Medicare, state Medicaid programs, and private insurers.

Meanwhile, more than a hundred emergency rooms around the country have closed in the past decade, victims in part of rising rates of uninsured patients appearing at their doors. At hospitals that have kept their emergency doors open, administrators have not been eager to add the additional ER beds that are often so desperately needed, because that would mean caring for more uninsured (and unprofitable) patients. Many cities now face a shortfall of emergency services, and hospitals routinely divert ambulances because their emergency departments are completely full. In Cincinnati, for example, diversions were so rare before 1998 that the city didn't even track them. By 2002, the total amount of time the city's hospitals were on divert status had jumped to 1,970 hours annually, and the problem just keeps getting worse. In the month of December 2003 alone, emergency rooms were on divert status for 1,935 hours. That's the equivalent of nearly eighty-two days.

I caught up with Patrick Campbell in June 2006, when he was living in Eugene, Oregon, pulling twelve-hour shifts as a hospitalist overseeing the care of patients admitted to Sacred Heart Medical Center. When I spoke with Campbell over the phone, he recalled the events shortly after the FBI's 2002 raid in a tone of voice that veered between incredulity and resignation. "I remember a day after the raid, I had to go see a patient over at [Redding Medical Center], and people were looking at me with hatred," he said. "Within a week, everybody in Redding knew who had talked to the government, even though I was identified on the FBI affidavit only as 'D1.'" Stories appeared in the Redding *Record Searchlight*, reporting expressions of outrage among the local citizenry—not at Moon and Realyvasquez's alleged perfidy, but rather at their persecution by the federal government. The paper quoted Rhonda Arnold, a medical assistant in Moon's office, saying, "I've never met a man as honorable as Dr. Moon." Colleagues of the doctors said it was an injustice, that patients would be "cardiac cripples" if not for Moon and Realyvasquez.

On November 8, 2002, nine days after the raid, Campbell filed a *qui tam* (whistle-blower) suit with the U.S. district court, in Sacramento. A *qui tam* lawsuit is typically filed by a private party, alleging fraud against a federal agency. If the Justice Department investigates and the fraud is proved, it enables the government to recover up to triple damages and substantial penalties from the defendants—while the whistle-blower can potentially receive a portion of the government's recovery. By then, Campbell was pretty sure he was going to need the money to start over in another town. Patients had left his practice; colleagues avoided him. The town of Redding was angry with him. The state medical board would initiate, and ultimately drop, disciplinary proceedings against him, putting his medical license at risk, after a patient complained that Campbell had given the patient's confidential records to the FBI without consent. His popularity did not improve when the hospital began laying off employees. At one point, a group of nurses threatened to sue him for loss of employment.

In June 2003, eight months after the raid, Campbell was stunned to learn that the Justice Department had moved to dismiss his whistle-blower suit in favor of another qui tam suit that had been filed just three days before his. The first-to-file whistle-blower was a Catholic priest named John Corapi, who had gone to Moon in June 2002 for what he thought was a routine cardiac checkup and had been told, like so many of Moon's patients, that he would die without immediate surgery. Unlike many patients, Corapi got a second opinion—in Las Vegas, where an old college buddy, Joseph Zerga, was an accountant. The doctors there told him that he had no significant coronary artery disease. When Corapi and Zerga complained to the Redding Medical Center CEO and got the brush-off, they went to the FBI.

The priest's legal standing as a whistle-blower was questionable. The Justice Department was suing Tenet Healthcare and the doctors on behalf of Medicare; Corapi, who was in his fifties, wasn't old enough to be a Medicare recipient. The priest's contribution to the FBI's investigation consisted only of his own medical records; he had no personal knowledge of any other cases, and his case involved only an unnecessary cardiac catheterization and a recommendation for bypass surgery. The sixty-nine pages of documents that Campbell plunked down on the desk of the FBI agent, by contrast, contained case histories covering a ten-year period; a record of Redding Medical administrators' ignoring multiple efforts to bring Moon and Realyvasquez's actions to their attention; names of physicians and a nurse who could corroborate his story; and even a glossary of medical terms. Even so, the Justice Department took the position that Corapi and Zerga were the sole whistle-blowers, because they beat Campbell to the courthouse.

In August, the court granted the Justice Department's motion to throw out Campbell's qui tam suit and subsequently enter into the $54 million settlement with Tenet Healthcare. Meanwhile, Corapi and Zerga stood to receive the entire 15 percent of the settlement owed to a whistle-blower, worth more than $8.1 million.

It would take more than two years for Campbell and his lawyer to get the
Justice Department's decision to remove him as a whistle-blower reversed.
In the meantime, Campbell's practice in Redding dried up completely. His
marriage foundered—"I wasn't the easiest person to live with," he said—
and in 2005, he left his wife and two children in Redding and moved to Eugene. When his lawyer filed an objection to the Justice Department's
decision, assistant U.S. attorney Michael Hirst, the prosecutor in the case,
accused Campbell of being "driven more by greed than indignation." The
prosecutor praised Corapi and Zerga, saying publicly, "Their willingness to
blow the whistle on fraud resulted in our putting a stop to the surgeries and
recovering $54 million." "That was a low point," Campbell told me. "It
played out in the local paper as a battle between competing whistle-
blowers, a doctor and a priest, duking it out in the courts."

In November 2005, the court reinstated Campbell's qui tam suit and he
agreed to settle for half of the whistle-blower bounty, giving him nearly
$4.5 million, before taxes and attorney's fees. Seven months later, in 2006,
his wife and kids were driving up from Redding for a visit over the Fourth
of July weekend. Campbell had not decided what he would do next. In the
weeks leading up to the settlement, he had imagined that it would bring
some sort of relief, a sense of closure, and maybe even a small measure of
vindication. But when I spoke with him, Campbell sounded tired. Some
days, he said, he thinks he will set up a new practice in Eugene or elsewhere; on other days, he wants to abandon medicine entirely and embark
on a new career.

Neither Moon nor Realyvasquez has ever admitted any wrongdoing. Shortly
after the raid, Moon appeared genuinely devastated by the charges, telling
reporters his only goal had been to keep his patients safe from heart disease.
He wept when a group of supporters strung up a banner that said, WE SUP-
PORT OUR DOCTORS! outside the courthouse. Maybe Moon and Realyvasquez and the hospital were deliberately bilking Medicare, as the Justice
Department's charges against them indicate. Or maybe, as Moon and Realyvasquez claim, they were making judgment calls within the wide latitude

permitted by the art of medicine, the uncertainty of cardiology. If that's the case, then the saga of Redding Medical Center points to the desperate need in medicine for clearer standards and better evidence for what works and what doesn't. The story of Redding also highlights the need for a new way to pay doctors and hospitals, a system that doesn't allow financial imperatives to propel clinical decisions.

FOUR Broken Hearts

At one o'clock on an afternoon not long after Christmas Day, 2006, in room 6 on the fifth floor of the Washington Hospital Center, in Washington, D.C., Dr. Jonathan Altschuler begins work on his sixth patient of the day, a seventy-year-old woman who is suffering from severe chest pains. A short, muscular man with close-cropped light brown hair and an angular face, Altschuler is a master of his craft. He's been in practice for twenty years and has performed perhaps ten thousand catheterizations, also known as angiograms. His patient—we'll call her Jean Crofton—is lying on a slim, ten-foot-long bed called a catheterization table, which is mounted on a mechanism that allows the doctor to move the patient back and forth under an X-ray machine. Crofton is awake but groggy from a sedative. She lies quietly as two nurses shave and scrub both sides of her groin before draping her entire body first in sterile blue paper and then a large plastic sheet. A Moody Blues melody fills the room from Altschuler's iPod speakers as he and a technician don gloves and paper gowns.

Before moving to his patient's side, Altschuler quietly rattles off the particulars of her case: "Elderly female, a smoker. Unstable angina. Abnormal nuclear stress test." Translation: Crofton has cripplingly intense chest pains that hit at odd moments—when she walks up stairs, gardens, or is at rest. The abnormal stress test suggests that she has at least one severe narrowing, or stenosis, in her coronary arteries, the vessels that supply the muscle of the heart with blood. The combination of unstable angina and an abnormal stress test indicates she's at high risk for a heart attack.

96

Standing at Crofton's right side, about even with her thigh, Altschuler palpates her groin to find the femoral artery, the pencil-thick blood vessel that runs right under the skin. "That's just my hand you're feeling. Now you're going to feel a big pinch and a sting," he says. Crofton groans loudly as Altschuler injects analgesic into her groin. He pauses for five seconds to let the drug take effect before slipping a needle fitted inside a plastic collar into her artery. Bright red blood pumps rhythmically out of the collar until he pulls out the needle and replaces it with a blue, hollow, flexible plastic tube, the catheter. A screen at eye level on the other side of the catheterization table shows an X-ray movie of Crofton's chest. On it, the catheter slides like a long, slender worm up the abdominal aorta until it reaches the top of her chest, where it follows the U-turn in the aorta down into the heart.

Leaving the catheter in place, Altschuler threads a thin, stiff wire into the opening. Once it reaches the heart, he says, "Puff, please," and a technician pushes a button that sends contrast, a fluid that shows up like dark smoke on an X-ray, through the catheter into the coronary arteries. Suddenly, the arteries appear momentarily on the screen, like gray, evanescent tree roots wrapped around the hazy, almost invisible shape of the heart. "Puff it," says Altschuler. "Puff it." Two more brief glimpses, each lasting no longer than two seconds, are enough to tell him where he is. He twirls and pushes the wire. Its flexible tip, no thicker than the hair from a horse's tail, probes the inside of the aorta in search of an opening that is perhaps twice the diameter of a pencil lead. After less than a minute, Altschuler says, "Okay, picture." A bigger dose of contrast flows up the catheter, and suddenly an entire section of Crofton's coronary arteries appear on the screen in black, with three main branches leading to smaller and smaller vessels.

"There's a lot of disease there," says Altschuler. Crofton's vessels narrow in several places where plaque, an accumulation of gunky, inflamed cells, has built up. The worst stenosis is blocking a main branch of an artery almost completely; blood can barely squeak by. This is the likely culprit in her angina, which occurs when tiny blood clots or bits of plaque get stuck in a narrow spot, temporarily blocking the flow of blood. Altschuler asks one of the technicians to bring him a stent, an expandable wire mesh tube no wider than a pine needle. In use since the late 1980s, stents have now nearly replaced balloon angioplasty as the preferred technique for opening a blocked section of artery. Altschuler takes a wire with the stent on one end and threads it up the catheter until it rests just inside the narrow spot in Crofton's artery.

Suddenly, the room goes still. All eyes turn to a monitor that shows electrical measurements of the patient's heart. The stent has completely occluded her blood vessel, and her heart's electrical activity is registering the possibility of an actual heart attack. On the screen that shows the blood vessels, there is a silver-dollar-sized blank patch of heart where the branches of her arteries should have been. No blood is getting past the stent.

Altschuler begins speaking quietly in the flattened-out, everything-is-going-to-be-fine tone that doctors use when a potential crisis looms. "The vessel's completely occluded . . . Puff," he says, as he moves the stent back and forth, millimeter by millimeter. "I can't tell . . . OK, yeah, yeah, yeah . . . I see it, I see it."

"Puff." On the screen, the stent is now in place inside the stenosis. "Inflate," Altschuler says sharply. The technician switches on a handheld hydraulic pump to inflate a tiny balloon inside the stent, expanding the stent to push against the vessel walls.

"Fourteen," says Altschuler. "Sixteen." He is counting out the balloon inflation pressure inside the stent.

"Down!"

The technician turns off the pump with a loud click, and Altschuler quickly extracts the balloon and wire from Crofton's blood vessel leaving the stent behind. At the next puff of contrast, everyone looks to the screen. In the spot where the last picture showed nothing, not a branch or a twig below the blockage, Crofton's arteries are once again filling and emptying rhythmically with each beat of her heart. Crofton's coronary artery is doing its job once again, supplying the heart muscle, that fist-sized pump that keeps us going, beat by beat, day in and day out, with life-giving blood. Technicians and nurses resume their activities around the room. The red line on the heart monitor that had been shooting up and down wildly is now oscillating within normal range. Without comment, Altschuler turns back to his task, rethreading the wire up the catheter into the next blocked artery.

Today, more than two million Americans a year find themselves lying on a catheterization table as a flexible wire is threaded through their femoral arteries and into their hearts. About eight hundred thousand of those catheterizations are performed on people in the throes of a heart attack, the patients who generally have the most to gain from an angioplasty or stent. But the vast majority of invasive cardiology procedures aren't aimed at saving lives. They are elective procedures, which means they are performed on patients who have symptoms of heart disease—stable angina, for instance, and shortness of breath—but aren't in imminent danger of dying. Of those 1.2 million elective cardiac procedures, at least 160,000 are "inappropriate," meaning they should not have been done, according to cardiologists' own rules for when to put in a stent or do an angioplasty. When outside cardiologists looked at the patient records from Redding Medical Center, they found hundreds of such inappropriate cases. Studies have found that half a million of the angioplasties and stents performed each year are of questionable value—not quite inappropriate, but not clearly called for either. The latest research, published in 2007 by scientists from the Veterans Health Administration, suggests that the vast majority of elective cardiac procedures are no more effective at preventing heart attacks and death than medical management, which involves giving patients drugs and counseling.

That's a lot of unnecessary invasive procedures, especially when you consider that rules for when to do these procedures have been clearly worked out. In many areas of medicine, far fewer data exist to guide physicians. Given the fact that invasive cardiologists should have the information they need in order to know when a catheterization is appropriate and when it isn't, you have to wonder why they perform so many unnecessary procedures. The answer to this question is complicated by several factors, not the least of which is the handsome compensation they receive for every stent, catheterization, and angioplasty they perform. But money isn't the only motivator here. Another reason invasive cardiologists do so many inappropriate procedures has to do with the art of medicine; when faced with a patient with symptoms of heart disease, a primary care physician or cardiologist must use her clinical judgment before sending the patient off to the catheterization lab. Once the patient is on the table, the invasive cardiologist who performs the procedure has his own decisions to make. Does the patient even need to be catheterized? If so, which narrowings actually need to be opened and which ones are best left alone?

But the third, less-obvious aspect of unnecessary cardiac procedures has to do with the perverse and poorly understood economics of American health care. Cardiac catheterization serves as a dramatic example of the law of supply-driven demand, an economic principle that may be unique to medicine. In this case, supply-driven demand means that when hospitals build more catheterization labs, cardiologists do more catheterizations.

Pump head

The chief of clinical cardiology at Johns Hopkins Medicine is a physician named Richard Lange, a tall man in his early fifties with a soft Texas accent and a large head topped with pure white hair. After doing his residency training in cardiology at Johns Hopkins, Lange spent twenty-five years at the University of Texas Southwestern Medical Center, in Dallas, before returning to Baltimore in 2004. On a bright spring day, he sits in his office and explains the history behind cardiologists' use and misuse of their invasive procedures.

"When I trained here in the early eighties, clot-busting drugs were not available. Angioplasty wasn't routinely available. Clopidogrel wasn't available. That's the antiplatelet drug we use to keep clots from forming. Defibrillators were just experimental," he says. All of these tools would soon revolutionize the treatment of heart attacks, but balloon angioplasty was especially gratifying for cardiologists, because they could actually see the effects of their handiwork. They could inflate the balloon in an occluded blood vessel, where it crushed the blockage against the sides of the artery, extract the ballon, and then watch the flow of blood. "Angioplasty seemed to be incredibly successful in certain patients," says Lange. "Over the last twenty years we've refined our efforts. The equipment we use for doing the procedure is better.

The radiological machines are better. The drugs we use are better. But the only way to know if your improvements are beneficial, if they really improve the outcome of patients, is to measure it in clinical trials."

That's where cardiologists have gotten into trouble. It was clear to them that they could save a heart attack patient's life with so-called primary angioplasty and stents, by opening a completely blocked vessel that was causing the attack. They also knew that angioplasty and stents could relieve the pain of angina and in some instances could help patients breathe more easily (because it improves the heart's ability to pump blood to the lungs). It seemed like an obvious, entirely logical extension to imagine that angioplasty and stents could also *prevent* heart attacks in patients with symptoms of serious heart disease, by keeping all of their blood vessels open. But when this idea has been measured in clinical trials, it hasn't panned out. "We know we can prevent heart attacks with aspirin, and with drugs called beta-blockers. We know that for certain," says Lange. "But it has turned out to be a little more mushy when it comes to the advanced technologies. Angioplasty and stenting have never been shown to improve survival. You can stent until the cows come home and not prevent a heart attack." This finding was supported most recently by a Veterans Affairs study published in the *New England Journal of Medicine*. And while the elective use of angioplasty and stents has skyrocketed over the past ten to fifteen years, there has been no change in the rate of heart attacks.

Only recently have cardiologists begun to understand why this is so. They once believed that plaque in the coronary arteries accumulated slowly over decades, like sludge in a pipe, until one day it finally blocked an artery completely and triggered a heart attack. By crushing the plaque against the walls of the artery, they reasoned, angioplasty or a stent ought to keep the blood flowing, at least for a time. Stents were seen as a more permanent solution, because they would actually hold the plaque up against the arterial wall. But it didn't work out that way. About a third of the time, stents clogged up with scar tissue in a matter of months, requiring another procedure. Now there are drug-eluting stents, devices that have been coated with drugs that seep slowly from the mesh and are supposed to prevent scar tissue from forming. The jury is still out on whether these stents will turn out to be superior. But even if they do prevent scar tissue from reblocking the artery, they still won't prevent heart attacks. That's because a heart attack occurs when a bit of plaque ruptures, triggering a blood clot that flows toward smaller and smaller arteries until it blocks the flow of blood. Most of the time, there's no predicting when or where a plaque will rupture, and just because a cardiologist installs a stent on one blocked artery doesn't mean an area of plaque that was in the process of forming on another won't be the one to burst and cause a heart attack. Studies have shown that in 75 to 80 percent of cases, none of the plaque that a cardiologist fixes with angioplasty or a stent ultimately proves to be the culprit in a heart attack.

It turns out that even bypass surgery offers a reduction in the chances of dying for only a tiny minority of patients. To perform a bypass, a surgeon takes a section of vein from the patient's leg and sews the ends above and below a blocked section of coronary artery, so that blood bypasses the blockage. Three large clinical trials looking at the survival benefit of bypass suggested that it helps only the sickest of the sick, about 3 percent of patients in the trials who underwent bypass. Dr. Nortin Hadler, a professor at the University of North Carolina and a vocal critic of many aspects of American medicine, points out that the potential benefit of bypass has to be weighed against the risks, including a 1 to 2 percent mortality rate during or shortly after the surgery. While some bypass patients are given a new lease on life, about 45 percent suffer from cognitive deficits like memory loss, confusion, or depression—"pump head" in the vernacular of cardiology, because patients undergoing bypass are generally put on a heart-lung machine, which pumps blood through the body while the heart is immobilized. These deficits can persist in many cases. "The healthy, active postsurgery patient is an urban legend," says Hadler. "An alarming number never return to the workforce or describe themselves as well again."

John Abramson tells the story of just such a patient. Abramson is a primary care physician who practiced for twenty years on the outskirts of Boston. He left his practice several years ago to research and write Overdo$ed America, a critique of drug research and pharmaceutical marketing. He now teaches at Harvard Medical School. His patient was an eighty-two-year-old man we'll call Henry Graydon, who had been diagnosed with metastatic prostate cancer. Graydon also suffered from heart disease, which Abramson was treating medically. While in Florida one winter, Graydon suffered a heart attack and underwent bypass surgery. Back home in Boston in the spring, he came to Abramson's office with a postsurgical infection in the sternum, the bone that runs up the middle of the chest.

Every day, for several weeks, Graydon and his wife came to Abramson for Graydon to have his wound drained. That meant removing a half-inch-wide, two-foot-long piece of gauze from the hole in Graydon's chest and then repacking the wound, inch by inch, with a fresh length of gauze. As he worked, Abramson noticed that Graydon and his wife, a previously happy couple who had been married for decades, were now bickering constantly. "If I had to leave the room for ten seconds, they would already be in an argument when I got back," says Abramson. "One day he came in without his wife, and I'm stuffing the gauze in, and it takes concentration not to hurt him. He said, 'Doc, I found out the secret to a happy marriage.' I stopped. He said, 'When my wife and I start to argue, I just let her think she's right.'" Graydon came in the next day, again without his wife, obviously agitated from another argument with her. Abramson was in the midst of repacking his wound when Graydon said, "Remember what I told you yesterday?" Abramson replied that he did. His patient said bitterly, "Just forget it."

Graydon died a year later of his prostate cancer. Abramson never understood how a harmonious marriage could fall apart so completely so late in life, until he began reading the literature on bypass surgery. Half of bypass patients over sixty-five, he learned, suffer from some form of dementia as a result of their surgery. "The reason he was fighting with his wife was he had a cognitive impairment," says Abramson. "He would ask her the same question over and over again. When they fought, she would say, 'Damn it, you just asked me that.' He had pump head."

Yet despite the potential for harm, physicians continue to give patients unnecessary bypass surgery, along with unneeded angioplasties and stents. In 2001, a group of researchers from Harvard and Brown universities published a study that looked at the medical records of nearly four thousand Medicare patients from 173 hospitals located in five states. Some of the patients had undergone a balloon angioplasty; others had had bypass surgery. The researchers wanted to know if the treatment given to this randomly chosen group of Medicare patients was appropriate, according to the set of rules that heart specialists have worked out. These rules are supposed to guide physicians when it comes to deciding whether to send an individual patient to the cath lab or the operating room or to treat him with medical management, which includes prescribing blood pressure medicine and blood thinners, like aspirin, to prevent his arteries from being blocked by plaque, and offering advice on improving his diet and exercise habits.

The researchers asked a group of outside cardiologists to use the established rules, which were already biased in favor of the treatments, to evaluate each case and decide whether or not the patient got the appropriate care. In the judges' estimation, about 75 percent of the bypass surgeries were clearly appropriate, while only about 30 percent of the angioplasties were. In 14 percent of the angioplasties and 10 percent of the bypass surgeries, the procedure was clearly not appropriate; surgery was entirely unnecessary for about 168,000 people who underwent angioplasty and 40,000 who had bypass surgery. The rest of the patients fell into a muddy middle ground, where the judges couldn't agree. In 15 percent of bypass cases and 54 percent of angioplasties, some of the experts thought the procedure might have been appropriate, while others thought it might not—they couldn't be sure.

The cost of all those unnecessary procedures and surgeries should be of obvious concern not only to the patients who may have been harmed by them but also to the people who pay for health care, which is to say, you and me. (We fund Medicare through our taxes. When we get our health insurance through our employers, most of us pay a portion of the premium directly; we also pay our employer's share indirectly in the form of lower wages.) The entire heart surgery industry is worth about $100 billion a year. Drug-coated stents alone cost U.S. taxpayers and insurers $3.4 billion. More than a billion dollars a year are being wasted by cardiothoracic surgeons who perform bypasses on patients whose symptoms could be controlled with medical management, using drugs, diet, and exercise, which are not only cheaper but also safer and far less invasive.

Before the most recent rigorous study published by Veterans Health Administration researchers, four large, randomized, controlled clinical trials had compared angioplasty to medical management of patients with serious heart disease, many of whom had already had a heart attack. All four studies found no difference in rates of subsequent heart attacks or death (and one found that mortality rates were actually higher in patients who were treated aggressively). The fifth study, from the VHA, confirmed those results. Why, then, do cardiologists persist in using an aggressive procedure or surgery when conservative, medical management is often an equally appropriate, if not a better choice? To be fair, deciding what a patient needs always requires a measure of clinical judgment, and a doctor's decision is complicated by many factors. What does the patient's EKG look like? How long has she had symptoms? Is she showing signs of heart failure or other potentially fatal complications? Even when faced with a heart attack patient coming through the double doors of the emergency room, physicians must use their judgment—the art of medicine—to make what can be a life-and-death decision about whether the patient needs a stent to open an artery or whether drugs alone will do the trick.

But that judgment, it turns out, can be influenced by more than just medical data. In an editorial published in the *New England Journal of Medicine*, Richard Lange and L. David Hillis, a colleague from Texas, place a portion of the blame for unnecessary procedures at the feet of heart disease patients and their families, who often expect and insist upon aggressive treatment. "In an era in which invasive cardiac procedures are a manifestation of high-technology," write Lange and Hillis, "the term 'conservative management' may project the impression (to physicians and patients alike) of obsolescence, inadequacy, and inferiority . . ."

But notice here that Lange and Hillis don't lay all of the blame for unnecessary cardiac procedures on patients; many of their doctors also think aggressive care is better, even though the scientific evidence says otherwise. When it comes to medical data, it doesn't get much better than four well-conducted studies all arriving at the same conclusion, yet some cardiologists, write Lange and Hillis, are skeptical that the results of these trials apply to their patients. Many doctors are happy to embrace the data that

confirm their preconceived notions about the effectiveness of invasive treatment, while ignoring studies that don't. Some simply lack the analytical
training to assess the evidence. More than one cardiologist has put in a stent
or two, patted a patient on the shoulder, and said, "You're as good as new,"
in the sincere belief that he has just fixed the patient's problem and prevented a heart attack.

Eric Topol, a prominent cardiologist at the Scripps Clinic in La Jolla, California, argues that there are both honorable and not-so-honorable reasons
for cardiologists to do this. A few years back, Topol, who was one of the pi-
oneers in the development of angioplasty, coined a phrase for cardiologists'
desire to fix every little blockage they see on the screen in a catheterization
lab. He called it the "oculostenotic reflex." Recently, he elaborated on what
he meant: "You see a stenosis, and you automatically think, 'We need to do
a stent.' Seeing is very powerful. So much of the work that's done could be
considered ornamental: Here's a narrowing; let's fix it up and make it look
pretty." (Seeing is indeed very powerful for physicians. Cardiothoracic surgeons talk about watching a heart "pink up" after bypass.) Yet most of the
narrowings that cardiologists feel compelled to treat with stents, says Topol,
are perfectly innocent. "They aren't tied to symptoms in the patient," he
says, and they don't pose a risk of causing a heart attack. Opening them up
with a stent almost certainly won't make the slightest difference in either
the patient's chances of suffering a heart attack in the future or his longevity
and quality of life. Yet once a patient is lying on the catheterization table and
the cardiologist has spotted a narrow place where blood ought to be flowing freely, it is incredibly hard to walk away. "You get on the train," says
Topol, "and you can't get off once it's moving."

Then there's the less-honorable reason for cardiologists to ignore the
data. Topol says, "The procedure can be done quickly; it is safe; and cardiologists find it relatively lucrative—and that's not helping matters." Medicare
pays the physician between $1,700 and $1,900 to catheterize a patient. The
doctor makes another $800 for the insertion of the first stent and $200
more for each additional stent, each of which generally takes no more than
a few minutes to slip into place. All those catheterizations and stents add up
to a median income for interventional cardiologists of more than $450,000

a year. (The hospital receives a separate fee that more than covers the cost of nurses' and technicians' salaries, equipment, supplies, and an overnight stay if the patient receives a stent. In total, the patient who walks out with one or more stents costs his insurer on average between $10,000 and $15,000, and as much as $50,000.)

Topol makes another important observation: Not all cardiologists are equally inclined to treat heart disease patients with aggressive intervention. In 1995, Topol led a study that looked at the treatment that heart disease patients received in different parts of the country. Just as Jack Wennberg had found variations in surgical procedures in Vermont and Maine, Topol's team of researchers discovered large differences in cardiac treatment in different locations. Patients were least likely to get angioplasty or bypass surgery in New England and on the West Coast; they were most likely to undergo an invasive procedure in Texas, Oklahoma, Louisiana, and other states in the south central region. Doctors in south central states were particularly quick to deliver elective angioplasties—the angioplasties that are done on patients who are not in the midst of a heart attack. The reverse was true for medical management, which was used far more often in New England than anywhere else in the country and far less often in places like Texas and Oklahoma. But here's the most important part of Topol's findings: Differences among regions were not linked to differences in health. The heart disease patients who received more-aggressive treatment in Texas and Mississippi weren't any sicker than the patients in Massachusetts and California; nor were they any more likely to benefit from angioplasty or surgery. Nonetheless, doctors in the south central states were far more enthusiastic about using invasive treatments.

Cardiologists' often-inflated beliefs about the curative power of their catheters undoubtedly contributed to the huge variation in rates of cardiac procedures observed by Topol. Some cardiologists cling to their belief in procedures, which certainly look miraculous on the X-ray screen, despite the data that say they won't make a bit of difference in the patient's outcome or they could cause harm.

This faith in the power of interventional cardiology and bypass surgery represents another kind of surgical signature, the varying degree of

aggressiveness that Wennberg first observed among physicians in Vermont
and Maine thirty years ago. In Elyria, Ohio, for instance, an aging industrial
city in the northeastern part of the state, a single group of thirty-one cardiologists has been responsible for thousands of invasive cardiac procedures
performed at the town's community hospital. In 2004, Medicare patients
around Elyria received angioplasties or stents at a rate nearly four times the
national average—about 42 procedures per thousand Medicare enrollees in
Elyria versus 11.3 in the rest of the country. In an interview with the *New York
Times*, Dr. John Schaeffer, the founder and president of the cardiology group,
the North Ohio Heart Center, said there's a simple explanation for Elyria's
high rate of procedures: Doctors in his group are quicker to put their patients on the catheterization table than other cardiologists, and quicker to
intervene. They believe in what they are doing. "With absolutely no exception," he said, "patients given aggressive treatment will come out with a
better outcome."

Yet aggressive cardiologists don't tell the whole story. One of the most
powerful drivers of geographic variation is the supply of catheterization
laboratories. Topol's group found an almost-perfect correlation between the
availability of catheterization labs in a region and the propensity for patients
to be given angioplasty or bypass surgery. There were lots more catheterization labs per capita in the south central region, where the rates of
catheterization and invasive cardiology were highest, and many fewer labs
per capita in regions where rates were lowest.* In other words, when hospitals invested in cath labs, cardiologists tended to fill them with patients
and perform lots of surgeries.

There are two ways to interpret these results. One explanation is that the
people of, say, Texas are getting the right number of stents because they
have plenty of cath labs available to them, and people in places like California, where the number of labs per capita is lower, are being denied procedures they need. The alternative explanation is that the extra cath labs in
Texas aren't doing Texans any good. In fact, maybe the mere presence of

---

*The only exception was New England, where there are lots of cath labs but physicians were less likely
to perform invasive procedures.

cath labs is leading to a lot of unnecessary procedures. (The United States as it happens, has more catheterization labs per capita than any other developed country, and its citizens undergo invasive procedures far more often, yet our mortality rates from heart disease are no lower.)

One way to decide which interpretation is correct is to look at the mortality rates in the different regions to see if fewer cath labs leads to more deaths. It doesn't. According to a recent study, there's no difference in mortality rates among regions with different numbers of cath labs. In other words, heart disease patients aren't dying on the West Coast because of a shortage of cath labs there. And Texas patients aren't any better off for the surfeit of labs in their region. In fact, it turns out that in places where cath labs are widely available and patients are getting more angioplasties and stents, cardiologists aren't necessarily performing the procedures on the right patients. Doctors in areas where there are lots of cath labs underuse their procedures on many patients who would likely benefit and overuse them on many others who are least likely to benefit and would have done just as well with medical management. In other words, these doctors have simply increased the number of total procedures they perform, without necessarily targeting the patients who really need it.

Party tricks

What all of these data suggest, aside from the observation that many cardiologists are either unaware of the scientific evidence or ignoring it when making their decisions, is that the supply of medical resources, rather than the underlying needs of patients, is determining how much medical care they get. Or to put it another way, supply is inducing demand.

Markets are not supposed to work this way. In most other industries, when supply exceeds demand, the product sits around on the shelves or in the showroom until the seller either reduces the price enough or ships it elsewhere to be sold. If your local car dealer has too many sport-utility vehicles on the lot, she either lowers the price or sends them to another dealer in an area where there's more demand for SUVs. If developers build too many apartments or charge too much for them, the apartments sit empty. If there are too many maid services in town, they must drop their prices in order to find new customers who were previously unwilling to pay for a maid at the higher price.

Medical markets, it turns out, often don't behave like other industries—despite the business-speak hospital administrators use to describe their profitable departments as "centers of excellence" and the care they provide as "product lines." If medicine did obey the rules of supply and demand in the same way as other goods and services, like SUVs or housecleaning, catheterization labs would sit unused when the number of labs in town exceeded the number of people in the population who really needed angioplasty or stents. If a hospital's lab sat empty too often, the hospital would need to shut it down, or lower the price of an angiogram to lure patients away from competing hospitals.

But that's not what happens in health care. Hospitals generally don't offer sales on catheterizations; they lower prices only under pressure from insurers and Medicare. Even if they did slash prices, it probably wouldn't attract more patients, since most people are insured and thus insulated from the price of their care, and in any case would undoubtedly view a cut-rate catheterization with some suspicion. (Using the cheapest maid service in town is one thing; getting inexpensive medical care could be bad for your health!) In any case, most patients base such serious medical decisions as where to undergo a catheterization not on the price of the procedure, which is generally unknown to them, but rather on the advice of their trusted doctor.

Yet even without lowering prices, cath labs rarely sit empty, because hospitals can employ a variety of methods for keeping them full. When they find their labs running below capacity, they may begin advertising the wonders of their cardiology departments ("Another day, another miracle"), or they may go out and recruit a hotshot cardiologist or two who can bring in more (paying) patients. When interventional cardiologists find appointments available in the lab, they too generally try to fill them—or as Wennberg might put it, they go hunting for moose. A readily available cath lab also lowers the barrier for other doctors to refer patients to an interventional cardiologist for an angiogram, because they know their patients won't have to wait weeks or months to get an appointment. And once that catheter has been slid into the patient's heart and the cardiologist has spotted a narrowing, the oculostenotic reflex kicks in, and the patient's chances of getting a stent or bypass surgery have just gone up.

This pattern of medical "demand" expanding to consume the supply of resources is so pervasive in medicine that it even has a name: Roemer's law. In the 1960s, Milton Roemer, a health services researcher from the University of California, Los Angeles, coined the phrase "A built hospital bed is a filled hospital bed." Twenty years later, Jack Wennberg set out to understand how Roemer's law actually worked. Why was it that more beds led to more hospital admissions (and more cath labs led to more catheterizations, stents, and bypass surgeries)? How were empty beds driving the clinical decisions of doctors? Weren't doctors making their decisions on the basis of the patient's needs? To answer these questions, he and several colleagues at Dartmouth looked at how often Medicare recipients in two different cities, Boston and New Haven, Connecticut, were hospitalized.

They chose Boston and New Haven because both cities were home to prestigious academic medical centers—the Harvard hospitals in Massachusetts and the Yale–New Haven Medical Center in Connecticut. There were 978 hospital beds in New Haven, versus nearly 3,000 beds scattered among several hospitals in Boston. When the number of beds was tallied according to the size of the population using them, Boston had 55 percent more beds per thousand Medicare recipients than New Haven. Just as Roemer's law predicted, Wennberg's team found that the elderly in Boston spent about 40 percent more time in the hospital than those in New Haven. It's worth pausing for a moment to think about what that really means. If a patient had gallstones in New Haven, he might be treated medically; if he lived in Boston he was 40 percent more likely to be hospitalized. Or if a patient had gall bladder surgery that required a single night at Yale–New Haven, the same surgery would have meant two nights at a Harvard hospital. Yet patients in Boston weren't any sicker than those in New Haven; they were just more likely to be hospitalized—and admitting them more often to Boston hospitals did not appear to improve their outcomes.

Then Wennberg took things a step further and began asking doctors in the two cities how they made their decisions about whether or not a patient was sick enough to be admitted. First, the researchers asked physicians in New Haven if they were being forced to ration care in any way, if they felt there weren't enough beds for their patients and they had to decide who was sickest and most in need of hospitalization. The doctors said no. They perceived the number of hospital beds available to them as being just right. When Wennberg went to Boston and asked physicians the same question, they gave the same answer. Then, as Megan McAndrew, the editor of The Dartmouth Atlas of Health Care, recalls, "Jack would do this little party trick and switch the data." Before showing a group of Boston physicians the results from his study, Wennberg would reverse the labels, so that the hospitalization rates from Boston were labeled "New Haven" and vice versa. He would then show his audience the mislabeled slides, which made it appear as if doctors in New Haven were hospitalizing patients far more often than their peers in Boston, rather than the other way around. Boston audiences "would come up with all these reasons for why those guys down in New Haven were admitting too many patients," says McAndrew. When Wennberg showed New Haven doctors the mislabeled slides, they would come up with reasons why their peers in Boston weren't admitting *enough* patients to the hospital. Then, says McAndrew, "Jack would say, 'Oops, my mistake. I had those switched.' "

The bottom line was that regardless of which city they were practicing in, doctors were blithely, astonishingly unaware that the supply of hospital beds was affecting their clinical decisions. They thought they were putting patients in the hospital entirely on the basis of what would help the patients—that medical demand, or how sick their patients were, was driving their clinical decisions. "Jack would talk to a doctor who had moved from New Haven to Boston and ask if he ever said to himself, 'I can admit anybody I want to up here!' " says McAndrew. The physicians reported they never even noticed a difference in the number of beds available to them. She recalls traveling to Sun City, Arizona, where she visited two hospitals with the fewest intensive care unit beds in the nation, relative to the surrounding population—and not surprisingly, the lowest rates for admitting Medicare recipients to the ICU. "I got into the ICUs and talked to the nurses and the doctors," says McAndrew. "I asked them, do you feel desperate here for more ICU beds? They said, no, in fact, we feel like some people who are admitted don't need to be here. Then I asked them if they knew they were at the rock bottom for ICU admissions in the nation. They were absolutely gob-smacked."

Wennberg came up with an allegory for how the supply of hospital beds can induce demand by influencing doctors' clinical decisions without their being conscious of it. Imagine a physician is standing in front of a conveyor belt that carries black, white, and gray marbles. The physician's job is moving the marbles from the belt to a shelf, according to a set of rules. White marbles, which represent the sickest patients, with conditions like heart attacks, strokes, and hip fractures, are always put on the shelf, which represents a hospital bed. Black marbles, which stand for the patients with mild complaints like colds and twisted ankles, are never put on the shelf. Gray marbles are the patients with serious but not necessarily life-threatening ailments, like pneumonia or gallstones, or chronic conditions like hernias, congestive heart failure, and angina. It is the decisions about these kinds of cases, the gray middle ground, that get doctors into trouble.

It turns out there are very few rules to guide physicians about how to treat many serious and/or chronic conditions. Does this pneumonia case really need to be hospitalized, or will she do just as well taking antibiotics at home? Is that patient's gall bladder disease bad enough to warrant surgery or will a change in diet do the trick? Any time there's any uncertainty about what's best for a patient, a doctor's decisions can be influenced by the supply of a medical resource, like beds. Physicians will tend to put a not-so-sick patient in a bed—provided there is sufficient room in the hospital—rather than find home nursing care or keep in touch with the patient by phone to monitor how he's doing or secure a bed in a nursing home, all of which can take a lot of time and trouble. Other researchers have confirmed this notion that physicians adapt their admission and discharge decisions according to the number of ICU beds available, admitting patients who are less ill and letting them stay longer when there is a place for them.

The consequences of these decisions are enormous. By admitting millions of patients who may not need to be in the hospital, or by putting them in more expensive beds than necessary, physicians are needlessly driving up the cost of health care (and more important, as we saw in chapter 2, needlessly exposing their patients to the dangers of being in the hospital, where errors, complications, and infection kill thousands of people each year).

This pattern of supply-driven demand, or supply-sensitive care, as Wennberg calls it, holds true not just for hospital beds but for all kinds of medical resources, even the number of specialists in a given area. In 2002, the *New England Journal of Medicine* published a startling study that found a fourfold difference in the number of neonatologists, the physicians who specialize in caring for sick newborn babies, in different regions across the country. The researchers looked at birth and death records for nearly four million babies born in 1995 to see if having more neonatologists in a region reduced the chances that an infant would die within the first month of life. They found that having about 4.3 neonatologists per ten thousand births in a region was best for reducing the chances of death. Any fewer specialists and the death rate began to climb among infants, particularly those born prematurely, at low birth weight, or with birth defects. Happily, there are only a few parts of the country that don't have enough neonatologists, or enough beds in a neonatal ICU, where the sickest babies are cared for. On the other hand, there are many areas of the country with extra specialists, beyond the 4.3 per ten thousand births—and excess neonatal intensive care beds because neonatal ICUs are profitable. Those additional doctors and beds do nothing to further reduce the infant death rate. They do, however, increase the chances that a relatively healthy baby will be placed in an expensive intensive care bed and cared for by a high-priced specialist.

Here, then, is an explanation for how a hospital's investments in technology, facilities, and physicians can lead to unnecessary care. A hospital constructs a cath lab, and all of a sudden cardiologists start doing more angioplasties and stents. When Redding Medical Center built the Tower and allowed Moon and Realyvasquez to recruit more cardiologists, the people of a rural, lightly populated area of northern California began getting even more unnecessary surgeries and cardiac procedures.

Once you begin to understand the concept of supply-driven care in medicine, all kinds of strange, seemingly inexplicable observations begin to make sense. For instance, think back to chapter 2, to Elliott Fisher's study of how much care patients with the same condition received in different hospitals. He found that patients who were hospitalized with a heart attack, hip fracture, or colon cancer got more care—but not better care—in hospitals where there were more specialists. And the extra care they got consisted of all sorts of discretionary tests and procedures that didn't improve their outcome—they increased patients' risk of dying. He was documenting the fact that the local supply of specialists drives up "demand" for care. Where there were more pulmonologists, patients in the hospital got seen more often by a pulmonologist, regardless of whether a pulmonologist was likely to help them get better. Remember, too, that Fisher also reported that patients were more likely to be put in the ICU in hospitals where there were more ICU beds.

This observation has many implications, probably none of them more unsettling than in the area of end-of-life care. When you ask Americans what kind of death they want, a vast majority say they would like to be at home, surrounded by loved ones. The last place they want to be is in an ICU, hooked up to machines, with tubes coming out of every orifice. But the ICU is precisely where huge numbers of frail, elderly, dying patients wind up—depending upon where they happen to live. For example, elderly residents of Los Angeles who are loyal to the University of California hospital, ranked among the best in the country for geriatric care, are likely to spend on average more than 11 days in the ICU in the last six months of their lives. But elderly residents of San Francisco who go to the aging but venerated University of California hospital there, high on a hill on Parnassus Street, are likely to spend only 3.3 days in the ICU. Same university hospital system, but wildly inconsistent treatment of elderly patients.

What's the difference between the two hospitals? Well, for one thing, more than fifty ICU beds per thousand Medicare beneficiaries at UCLA, versus twelve at UCSF. In a recent study, the Dartmouth group found wide variations in the way two hundred hospitals in California treated dying patients. At Garfield Medical Center, for example, a hospital in Los Angeles, the average Medicare recipient cost taxpayers more than $104,000 over the last two years of life. In the last six months of life, that average patient saw a doctor nearly ninety-three times and spent twenty-three days in the hospital, eleven of them in the ICU. That sounds a lot like the kind of death most Americans dread. At UCSF, by contrast, that same patient would have racked up only half as much in expenses, about $57,000 in the last two years of life. He would have had thirty doctor visits during his last six months and spent only eleven days in the hospital. The huge variation between these hospitals makes no sense—until you look at the resources each hospital has invested in. With sixty-one beds per thousand Medicare beneficiaries and the equivalent of about twenty-five full-time doctors per thousand, UCSF seems positively frugal when compared with Garfield Medical Center, which has double the number of per capita beds and doctors.

With the concept of supply-driven care in mind, you can see how the decisions that hospital administrators make—about the doctors they contract with, the CT scanners they buy, the neonatal ICUs they build—influences not only the kind of care their patients receive but also how much money they cost Medicare and other payers. This changes the way we ought to be thinking about health care reform. What we want are efficient hospitals, places where patients can be sure they will get high-quality care, care that gives them the procedures and tests and drugs they need—and doesn't give them what they don't need—for the most reasonable cost. That's what markets are supposed to do—create efficiency. But we can't achieve efficiency through market forces when normal economic rules don't apply to large swaths of American health care, when the supply of many resources is dictating what kind of care patients receive, and how much of it, rather than what's best for them.

FIVE The Desperate Cure

In 1981, William P. Peters was still on the upward slope of his life, rising with the unerring directness of a missile. Only twenty-eight years old, he had begun his formal training in cancer research as a summer intern at the age of fourteen, at Roswell Park Cancer Institute, near his hometown of Buffalo, New York. He took his bachelor's degree in biochemistry, biophysics, and philosophy from Penn State and both a medical degree and a Ph.D., in medical genetics, from Columbia University. He served his internship and residency at Harvard. Now a fellow at the world-renowned Dana-Farber Cancer Institute, in Boston, he was about to administer the experimental breast cancer therapy that would be linked with his name and would come to be considered one of the most controversial treatments in all of medicine.

His patient's name was Diane. A truck driver who was only a year older than Peters, Diane had an enormous breast tumor. It was erupting from the skin of the upper right quadrant of her right breast and simultaneously penetrating deep between her ribs and into her right lung. One of the largest tumors Peters would ever see in his career, it was far too big to be removed surgically. "It was the size of a muskmelon," Peters would later recall. "It was a terrible circumstance." Diane would almost certainly be dead in a matter of months.

Peters described for his new patient the outlines of the bold experiment that he hoped she would be willing to try. He wanted to give her extremely high doses of several chemotherapy drugs, doses toxic enough, he believed,

117

to deal her cancer a mighty blow. Unfortunately, the chemo might also kill Diane. Such high doses of the drugs would wipe out her bone marrow, which makes the immune cells of the blood, leaving her vulnerable to dying from the least little infection. Peters explained that he would attempt to "rescue" her once the chemotherapy was finished, with an infusion of her own bone marrow, which he would extract from her hip bone before starting the chemotherapy. If all went as planned, Diane's marrow cells would find their way back into her bones over a period of weeks and begin churning out immune cells, so she could fight infection once again.

The treatment, which was called high-dose chemotherapy with autologous bone marrow transplant, or sometimes simply bone marrow transplant, was a long shot at best. "We knew the treatment was going to kill some people along the way, to be quite honest," Peters recalls. "But we knew the disease killed everybody." Or at least, many women with late-stage breast cancer would die. The possibility that Peters and his colleagues might be able to cure even some patients with advanced breast cancer seemed worth the risk. "We were going to change the horizon; we were going to swing and go for the ring," Peters says. "That drove us. You had to believe you were going to pull off something that was going to change history."

Peters scheduled the operating room at nearby Brigham and Women's Hospital for a Monday morning. Diane was put under general anesthesia, and Peters began the procedure of plunging a needle through the flesh of her hip into the bone and drawing out aliquots of marrow. Partway through the procedure, the needle broke off, its tip embedded in her bone and the top buried somewhere in her muscle. Cursing, Peters frantically searched the operating room for pliers to grasp the hidden needle, but Brigham and Women's was not set up for bone marrow work, so there were no pliers to be found. A nurse was sent out of the operating room to fetch a pair.

By evening, Diane had been wheeled back to the Dana-Farber, where she would receive her first doses of chemotherapy. "We were being watched like a hawk," Peters recalls. Other doctors at the Dana-Farber were dubious that a woman could stand the punishing doses of chemotherapeutic drugs—roughly ten times the standard dose—but Diane proved them wrong. She weathered the side effects of the chemo, even as it wiped out her bone marrow. But the treatment's effect on her monstrous tumor seemed nothing short of miraculous. "Within a week, this huge mass, this ten- to twelve-centimeter mass, disappeared," says Peters. "I mean, you could literally come in every day and watch this thing melt away. Bingo."

Despite her early improvement, Diane's tumor returned soon after the treatment ended. She died a few weeks later. Peters remained undaunted. He transplanted a second patient, a thirty-one-year-old woman named Cheryl Shapiro, whose tumor had metastasized, or spread, to other parts of her body. The doctors were elated when Shapiro recovered fully, with no signs of cancer. They had demonstrated they could administer high doses of chemotherapy and then rescue the patient with a transplant of her own marrow. Within a year, they had transplanted a dozen more women, all of whom responded almost as well as Diane and Shapiro, at least at first. Three made complete recoveries; Shapiro's case was followed for more than twenty years, and she may still be alive today. "We really thought we were going to solve the cancer problem," says Dr. I. Craig Henderson, a colleague of Peters's during the early days at the Dana-Farber. "We thought we had a cure for cancer."

Over the next two decades, Peters would become the treatment's most ardent and tireless advocate. Some colleagues took to calling him Elmer Gantry, and the name fit. A true believer in the power of high-dose chemotherapy, Peters was like a Bible-thumping evangelist, crisscrossing the country, extolling the promise of his experimental therapy. A short, dapper, energetic man with small, soft hands, a quick wit, and a manner that could veer wildly between genial physician and salesman, he would pace to and fro across the stage at scientific meetings, carrying the mike in one hand and gesturing toward charts and graphs projected on a screen with the other. He appeared on television programs like *60 Minutes* and *20/20*. Newspaper articles quoted him saying, "This saves more lives than any form of chemotherapy."

Paul Goldberg, editor of an industry newsletter published in Washington, D.C., called the *Cancer Letter*, remembers the show Peters put on at a luncheon with members of Congress. Peters was urging Congress to pass legislation that would force insurers to cover high-dose chemotherapy, which was not only experimental but exorbitantly expensive. Goldberg recalls, "Bill took the microphone and said, 'I could give you a lot of statistics about the effectiveness of this treatment protocol, but I think it would be easier to do this with a simple demonstration.' Then he asked the seventy or so breast cancer patients who had accompanied him to the lunch to stand up." Peters turned back to his congressional audience and announced that at least half of the women would be dead had they not undergone his lifesaving treatment. "Then he delivered his punch line," Goldberg recalls. "He said, 'As you look at a woman across the table from you, ask yourself, is the price of this woman's life worth the price of a luxury car?' "

The real question, however, was not the worth of a woman's life but whether high-dose chemotherapy followed by a bone marrow transplant could actually cure breast cancer. That question would not be fully answered until 2001. Based on only the slenderest threads of evidence, tens of thousands of breast cancer patients would undergo the terrible rigors of the treatment in the intervening decades between the moment Peters and his colleagues administered the first dose of chemo to his patient Diane and the publication of clinical trials that would show the treatment wasn't a cure for breast cancer. Even when the evidence was in and it was finally clear that high-dose chemotherapy was no better than standard treatment, some doctors continued to argue that it could benefit some women.

How is it that a dangerous, highly experimental treatment came to be given to thousands of women before it had been adequately tested? The story of high-dose chemotherapy's rise and subsequent fall involves the courts, insurers, hospital administrators, and proselytizing doctors like Bill Peters, as well as the desperate women who were led to believe, by their doctors and the press, that going through the ordeal of a transplant would save them from cancer. Among those who know it, the story of high-dose chemotherapy has come to symbolize everything that's wrong with the way many new, unproved medical treatments are swiftly embraced by physicians and patients—often with only minimal evidence to suggest they actually work. Why were doctors so willing to believe that giving women with breast cancer near-lethal doses of chemo would work? And why were women willing, even eager, to be subjected to it? The answers to these questions speak volumes about why doctors deliver much of the unnecessary care that plagues American medicine.

If a little chemo is good...

High-dose chemotherapy was the brainchild of Dr. Emil "Tom" Frei III, the director of the Dana-Farber and a towering figure in the field of cancer. Frei was a father of one of the few cancer cures, so-called combination chemotherapy, the lifesaving technique that involved giving lymphoma patients several different chemotherapeutic agents together. A tall stork of a man who liked to tell jokes even a six-year-old would get, Frei crackled with new ideas and enthusiasm. Peters and Craig Henderson delighted in working for him. As Henderson recalls, "Frei was a pied piper. He was just unbelievably exciting to be around."

It was Frei's idea to use combination chemotherapy in high doses on breast cancer. Doctors were having only limited success treating advanced breast cancer with chemotherapeutic drugs. The tumors would respond to the drugs at first, and sometimes even disappear, only to come roaring back once the drugs were stopped. That told them that the chemo had not wiped out every last cancer cell. The few that remained in the body were able to grow once again as soon as the treatment ended. Doctors wanted to give higher doses, and there was good science behind their reasoning. "Chemotherapy shows what's known as a dose-dependent curve," says Henderson. "The higher the dose, the more cancer cells are killed." But the higher the dose, the greater the toxicity to normal cells and the more deadly the side effects. The doctors believed that breast tumors resisted being cured by chemo because doctors simply could not give their patients high-enough doses without causing them serious harm.

Frei reasoned that combination chemo could get around that problem because each drug had a different side effect. Besides causing hair to fall out in clumps, Adriamycin also damages the heart when given in high doses. The drug BCNU harms the liver. Giving three or four drugs in combination would allow doctors to increase the total dose of chemotherapy while spreading around the collateral damage to healthy organs. Of course, the drugs were still going to destroy the patient's bone marrow, which is acutely sensitive to chemo. Frei solved this problem by coming up with the idea of giving the patient a restorative transplant, using her own marrow. In the 1970s, transplants—using bone marrow taken from a healthy donor—had brought about some of the first cancer cures, in leukemia and lymphoma. Why not apply the same principle to a solid tumor, such as breast cancer? Using the patient's own marrow, Frei reasoned, would avoid the problem of rejection, making the transplant that much easier. "Intuitively it made sense," says Henderson. "If a little chemo is good, more is better."

The idea made sense to leukemia doctors, who had been using bone marrow transplants on their patients for more than a decade. Hope Rugo was a young transplanter at UCSF in 1989 when she heard Peters speak at a medical meeting. His results with breast cancer patients seemed to her to be both credible and extraordinarily promising. "From the transplanter's standpoint, it made sense," she recalls. "More chemo is better. His data said even patients with metastatic disease could have a response." That jibed with Rugo's experience transplanting patients with leukemia and other blood cancers. "You could take people who had relapsed [from leukemia or lymphoma], and you could cure them," she says. "Not everybody, but some could be cured. We thought, wow, we've got to try this. If Bill Peters could give people a whole lot of chemotherapy, maybe we could too."

Rugo began using Peters's protocol on breast cancer patients and was not disappointed by the results. She watched in astonishment, just as the Dana-Farber team had done a little less than a decade earlier, as her patients' breast tumors seemed to melt away practically before her eyes. "We looked at eighteen-month survival, which is what you do in leukemia, and 80 percent [of breast cancer patients] were disease free at eighteen months," she says. Such results seemed like a cure to Rugo and other blood cancer specialists, who knew that when leukemia patients lived that long after a transplant, it often meant their cancer was gone for good. The word spread among transplanters, who began trying the technique on breast cancer patients around the country.

Forced to pay

By the time Alice Philipson's first breast cancer patient came to her law office in Berkeley, California, in 1991, she had learned a thing or two about building a case against health insurers who refused to pay for medical treatments. A blunt, handsome woman with short-cropped white hair, Philipson pioneered the legal specialty of suing insurers for denying AIDS patients coverage for medical care in the 1980s. Back then, it was a branch of law that few lawyers had mastered, or indeed wanted any part of, because of a Supreme Court ruling that limited the amount the courts could award patients who sued their insurers for denial of coverage. "There was no pot of gold for the lawyer," says Philipson, "and most people don't have the money to pay you. You have to go to the courts to get paid."

Her new client's name was Ricki, a forty-eight-year-old psychologist with a child still in high school and an advanced case of breast cancer. When Ricki was first diagnosed three years earlier, she underwent a double mastectomy and chemotherapy. Now, the cancer was back, and Ricki was looking to high-dose chemotherapy and a bone marrow transplant as her only hope. But her insurer, a Blue Cross affiliate, did not want to pay for it.

The company's reluctance was not surprising. The bill for high-dose chemotherapy began at $150,000 and could hit $500,000 if the patient suffered complications. The chemotherapy drugs alone ran into the tens of thousands of dollars. Women spent at least three weeks in an isolation room in the hospital, protected from the infections that teemed in the outside world and racking up charges while waiting for their bone marrow to regrow. Publicly, insurers argued that the treatment was still unproved and experimental, and thus not something they were compelled by law to cover. They knew that high-quality scientific studies—well-designed, randomized, controlled clinical trials—had not yet been done, and the observational reports, no matter how promising, could be wrong. Privately, insurers worried that if they agreed to pay for one expensive, experimental procedure, there was no limit to the questionable therapies desperate patients might demand.

Philipson was sympathetic to Ricki's plight, but she was not about to take the case unless Ricki could provide scientific evidence that demonstrated the value of the treatment she was seeking. She knew Ricki's case would not have a prayer if the treatment was truly experimental—or worse, a crackpot cure like laetrile. "I put my life into these cases," says Philipson. "I pour my heart into them. The emotional price for me is high, but the emotional price for patients . . . they are looking to me to get them something they think will save their lives." She told Ricki she would represent her, on the condition that they find published, scientific evidence that high-dose chemo was not experimental but established therapy.

Within a week, Ricki delivered a stack of medical articles that persuaded Philipson they had the evidence they would need. By the early 1990s, doctors around the country who had begun to try Peters's desperate treatment were publishing their results. Hope Rugo, just across the bay from Philipson's office, had written up several cases of breast cancer patients. As Philipson sifted through observational reports in the medical literature, she began to believe she and Ricki had a case. "The way [the research papers] portrayed it, bone marrow transplant was the best thing since sliced bread," she recalls. "They were saying this is a cure."

At the same time, Philipson also learned that the cure Ricki wanted to undergo came at a dreadful price. Her client's ordeal would begin even before the first dose of chemo, with the arduous process of extracting bone marrow from her hip. Then came the drugs, which destroyed the lining of the entire intestinal tract, from mouth to anus, making both swallowing and eliminating unbearably painful. Women who underwent high-dose chemo suffered waves of nausea and vomiting alternating with racking bouts of diarrhea. Some women became disoriented, others agitated and angry, pacing their isolation rooms as they waited for their bone marrow to regrow.

For many women, the loneliness was crushing. Others succumbed to infection before their bone marrow could reconstitute itself. One in five women, fully 20 percent, Philipson learned, died not from their cancer but during or soon after the treatment. High-dose chemotherapy killed the patient before it killed her tumor. And the chemo left many women who survived with permanent, sometimes debilitating damage to the heart, kidneys, lungs, liver, or nerves.

Going through high-dose chemo, suffering the side effects, and even risking death seemed like a chance worth taking to women like Ricki. As late as 1989, a woman with stage III breast cancer—cancer that was two inches across and had spread to the lymph nodes—had a 50 to 70 percent chance of relapsing after standard chemotherapy. Once she had progressed to stage IV, meaning her cancer had metastasized or spread to other organs, as Ricki's had, her chances of dying from her disease were overwhelming. Given such odds, many breast cancer patients were not merely willing to undergo a transplant, they were eager.

If Ricki was prepared to try high-dose chemo, then Philipson was prepared to argue her case. Her job was to show that the insurer was obliged contractually to cover the procedure. She bombarded the company with scientific papers and letters from cancer experts saying the procedure was standard practice. Meanwhile, Ricki paid out of her own pocket to have her bone marrow harvested, the first, and least expensive, phase of the treatment. "We were working against the clock," Philipson recalls. "If her tumors get too big, she can't have the treatment. I'm telling the insurer this is urgent, this is part of their duty." In the end, the company agreed to pay for Ricki's transplant. Her case was one of the first ever that successfully forced an insurer to pay for a bone marrow transplant for breast cancer.

It would not be the last. As Philipson's name circulated among breast cancer support groups in California, more women came to her, hoping to get their transplants covered by their insurers. Over the next two years, she won three more cases. Then, in 1993, Philipson assisted in a landmark trial that threw open the legal floodgates and forced insurers to begin paying for increasing numbers of transplants around the country. That year, a Southern California lawyer named Mark Hiepler sued Health Net on behalf of his sister, Nelene Fox, who had died from her breast cancer while trying to persuade the insurance company to cover a transplant. A loophole in the law allowed Hiepler to sue for damages, and Health Net decided to fight. Philipson advised Hiepler to comb through the company's records for evidence that the decision to deny his sister coverage was made in bad faith. He soon discovered that the company doctor who made the decision got a bonus at the end of the year if Health Net saved

money. "It sounded terrible," Philipson recalls. "The [insurer's] defense attorney says, 'It's no different from John Deere or any other American company.' The jury comes back and says, 'The hell it isn't different. John Deere
makes tractors and you decide on people's lives.'" The jury awarded the
Fox family eighty-nine million dollars in damages, a record judgment
against an insurer.

Ricki didn't live to see the end of the Health Net case. She had survived
the transplant, and her cancer had stayed away for nearly two years. Then, in
1993, it came back more aggressively than ever. She was dead in a matter of
weeks. The cure had failed. Philipson was saddened by the news of Ricki's
death, but she was too busy with other breast cancer cases to focus on it.
Within a year of the Health Net judgment, record numbers of women were
filing suit against their insurers. The strategy was always the same. The plain-
tiffs argued that the insurer was refusing to pay for a treatment that was accepted medical practice. Transplant doctors served as expert witnesses,
testifying to that effect. Peters himself often served in that capacity, telling
the courts, as he did in a 1990 case against a Blue Cross affiliate, "[T]he regimen prescribed is neither experimental nor investigational, as all elements
of the treatment are well established and the treatment has over the years
proven itself to be an effective cancer therapy."

To much of the cancer community, high-dose chemo certainly seemed
well established and effective. Besides the articles by transplanters like
Rugo, reporting that their breast cancer patients were still alive as long as
two years after their treatment, Peters had published results of a more-
formal study in 1993, claiming that high-dose chemo was far superior to a
standard regimen. Peters compared the outcomes of his transplant cases to
the outcomes of breast cancer patients who had received standard treatment
from other doctors in the past. Approximately 70 percent of his transplant
patients were cancer free forty-eight months after his treatment; only 35
percent of women were alive after standard treatment. In the field of cancer,
the difference was huge. "That paper drove the field," says Craig Henderson.
"Every transplanter, every cancer doctor had a copy."

By then, Peters had left the Dana-Farber to build a prestigious breast cancer clinic at Duke University Medical Center, where he would train the next

generation of transplanters. As more and more doctors began trying their hand at high-dose chemo, stories began appearing in the media, adding to the growing sense of hope in breast cancer support groups. Nearly all of the stories followed the same format. The dying patient was cast as a victim of both her breast cancer and her insurance company. Women were in a "desperate struggle to buy more time," as the *Dayton Daily News* put it, and the only thing standing between them and a possible cure was their greedy insurers. Soon breast cancer advocacy groups, like the Susan G. Komen Breast Cancer Foundation, which sponsors the annual "Race for the Cure," took up the cause. With the help of transplant doctors like Peters, they lobbied state legislatures and the federal government to mandate insurance coverage for the procedure.

Insurers were in a bind. Paying for transplants could cost them millions of dollars a year. But if they refused to cover them, they faced court cases like *Health Net* or irate legislatures. Most chose to pay, and as the insurance money flowed, the number of breast cancer patients who were transplanted soared. In the 1980s, fewer than a hundred transplants a year were being performed on breast cancer patients. By 1994, the number had jumped to nine thousand transplants annually.

The money pours in

Hospitals were only too happy to have their doctors performing transplants. High-dose chemo followed by a bone marrow transplant was one of their few sources of profit in the 1990s, a time when hospitals were being squeezed financially by managed care. Transplanting breast cancer patients was good business. It came to be even better business with the appearance of new drugs called growth factors, which made transplants a little less risky and shortened a woman's stay in the isolation ward. Growth factors stimulated the proliferation of bone marrow cells in a woman's body, making it possible to harvest marrow cells from the blood, rather than having to extract them from her bone. The new drugs also helped marrow cells regenerate once they were returned to the woman's body after her chemotherapy. Eventually, it was possible to administer high-dose chemo and a transplant on an outpatient basis. The drugs also cut the death rate, so that by 1995, transplants were killing less than 10 percent of patients.

Best of all, growth factors increased the profit on a transplant, bringing the cost down to under sixty thousand dollars. Hospitals continued charging insurers between eighty thousand and one hundred thousand dollars per patient. Under Peters, Duke University's breast cancer transplant program *netted* fourteen million dollars one year. Soon, community hospitals wanted their share of the profits. "Performing transplants on breast cancer patients filled up our transplant wards," says Hope Rugo. "And when we started making money, all the little hospitals said, 'I can do this too.' " Soon, hospitals large and small were converting entire wards into transplant units. Many hospitals turned to Response Oncology, a company based in Memphis, Tennessee, that franchised bone marrow transplants. Hospitals hired Response Oncology to teach teams of nurses and oncologists, in two-day sessions, how to administer high-dose chemo and perform a transplant. The company also advised hospitals on how to build new wings and then handled the insurance claims.

While hospital administrators wanted their share of the profits, oncologists wanted their share of the glory. Transplantation was a medical high-wire act, a daredevil procedure that brought a patient to the brink of death and then snatched her back at the last moment. "Transplanters became gods at hospitals," says Henderson—gods whose belief in their own omnipotence seemed to expand with every patient they treated. Some transplanters began treating ovarian cancer with high-dose chemotherapy, although there was no valid scientific evidence that it improved a patient's odds. Others subjected women with smaller, less-advanced breast tumors to the rigors of high-dose chemo. Peters seemed equally caught up in the excitement. At a lunch with colleagues at a scientific meeting, he announced cheerily that he was going to begin transplanting patients with advanced prostate cancer. His colleagues sat in stunned silence until one of them pointed out that advanced prostate cancer rarely responds to chemotherapy, no matter how high the dose.

And the trouble was, high-dose chemotherapy wasn't a cure, even for breast cancer. Alice Philipson knew it by 1995. She had not thought to question the treatment when Ricki died. Medicine, she knew, was an art, and no cure worked every time. But then another former client died, and another. One day, Philipson realized that every woman she knew who had received a transplant was dead. "Nobody got cured," she says. "I put them through litigation when they were dying. Then if I won, they got to have a bone marrow transplant. You can't raise your head, you are so sick, and it's so horrible and so hard, and you don't have time to say good-bye to the people you love. I had to decide for myself whether I was going to take these cases anymore, and I decided not to. It was a cure that didn't work."

Craig Henderson knew it too. He had grown increasingly skeptical of high-dose chemotherapy since the first, heady days at the Dana-Farber. He knew that Peters's seminal 1993 paper, which compared his transplant patients with women who had received standard treatment in the past, was not proof that transplanting saved more lives. The stellar results from that study could be explained by selection bias: the possibility that the women who got transplants started out healthier, and had less-advanced disease, than the women who had received standard therapy from other doctors. Peters's subjects might have done just as well on conventional therapy as they did with a transplant. The only way to show for certain that high-dose chemotherapy was more effective than conventional treatment was to perform a randomized, controlled trial, the gold standard of medicine. Researchers needed to take a group of breast cancer patients and randomly assign them to receive either standard treatment or high-dose chemo, and then see which group had the largest number of survivors after several years.

Such arguments went right over most oncologists' heads. Most doctors, says Henderson, have little training in statistical analysis or the design of clinical trials. They took Peters's paper as proof that high-dose chemotherapy worked. What's more, Rugo and other transplanters didn't seem to realize that breast tumors are not like blood cancers, in that they don't respond to high doses of chemotherapy in the same way. The slower a tumor is to grow, the less susceptible it is to chemotherapeutic agents, which work by interfering with the biochemical process of cell division. The faster cells are dividing, the harder chemo hits them. That makes blood cancers, which grow at lightning speed, acutely vulnerable to chemotherapy. By contrast, high doses of chemotherapy can't kill every last breast cancer cell as effectively, because they grow much more slowly.

Transplanters were also fooled when it came time to look at how their breast cancer patients fared over the long term. Compared with leukemia, which can come charging back in a matter of weeks after a transplant, breast tumors can take several years to reappear. But the blood cancer doctors didn't wait that long to declare transplants a success for breast cancer patients. They looked at survival at eighteen months, which was standard for blood cancers. When they found no evidence of breast cancer, they assumed their patients were cured.

Henderson warned his colleagues against accepting high-dose chemo as an article of faith. By the time he left the Dana-Farber in 1992, to head the division of oncology at UCSF, Henderson had already gained a reputation as a critic. Many of his colleagues scorned him, calling him a naysayer and snubbing him at medical meetings. High-dose chemo had become a medical juggernaut, and nobody wanted to hear that it might not work.

But Peters himself knew that Henderson was right. He knew he had to subject high-dose chemo to the ultimate test, a randomized, controlled clinical trial. A randomized trial was the only way to avoid being fooled into seeing merit in the treatment when there was none, to prove that high-dose chemo was better than conventional therapy. By 1991, he had persuaded the National Cancer Institute to fund a trial. Peters and other doctors needed to enroll approximately one thousand breast cancer patients, who would have to be followed for five years after they received their treatment. Physicians around the world were organizing smaller clinical trials, but Peters's was by far the most ambitious. Patients were eligible if their breast cancer had not yet metastasized but was nonetheless likely to recur. Each woman would be randomly assigned to one of two treatments: Half would receive a moderately high dose of chemotherapy and no more. Those patients would form the control group of the trial, the equivalent of aggressive standard therapy. The other half would get an additional, even higher, dose and then a restorative transplant. The plan was to get the majority of transplanters around the country to include all of their patients in one of the randomized trials.

But by the time Peters had organized his trial, neither doctors nor their patients wanted to participate. Transplanters were already convinced that they could cure at least some patients with a transplant, a conviction driven in part by Peters's own enthusiasm and his 1993 paper. Why would they ask half their patients to accept anything less than a possible cure? Henderson remembers an interview with a transplanter at UCSF. "He pulled out [Peters's] '93 paper," Henderson says, "and he said, 'I don't see how with these data it's even ethical to do a randomized trial.'"

"We didn't want to randomize patients," Rugo recalls. "They came to us in great shape, basically healthy women. These were young women with kids, and they were desperate. We believed standard chemo did not provide much benefit. We gave up on the randomized trial."

Certainly many patients themselves had no interest in participating in a trial. That would mean risking *not* getting a transplant, their "one chance to live," as more than one patient put it. They'd read the newspaper accounts. Even their doctors were telling them they might be cured by high-dose chemo. More than that, high-dose chemotherapy made sense—if a little chemo works pretty well, more will work better. The treatment's terrible rigors only added to the perception that it might be a cure. "A lot of it had to do with psychology," says Marilyn McGregor, a breast cancer survivor and activist in San Francisco. "Women, especially younger women with children, will do anything to save their lives, so they did not hear the statistics [about being disabled or dying from a transplant]. Or they made their bargains with God that they would go through this treatment if only they could be allowed to live. They just wanted to believe." Why on earth would they want to enter a trial that might randomize them to get standard treatment?

Instead of having results in five years, the randomized trials took nearly a decade to complete. Not until the summer of 1999, at the annual meeting of the American Society for Clinical Oncology, the premier professional organization for cancer specialists, would results from five different clinical trials of high-dose chemotherapy finally be presented. For all of the hype surrounding high-dose chemo, and all of the hopes that had been hung on it, four of the five clinical trials found no advantage over conventional treatment. Peters's trial, the largest by far, with data from nearly eight hundred patients, showed that women who received a transplant were slightly more likely to be cancer free after five years than women who received conventional therapy—but the advantage was wiped out by the fact that they were also more likely to die from the treatment.

Peters argued that his data were preliminary and that it would be a rush to judgment if oncologists stopped doing transplants before his trial was completely finished. "It's too early to draw conclusions," he said repeatedly to colleagues and reporters at the meeting. Many transplanters agreed, pointing to the single clinical trial that had shown positive results. It was a small trial, to be sure, only 154 patients, but the results were spectacular: Only nineteen of seventy-five women who had received a transplant had relapsed, while another eight died. That was far better than the seventy-five women in the trial who received conventional treatment. The results were presented at the meeting by the researcher himself, Dr. Werner Bezwoda, South Africa's premier breast cancer specialist. Bezwoda's paper and Peters's boundless optimism gave transplanters reason to keep performing the procedure.

But Bezwoda's paper would turn out to be a fraud. When a team of cancer specialists from Washington, D.C., traveled to South Africa to audit Bezwoda's data in 2000, they discovered a jumble of incomplete records, missing patients, and deviations from standard scientific practice. Out of 154 patients reported in his paper, Bezwoda had charts for only sixty-two cases. Medical researchers are required by scientific convention to keep meticulous records when they conduct clinical trials. When the team asked Bezwoda's wife, who had served as his assistant, where the rest of the charts could be found, she told them they were in a room mixed with those of thousands of other patients who were treated at a now-defunct hospital. The records Bezwoda did have on hand contained only the sketchiest of information. The South African's protocol, or description of how he planned to treat patients in the study, appeared to have been written not before he began the research, as it should have been, but just before the auditors arrived. Three days after the auditors returned to the United States, Bezwoda sent a letter to his university, admitting he had committed a "serious breach of scientific honesty and integrity." The results of the study, he wrote, had been "a misrepresentation." The letter was forwarded to the American Society for Clinical Oncology, which sent out an advisory to its members and a press release, announcing the fraud. Bezwoda would later claim his work wasn't fraudulent after all. A year later, the society issued a second statement after an audit of another study by Bezwoda, saying that his results "should not be used as the basis for the treatment of any patient."

That warning came too late for four women in Seattle. Two researchers at the University of Washington, in Seattle, had already begun a trial using Bezwoda's special high-dose regimen for women with metastatic breast cancer. They copied his published formula faithfully, administering it to four breast cancer patients, all under the age of fifty. Two died of congestive heart failure brought on by the chemo a few months after their treatment. One woman lived with acute cardiac damage until she succumbed to her breast cancer. A fourth patient was still alive a year later, though she suffered from serious heart trouble brought on by the treatment. The researchers halted the study. The use of high-dose chemo for breast cancer had already declined dramatically after 1999. With the Bezwoda results discredited, it was abandoned.

Spinal fusion

The memory of high-dose chemotherapy has already begun to fade, but it still matters for the simple reason that most of medicine remains just as experimental as high-dose chemo was, and just as untested. High-dose chemo ranks among one of the most brutal treatments ever devised, yet patients and doctors embraced it readily, in part, perhaps, because of the ancient dictum, that desperate diseases require desperate measures. High-dose chemo made too much sense not to work—if a little chemotherapy kills most breast cancer cells, more will kill the rest. All of which makes the saga of high-dose chemo more understandable, if not easier to forgive.

Unfortunately, it represents just another treatment among many that are based more on sound reasoning than on sound evidence, on hope rather than real cures.

Most of us cannot imagine this to be the case. We live in the age of science, after all. We think the difference between experimental and standard care is well defined; that doctors adopt new medical advances on the basis of valid evidence; that new treatments represent improvement over the old. We look back at the history of medicine and its litter of discarded treatments with a sense of superiority, smug in our belief that superstition and ignorance have been banished from medicine. Until only a few generations ago, disease was thought to arise out of either an imbalance among the four humors or a contagion in the blood. Treatments were based on this faulty paradigm, and thus it seemed to follow, for example, that cutting a vein and letting the blood run out would rid the body of what ailed it and restore balance. Patients often did feel better after a bloodletting, or at least different, while the doctor could feel the satisfaction of having done what was right according to prevailing conceptions of disease. We now know that bloodletting at best did nothing and at worst hastened death, thanks to a Parisian doctor named Pierre Charles Alexandre Louis, who performed an experiment in 1836 that is now recognized as one of the first clinical trials. He treated patients who had pneumonia with either bloodletting or less-aggressive measures. As physician Kevin Patterson writes, "At the end of the experiment, Dr. Louis counted the bodies. They were stacked higher over by the bloodletting sink."

You don't have to look very hard for more-recent examples of discredited treatments. Until the 1980s, breast surgeons were still recommending the radical mastectomy, the removal of the entire breast and underlying chest muscle of women with breast cancer. The idea was to slam the door in the cancer's face by removing every last possible tumor cell in the vicinity of the primary tumor. But this was based on an incorrect view of cancer, which can spread to the rest of the body via the blood and the lymphatic system, even when the tumor is still quite small. Clinical trials would finally show that lumpectomy with radiation was just as effective as mastectomy, and far less traumatic for many women. Other examples of widely accepted medical treatments that have been shown not to be effective and frequently harmful when valid studies are done include routine episiotomy, brain bypass surgery for patients with warning signs of stroke, and hormone replacement therapy to prevent a second heart attack in women. The list goes on.

Today, doctors routinely prescribe drugs, perform procedures, and use medical devices and tests on the basis of evidence that sometimes has only a little more science to support it than the contagion theory. They recommend the prostate-specific antigen, or PSA, test, even though there is little to suggest that it reduces a man's chances of dying from prostate cancer prematurely. Much of the discretionary care, "the small stuff," as Elliott Fisher put it in his study of hospital spending patterns—the vena cava filters, the laryngoscopies, the pulmonary artery catheters—has never been shown to improve survival, much less comfort, in many of the patients who receive it. Even many big-ticket procedures and surgeries have never been subjected to rigorous scientific inquiry. Spinal fusion for low-back pain is one such surgery. In the view of Jerome Groopman, a noted oncologist and author of How Doctors Think, "Spinal fusion may be the radical mastectomy of our time."

In 2004, approximately 303,000 lower-lumbar spinal fusions were performed in the United States. The surgery involves removing the cartilaginous disk that sits between two vertebrae and filling the space with bone chips harvested from cadavers or the patient's own hip, which eventually fuse to the vertebrae so they don't collapse together and squeeze the spinal cord. Sometimes surgeons use devices called pedicle screws, which attach to the vertebrae above and below the space emptied by the removed disk, in order to hold them apart. The surgery can offer tremendous relief to patients suffering from spinal fractures and tumors of the spine, where vertebrae have been displaced and threaten the spinal cord. But such cases make up a tiny fraction of the spinal fusions that are performed each year. The vast majority are given to patients suffering from chronic lower-back pain.

Roughly two thirds of Americans will suffer from back pain at some point in their lives, often as a result of a minor injury or strain. The human back seems poorly designed, given how often and how easily it can be hurt—just scooping up a small child from the floor or twisting to reach an item on a high shelf can be enough to send one's back into spasms of agony. Sometimes back pain involves sciatica, a particularly unpleasant tingling, burning sensation that runs down the sciatic nerve from the buttocks into the leg. One in four Americans claims to suffer from severe, chronic back pain.

Given how frequently it strikes, you would think doctors would have a clear idea of what causes back pain and how best to treat it. But there's not much agreement there, and doctors who have trained in different disciplines often view it through different diagnostic lenses. In a paper titled "What You See Is What You Get," back expert Dr. Richard Deyo and his colleagues at the University of Washington found that rheumatologists, for instance, tended to give back pain patients blood tests, to look for rare immunological disorders to explain their condition. Neurologists performed tests of how well nerves conducted impulses along the spine. Surgeons ordered MRIs and CT scans, which show the anatomy of the bones and soft tissue in the back.

CT scans and MRIs are often used to make the case for surgery, especially when they show damage to a disk. You can think of a disk as a jelly doughnut, which will bulge when squeezed between the vertebrae. Squeeze the disk hard enough, and the outer sheath, called the annulus, may rupture, allowing bits of jellylike material to break through and press on nerves in the back. Back surgery is frequently performed because a patient shows a ruptured, or herniated, disk on an MRI or CT scan, but the disk may not necessarily be the source of the person's pain. Studies of CT scans have shown that 27 percent of people over the age of forty have a herniated disk but no back pain. In a study using MRIs, 36 percent of people over sixty had herniated disks, and 80 percent had disk degeneration, bulges and narrow bits. Yet none of them had significant back pain. CT scans and MRIs also turn up other anatomical anomalies that appear significant on the scan but don't cause the patient any problem. If herniated or degenerated disks aren't necessarily the problem, then what causes back pain? The back is a complicated structure, with ligaments, tendons, and muscles, all of which can be injured or strained. About 85 percent of patients with lower-back pain can't be given a precise diagnosis.

Sometimes a ruptured disk coincides with the sudden onset of pain. But that doesn't necessarily mean surgery is called for. Studies have found that about 80 percent of people who rupture a disk will recover within a few weeks if they take anti-inflammatory pain medication like ibuprofen, rest for a short period, and get physical therapy. The disk shrinks a bit over time, and the jelly that has leaked out gets reabsorbed. A simpler surgery, called diskectomy, which involves trimming the bulging bits from a disk, can relieve pain in some cases where the disk fails to heal on its own. But the first well-designed, randomized, controlled trial of diskectomy, called the Spine Patient Outcomes Research Trial, or SPORT, which was completed in late 2006, found virtually no difference between patients who underwent surgery and those who chose more conservative treatment.

Of course, not all back pain and sciatica go away with conservative treatment, and a lot of people wind up having spinal fusion surgery. Some opt for surgery within a few weeks of the onset of pain, without giving other forms of treatment a chance. A few find complete relief; their pain is wiped out. But does surgery usually help most patients? And is it any better than more-conservative treatment, like physical therapy? Nobody knows, because surgeons, though they have been performing back fusions for decades, have never actually done the correct research that's necessary to find out. The best that can be said for spinal fusion is that one in four patients are helped by surgery. But even that number isn't based on very good science, and many patients wind up going back to their surgeons. A study of workers injured on the job in the state of Washington who underwent fusion for degenerative disk disease found that 22 percent were still in pain and had opted for more surgery. Surgeons themselves reported that many of their patients remained in chronic pain even after multiple fusions.

If they don't know which patients are most likely to benefit, or if it even works at all, why do surgeons continue performing fusions? Fusion surgery is one of the more lucrative procedures in medicine. According to the Agency for Healthcare Research and Quality, average hospital charges come to forty-two thousand dollars per case. The surgeon's reimbursement from Medicare is about four thousand dollars, and private insurers may pay more. Back surgeons can easily make one to two million dollars a year. But money is only one of the factors driving the large number of fusion surgeries. Many, if not most, surgeons believe they are helping their patients, and they think that the research that's been published supports their belief. Just as the transplanters did not know that valid evidence for high-dose chemotherapy was lacking, back surgeons often don't understand the meaning of good medical research. They are untroubled, for the most part, by the fact that there have been no well-conducted, randomized, controlled clinical trials, the sine qua non of high-quality evidence, that can say with any certainty that fusion is better than nonsurgical treatments.

Dr. Michael Stuart was a family practitioner for twenty-five years with Group Health Cooperative of Puget Sound, in Seattle, before he embarked on what has become something of a mission to educate his fellow doctors. A lecturer at the University of Washington School of Medicine, Stuart is a round-faced man in his fifties, balding, with wire-rim glasses and a laid-back, Puckish manner. Five years ago, he quit his practice to form the Delfini Group, which consists of Stuart and Sheri Ann Strite, a former research coordinator at Group Health with extensive experience designing clinical research protocols. Together, the two travel the country, teaching doctors to think more analytically about medical science. "Doctors have no idea how to evaluate the medical literature," Stuart says, "because they were never taught." Pressed for time, physicians often skim the journals, reading only the abstracts and conclusions of articles and missing the clues buried inside that a piece of clinical research was poorly designed, or that the results were incorrectly interpreted. But even doctors who want to be more discerning, says Stuart, can't always tell the difference between a good study and a bad one, because they don't know how.

In June 2006, Stuart and Strite spent three days with a group of back surgeons in Boise, Idaho. They were called in by the medical director of a local insurer, who was alarmed by the number of back surgeries that the patients covered by his company were undergoing. By 2003, Boise was already on the radar of Jack Wennberg's group at Dartmouth, which noted in

The Dartmouth Atlas that the city of not quite two hundred thousand had a per capita back fusion rate that was more than twice the rate found in the rest of the country. Dr. Douglas Dammrose, medical director for Blue Cross of Idaho, says that many of the spinal fusions his company is paying for are repeat surgeries—patients who were still in pain after a first surgery and returned to the surgeon for another. Dammrose also notes that the ratio of back surgeons to other kinds of doctors in Boise is higher than in most places. In a recent phone conversation, he told me, "I think the whole mountain region has a lot of orthopedists and spine surgeons. They're outdoorsy types. They like to ski."

Over the course of three days, Stuart and Strite led a group of spine surgeons and physiatrists, doctors who specialize in physical therapy, through a course intended to teach them how to pick apart medical research. They started the group out easy, on medical topics that had nothing to do with backs, pain, or surgery and with studies that were clearly biased, or that did not include enough patients to come to a statistically significant result. The surgeons learned quickly and were ready by the third day to pick apart the studies they themselves chose, from their own field, as the best evidence available for spinal surgery.

None of the studies, it turns out, was scientifically rigorous enough to be considered valid evidence that spinal fusion is superior to nonsurgical remedies. "It was quite an eye-opening experience for them that not a single article they selected was valid," says Stuart. In one of the studies the surgeons chose, for instance, when they reanalyzed the data in the article, they found that 55 out of 109 patients who received surgery felt better after one year; 54 out of 109 who got nonsurgical treatment were also in less pain. After dissecting the studies, the surgeons sat for a moment in stunned silence, says Stuart. "Somebody said, 'Wow, we've gone through everything we've relied on.' Then one doctor threw up his hands." It almost seemed as if the physicians, in recognizing that the evidence for their craft was lacking, were going through the stages of grief. One surgeon seemed sad; others expressed disbelief. Later, a doctor confronted Stuart, saying angrily that he didn't have time to read the journals, and that it was unreasonable to expect doctors to spend their weekends critically evaluating the literature.

Regret

In 2001, I flew to Detroit to meet Peters at the Barbara Ann Karmanos Cancer Institute, where he had recently stepped down as CEO. He came out from behind his administrative assistant's desk and extended his hand. Not yet fifty, Peters still exuded the same energetic enthusiasm that had helped persuade so many of his colleagues in cancer to try his bold experiment on their own patients. The interiors of the cancer institute's executive offices looked like they might belong to an architectural firm, not a hospital, with sleek wood paneling and richly colored fabric on the chairs. Peters wore a tie with an abstract pattern that appeared to echo the carpeting. He seemed delighted when I noticed the similarity. "I designed the interiors myself," he said.

I asked him if he had any regrets, if perhaps he felt he deserved some of the blame for how events turned out. Precisely twenty years elapsed between the bold experiment that he, Frei, and their colleagues first envisioned back at the Dana-Farber and the Bezwoda investigation's ignominious conclusion. Over the course of that time, transplanters subjected roughly forty-two thousand women, thirty thousand in the 1990s alone, to the risks of an entirely experimental treatment. All told, the nation spent $3.4 billion paying for it, and at least nine thousand women died not from their cancer but from the treatment they hoped was a cure. Yet Peters seemed genuinely baffled at the thought that his own evangelical enthusiasm for high-dose chemotherapy, the impassioned talks he gave to colleagues around the country, the quotes he gave to newspapers, might have made it more difficult, if not impossible, at times for doctors to recruit women into the randomized clinical trials. "My interest was to get [colleagues] to put patients on the randomized trials," he said. "What happened was people said, 'Huh, we don't have to send our [patients] to a randomized trial; we can do it ourselves.' On top of that, people made money."

High-dose chemotherapy also arrived at a pivotal moment in the history of breast cancer and American medicine, which is particularly prone to embracing excessive treatments. It's a system that values innovation at the expense of caution, that is often swayed more by personality than by science, and that sometimes rewards daredevil doctors at the expense of patients. In the case of high-dose chemo, insurers unwittingly made the treatment a feminist cause by refusing to pay for it. Breast cancer advocacy groups, which had only recently learned to flex their political muscle, threw their weight behind the embattled women who were fighting both cancer and their insurers. Under pressure from HMOs, hospitals welcomed the profits that high-dose chemo provided. When transplanters like Peters testified in court that the procedure was established practice, when in fact it was not, they stoked the perception among patients that high-dose chemo offered a shot at a cure.

Hope Rugo stopped performing transplants on breast cancer patients in 1999, shortly after the data from the five randomized trials came out. When I asked her the same question I asked Peters, if she had any regrets, she paused for a moment. Then she said, "We believed in it so passionately. Now I think about all the women who died during transplant, who would have lived much longer without it."

SIX The Limits of Seeing

FOR MORE THAN a century, doctors have gathered in hospital auditoriums once a week for grand rounds, a kind of Socratic master class in the art and science of medicine. In the days when doctors knew little more about a patient's condition than what they could glean from a physical exam, grand rounds served as a showcase for top clinicians. Onstage there was usually a patient, sitting in a chair or lying on a gurney, along with the senior physician and a doctor-in-training. Sometimes junior doctors picked a difficult case to see if they could stump the teaching clinician. Often they looked for patients with highly visible symptoms: a swollen joint, a distended belly, or a peculiar rash, anything that could easily be seen by the audience. Each case would generally begin with the younger doctor reciting the patient's history. Then the senior clinician would ask the patient a few questions and perform a physical exam before turning to the assembled white coats to discuss his diagnosis and what was known about the patient's condition.

Today, older physicians sometimes lament that grand rounds are no longer grand. All too often, the give-and-take between teacher and audience has given way to didactic lectures on some minute aspect of biomedical research, and PowerPoint has replaced actual cases involving real patients. But the Socratic spirit of grand rounds lives on in some hospital departments.

At five minutes to one on a Tuesday afternoon, a classroom on the fifth floor of the main hospital of the University of Medicine and Dentistry of New Jersey has already filled to capacity with about three dozen doctors and technicians. Everyone in the radiology department is expected to attend grand rounds. The residents and interns sit at desks in the middle of the room. A fidgety bunch, the interns flip through notes pulled from their pockets, while the residents chatter among themselves. The attending radiologists and technicians, in their long white coats, lean nonchalantly against the back wall of the room, while the most senior doctors sit in a cluster near the door, middle-aged men and women dressed in somber suits and skirts.

The chatter stops when Dr. Stephen Baker enters the room and strides toward the front of the class. Chairman of the department, Baker is a short, intensely intelligent man in his sixties, with stiff black hair that sometimes stands out from his head at odd angles and startling green eyes. He stands to one side of a large screen suspended from the ceiling as a series of radiological images flash beside him. Each image on the screen reveals a body part of a patient who was recently in the hospital's emergency room—and each case was chosen by Baker to teach a particular lesson.

Baker asks an attending radiologist to recite the patient's particulars for the first case: "Thirty-seven-year-old female, HIV positive, left chest pain, dypsnea [shortness of breath], and a history of illegal drug use, PCP. Pneumonia on chest X-ray." The patient is now being treated for the pneumonia. Baker peppers the radiologist with questions: "When do you repeat the chest X-ray?"

"I'm not going to," he says. Right answer.

"How long will she be here?" Baker asks. A while, says the radiologist; an infectious disease specialist wants to rule out meningitis by doing a lumbar tap on the patient, an often-painful procedure that involves plunging a long needle between two vertebrae in order to extract an aliquot of cerebrospinal fluid. Baker asks if the woman is showing the signs or symptoms of meningitis.

"No," says the radiologist.

"Then why do a spinal tap?" Baker grouses. "To tap a patient like this seems intrusive."

When Baker gives grand rounds, the lessons more often than not focus on when not to do things to patients, especially when not to perform imaging tests—CTs, X-rays, MRIs, PETs, the tools of the radiologist's trade. This might seem counterintuitive—a chief of radiology encouraging the members of his department to perform fewer radiological studies—but Baker belongs to an increasingly vocal minority of radiologists who believe that their tools are being misused and overused.

Seventy-six million computed tomography scans were performed on American patients in 2005. That's up from forty million CTs in 2000 and sixty-five million in 2004. At that rate, radiologists will be running patients through a CT scanner one hundred million times a year by 2010, or an average of one CT a year for every third citizen—a "ridiculous" number, in Baker's view, because in his opinion, many of the scans being done today are already unnecessary. These days, utilization rates of all kinds of imaging tests—MRIs, ultrasounds, PETs—are going up faster than those of any other medical technology. The use of images is rising in lockstep with the supply of increasingly sophisticated imaging machines—without much evidence that they are helping patients. The only imaging test whose rate of use is going down is the lowly X-ray.

The next case on the screen is a chest X-ray of a forty-eight-year-old man with a history of an abdominal aortic aneurysm. In other words, he has a weak spot in the wall of his aorta. The man's aneurysm has remained stable for some time without threatening to balloon outward, or dissect. He came into the emergency department earlier in the day, complaining of a sharp, burning pain in his chest, a sign that his aneurysm may finally have begun leaking blood into his abdominal cavity. If that's the case, the man needs surgery right away, or he could be dead in a matter of hours. When Baker asks for the patient's history, an attending radiologist says a chest X-ray has been done and she is about to do a CT scan on the patient.

Baker tends to talk at warp speed, and his mild Long Island accent gets more pronounced the more agitated he becomes. He chides the young doctor for bothering with the chest X-ray, which can't show if a patient's aneurysm is dissecting. "Why do an X-ray you didn't need?" he says. "This patient should have gone to CT immediately. All you did by sending him to X-ray was take him away from anybody who was capable of observing him except an X-ray technician." And so it goes through half a dozen more cases.

Grand rounds at any hospital can be awkward, sometimes even painful, to watch. Details about patients are delivered in a staccato shorthand that can leave medical students scrambling to follow what's going on. Department chiefs may single out individual attendings and residents for a grilling, hurling questions at them in order to trip them up before moving on to the next victim. Baker doesn't go in much for public humiliation, but he is not above asking a misleading question that lures a doctor into an incorrect answer if it will help him make a larger point.

The last case for the day is an elderly man who is dying of prostate cancer. Dr. Curtis Bakal, one of the senior radiologists in the department, switches the image on the screen to the man's chest X-ray and briefly describes his case: "Seventy-eight-year-old male, history of prostate cancer, brought to the ED from a nursing home with shortness of breath. He's a DNR." Translation: Sometime in the past, the man recognized his condition was terminal, and he signed a "do not resuscitate" order, which means he did not want any heroic measures taken as he neared death.

Baker points to the man's chest X-ray and challenges the students in the middle of the room to diagnose the cause of the man's shortness of breath. The bones show bright white on the X-ray against the dark shadows of his lungs, the image indistinct and hazy.

"Does he have pneumothorax?" demands Baker. This is a condition in which air leaks from the lungs into the chest cavity, where it can compress the lungs and make breathing difficult. Pneumothorax is relatively easy to treat, and even though the man has a DNR order, his emergency doctor would undoubtedly insert a chest tube to correct the condition and spare him the anxiety of being unable to breathe. None of the residents or medical students raises a hand.

"How many vote for trick question?" Baker asks playfully. Again, no hands go up, but the students' eyes are now swiveling back and forth to see if anybody else knows the answer. Above all, medical students do not want to be caught without an answer, or worse yet, giving the wrong one.

"How many of you have sudden deltoid weakness and can't raise your hand?" A few giggles erupt, but still no hands go up.

It was indeed a misleading question: The man doesn't have pneumothorax. Baker points to a white line on the X-ray, a fold of skin on his chest that left a shadow on the image, making it appear as if there is air in his chest but outside his lungs. The next question is for attending radiologist Bakal: "Mental status?"

The patient, says Bakal, is "arousable." That means he is barely conscious, able at most to move his hand when prodded or open his eyes when his name is called. The man has been in this state for some time, even before his breathing problem began.

Bakal recites the rest of the man's history. After a radiologist reported back to the emergency department that the patient did not have a pneumothorax, an emergency physician ordered an MRI of his brain. The reason for the MRI was to determine if a stroke was interfering with the man's breathing or, more likely, if metastatic tumors had migrated from his prostate into his brain, where they were causing his brain to swell and putting pressure on his breathing center.

Baker is visibly annoyed that the emergency physician has ordered an MRI. "This man is a DNR," he says. "Do not resuscitate." DNR should also mean do not test, says Baker, unless the test will help the patient. There is little to be done for a near-comatose man as frail and sick as this one. The results of the MRI will not make a difference in the patient's condition, or his treatment. The emergency doctor could give him steroids to reduce brain swelling and maybe temporarily ease the patient's labored breathing, but there is no stopping his inexorable march toward death. "Why should we subject him to the indignity of an MRI?" says Baker. "He could croak in there. Would you want to spend your last hour practically naked inside an MR scanner?"

There's no denying the fact that imaging technology has revolutionized the practice of medicine since General Electric's first medical CT scanner was introduced in 1978. A primitive version of today's sophisticated machines, with only a single X-ray source and a single X-ray detector, the scanner was so slow that patients had to lie perfectly still and hold their breath for up to twenty seconds to create a single image, or slice, and the device's usefulness was restricted largely to looking at the brain, the only part of the body that stayed still long enough not to blur an image. Even so, head CTs transformed the practice of emergency medicine and neurology. Before

CT, patients who came into the emergency department with trauma to the head were X-rayed, which could show skull fractures but not bleeding inside the skull. By the time doctors realized the patient was bleeding and sent her in for surgery, it was often too late to prevent devastating brain damage, or even death. Similarly, before the advent of CT, neurologists had no way of knowing if a patient's neurological symptoms, such as slurring of speech, difficulty walking, or cognitive deficits, were due to a stroke or a brain tumor until they went in for exploratory surgery. CT scans allowed doctors to peer inside the skull and spot tumors, or catch bleeds in time to make a difference. *Time Magazine* noted that medicine's new "wondrous machines" were expensive, but in the end they would save billions of dollars by eliminating unnecessary surgery and catching diseases early, when they were easier to treat. *Newsweek* hailed the new imaging technologies for their ability to render the human body "almost as transparent as a jellyfish."

Today's CT scanners, along with MRI (magnetic resonance imaging) and PET (positron-emission tomography), truly are wondrous machines that have made the diagnosis of many conditions far faster and simpler for physicians, and less risky for patients. A CT scan of a lung or kidney can reveal a tumor no bigger than the period at the end of this sentence, while MRI can peer into joints and illuminate tears in soft tissue and cartilage. As images have become swifter and sharper, physicians have grown ever more dependent upon them.

A young emergency physician who practices in a small town in Maine told me a story that typifies how most doctors view imaging tests. An older man came into the emergency room in the wee hours of the night complaining of sharp pain in his neck and his back. The man had been to the ER two weeks before with the same complaint. Another physician examined the patient at the time, found nothing wrong, and sent him home with instructions to take some Motrin. The man's pain got better for a few days, but then it came back. When the young emergency physician—we'll call him Dr. Brown— examined the patient, he could not put his finger on a diagnosis. Nevertheless, Brown ordered a chest CT with contrast. "I had to wake up the CT tech to do the scan," the doctor told me. "She wasn't too happy. She said, 'You want me to do a chest CT and you can't tell me why?' I didn't really know why.

The guy was basically healthy. But the fact that the pain was bad enough, and it couldn't be explained by neck strain, and the history he gave me . . . it all added up to a hunch." Brown's instincts were correct: The CT showed the man's aorta was dissecting; a section had ballooned out like a weak spot in a bicycle inner tube and was stealthily leaking blood into his abdominal cavity. The patient was sent directly to the operating room, where a surgeon clamped the dissection, repaired the man's aorta, and saved his life.

Doctors tend to remember triumphant moments like this one, their hunches that saved a patient's life. When an imaging test is involved in their memories, it reinforces their already implicit and profound belief in the power of technology to reduce the terrible, wearing uncertainty of medicine. We patients have also come to believe that high-tech images represent high-quality care. Think of any medical show on television—*House*, *Grey's Anatomy*, or ER. TV doctors are constantly peering at computer screens of CT images or throwing plain X-ray films up on a wall-mounted light box in order to figure out what's wrong with their TV patients. Imaging tests provide all of us, doctors and patients, with a welcome sense of sureness that the body and its diseases are knowable, that by gathering enough information, our doctors will come to a correct diagnosis and effective treatment.

But our image of imaging, our belief in its power to help doctors heal, may be ill founded. Imaging tests should be saving lives by reducing the rate at which doctors incorrectly diagnose and treat their patients. That is, after all, the whole point of using an image—to improve the physician's ability to see inside the body and know as precisely as possible what's going on so she can decide on treatment that will actually help the patient. Yet, as Baker was trying to drive home to his young doctors, a healthier patient isn't always the outcome. Even as the number of imaging tests is going up, numerous studies suggest that all those pictures are not nearly as effective at improving diagnosis as many doctors—and patients—tend to think.

Take studies of autopsies, the most reliable, not to mention the oldest, tool for determining whether physicians were correct in their diagnoses—and treatment—of patients. Autopsies have been performed for more than two thousand years, but it wasn't until the late 1800s that physicians came to see them not just as a method for learning anatomy but also as a means for tracking medical missteps—the rates of which are shockingly high. Studies of autopsy results dating back to 1938 have consistently found high rates of diagnostic error; in 25 to 40 percent of cases where an autopsy was performed, the patient died of an undiagnosed cause. In other words, the doctors had misdiagnosed the patient and were treating him for the wrong condition—giving him drugs for chronic heart failure, for instance, when he was in fact suffering from pneumonia. Incredibly, the rate of misdiagnosis has remained virtually unchanged since researchers began tracking autopsy results, back in 1910.

What that says to George Lundberg, a noted pathologist, ardent champion of the autopsy, and former editor of the *Journal of the American Medical Association*, is that imaging tests have not done much, on average, to improve doctors' powers of diagnosis. In a *JAMA* editorial accompanying a large autopsy study published in 1998, Lundberg wrote that the low-tech autopsy "trumps high-tech medicine in getting the right answer again and again, even during the 1990s and even at academic medical centers." Actually, the autopsy doesn't so much trump high-tech medicine as it reveals some of its limitations. A more-recent paper, published by a group of researchers at the University of California, San Francisco, in 2003, looked at fifty-three separate studies of autopsies performed since the 1960s, the period of time that spans the meteoric rise in the use of imaging tests. The authors found only a tiny drop in the rate of misdiagnosis. They estimated that among the 850,000 or so Americans dying in hospitals each year, nearly 35,000 might have survived if they'd been given the correct diagnosis and treatment.*

All of this research suggests that for every scan that helps a physician come to the right decision, another scan may cloud the picture, sending the doctor down the wrong path. But how can this be? If imaging is providing so much information, if it can make the body as "transparent as a jellyfish," why aren't doctors getting better at figuring out what's wrong with their patients?

----

* To be fair, the rate of autopsies has dropped precipitously in the last two decades, and many of those that are done today are in cases where the cause of death is unclear. That would suggest that their estimate of the rate of misdiagnosis may be exaggerated at least a bit.

In a brilliant essay on mammography and the limits of seeing, *New Yorker* writer Malcolm Gladwell tells a story that illustrates how high-tech images can be deceiving. When the first Gulf War began, the U.S. Air Force employed two squadrons of F-15E Strike Eagle fighter jets to find and destroy Scud missile launch sites in the Iraqi desert. After a Scud was airborne, it would leave a light trail in the night sky, allowing the fighter pilots to narrow down the site of the launch to a few square miles. The Iraqis were using modified flatbed trucks as their launching sites, moving them around so they could launch from a different spot each night. Once the missile was dispatched, they would hide the truck in one of the many culverts under the highway between Baghdad and Jordan. The U.S. pilots employed a state-of-the-art, $4.6 million device called a LANTIM navigation and targeting pod, which took high-resolution infrared photographs of the desert floor below the plane, allowing the pilots to spot a launcher and bomb it into oblivion. The air force boasted to the press that it had destroyed about one hundred launch trucks. Military officials, writes Gladwell, "were not guessing at the number of Scud launchers hit; as far as they were concerned, they knew." Yet when the hostilities ended and the air force sent a team in on the ground to verify the effectiveness of its air campaign, the team discovered the actual number of Scud launchers destroyed was zero. Looking at a black-and-white screen that measured six inches by six inches at a patch of desert from twenty thousands feet up, pilots weren't able to correctly identify missile launchers with any accuracy. They couldn't tell the difference between a real Scud sitting on its launcher, a tanker truck transporting oil to Jordan, and a decoy constructed by the Iraqis out of old trucks and spare missile parts.

Just like high-tech infrared photography, medical imaging can trick physicians into thinking they know more than they really do. Doctors routinely dismiss possible diagnoses because their high-tech tools show a negative result. False-positive results—a scan that indicates there's something wrong when there isn't—can lead them to perform even more unnecessary tests, some of which can be invasive and potentially dangerous, in an effort to confirm the (incorrect) diagnosis.

The power of imaging tests to fool doctors can be seen readily in appendicitis. One of the most prevalent conditions an emergency room physician encounters, a suspected appendicitis case, or "appy," in ER slang, is also the most common reason for an abdominal CT scan. Each year, physicians order more and more abdominal CTs for suspected appies, about 250,000 of which result in surgery. Surgery for appendicitis is the most frequently performed emergency operation in the world, and over the course of a lifetime, 12 percent of men and 25 percent of women will have their bellies sliced open because of suspected appendicitis.

While appendicitis is common, it isn't always easy to diagnose, and emergency room doctors are constantly walking a fine line between missing an appy, on the one hand, and sending a patient for unnecessary abdominal surgery, on the other. Either way, it's a big error in emergency medicine. Missing an appy can mean a burst appendix, which can lead to all sorts of nasty complications, even death. Yet doctors don't want to send a patient off to an unnecessary, or "negative," appendectomy. For one thing, they might get an earful from a cranky surgeon who has just opened a patient and found nothing wrong. For another, unnecessary abdominal surgery is not something any physician wants a patient to undergo. An appendectomy means spending an average of more than three days in the hospital at a cost of nearly eleven thousand dollars, whether or not your appendix needed to come out.

Despite physicians' best efforts, about 15 percent of people who go under the knife to have their appendix removed don't actually have appendicitis. Sometimes the surgeon goes in and finds not a swollen appendix but a burst ovarian cyst. Other conditions that can mimic the pain of appendicitis include an intestinal blockage, constipation, menstrual cramps, and even a bad case of gas. In women of reproductive age, one in four appendectomies is negative or unnecessary. In people older than eighty, the negative appendectomy rate is a whopping 35 percent. (Surgeons generally remove the appendix once they're inside the belly.)

You would think that the advent of CT scanning would have significantly reduced the chances that emergency room doctors will misdiagnose appendicitis. A doctor can generally recognize an infected appendix on a CT of the abdomen by its swollen size and the "fat stranding," or striations in surrounding fatty tissue caused by the inflammation—provided those signs are present. Astonishingly enough, however, the rate of negative appendectomies probably hasn't budged in the two decades since belly CT scans became commonplace. In 2001, a surgeon at the University of Washington named David Flum published a study looking at rates of misdiagnosed appendicitis between 1987 and 1998, precisely the period when CT scanning became widely available and widely used around the country. Flum and his colleagues examined 63,790 records of appendectomies to see whether the rate of mistakes had changed over the eleven-year period. It hadn't. It was 15.5 percent in 1987 and 15.5 percent in 1998.*

That's not to say that a CT scan can never help catch a suspected appy or protect a patient from a negative appendectomy. CT scans may provide greater certainty when doctors are faced with a confusing case. But a CT scan, clear as it may seem, is only one piece of information—and a potentially misleading one at that—which can fail to add much to a careful clinical exam. Even newer CT scans, which offer higher resolution, will not always reveal to the doctor what the right course of treatment is, because, as Malcolm Gladwell puts it, "the human task of interpretation is often a bigger obstacle than the technical task of picture taking."

Here's how CT can muck things up in the ER. The patient, often a young woman, comes in with pain in the lower right quadrant of the belly, an elevated white blood cell count, and a fever. As the emergency physician palpates, or touches, her belly, fingers pressing closer and closer to the spot where the appendix is located, he can feel the telltale "guarding," or involuntary tightening of her abdominal muscles. All classic signs of appendicitis. The doctor thinks this is almost certainly an appy, but he knows that an ovarian cyst can sometimes mimic the pain of appendicitis in young women, so just to make sure, he orders an abdominal CT scan. (Or, as is often the case, the surgeon demands a scan before she will even see the patient.) Whatever the reason for the CT scan, it comes up negative. Maybe this patient's infection isn't causing any fat stranding. Maybe her appendix

---

* This study looked only at patients in Washington State, but there's no reason to think that misdiagnosis rates in that state are any higher than anywhere else in the country.

hasn't become terribly swollen yet. So now the emergency physician must look for another explanation for the young woman's pain. The doctor pulls out the ultrasound machine, but there's no trace of an ovarian cyst. Instead of trusting his initial clinical judgment, which told him the patient almost certainly had appendicitis, the ER doctor goes with the negative CT scan and sends her home. Two days later, she's back in the emergency room, and this time, the appy shows up bright and clear on another CT. Only now she's had two belly CTs and two extra days of pain, and worse yet, her appendix has burst and she has a serious abdominal infection.

This is not an uncommon story. In fact, it's the precise story recounted to me by an emergency physician I happened to fall into conversation with while standing in line at an airport, and it's not unlike the cases other physicians have described concerning the use of imaging tests for a variety of conditions. Dr. Jerome Hoffman, an emergency physician at the University of California, Los Angeles, has seen his share of appendicitis cases. He's also an expert in critically appraising medical evidence and how doctors use evidence to make clinical decisions. He says, "Say I see ten patients with belly pain. Three of them I know have appendicitis. Six I know don't have it, and one of them, I'm not sure. If I do a CT scan on that one, it will help me decide most of the time. That way, if I use a CT when I'm in doubt, I'm going to be right more than nine times out of ten. But if I slavishly believe whatever a CT tells me, and I do it on all ten patients, the CT is going to be wrong at least one time out of ten, and now I'm down to being right only nine times at the most, maybe less." That means that more patients will either have their appendicitis go untreated or wind up getting an unnecessary appendectomy, all because their doctors put more faith in an image than in their clinical judgment.

An article of faith

Why are doctors ordering so many imaging tests? If tests can cloud their judgment and lead to the wrong diagnosis, why do they persist in relying so heavily on high-tech scanners? In 2005, the *Journal of the American Medical Association* published a survey of 824 Pennsylvania doctors in high-risk specialties, including obstetrics, neurology, and emergency medicine; 59 percent of those surveyed said they routinely ordered unnecessary tests, including imaging tests. Doctors know perfectly well they are ordering useless imaging tests, but when you ask them why they do it, they offer conflicting reasons. Some emergency physicians admit that they will occasionally send a patient off to radiology for "bed control"—to free up an ER bed that can be filled with a patient from the crowded waiting room. Radiologists say they run patients through scanners even when they know they shouldn't because other physicians asked for the test. It's not their job to reason why; they just provide the radiological services that are requested. (Stephen Baker points out that radiologists make money on every image they read, so they have little incentive to argue with ordering physicians.) But the two reasons doctors give most often for why they do so much excess imaging are patient demand and worries about malpractice suits.

Many physicians, but especially those who work in high-wire specialties like neurology, emergency medicine, and radiology, live with the quiet but persistent fear that they will be sued for failing to order an imaging test—or failing to correctly diagnose a disease on a scan that's been performed. An emergency doctor's worst nightmare is the patient who presents with atypical chest pain that gets diagnosed as heartburn, but who actually has a dissecting aneurysm or a heart attack. A really paranoid doctor might order a CT scan on every patient with chest pain to rule out an aneurysm, even when he is virtually certain it's nothing worse than heartburn. Next in line for ER doctors to fret about is the patient who is sent home after coming in with a head injury, only to return to the hospital in a coma with a brain bleed. Radiologists, on the other hand, worry they will be accused of missing a cancer—a concern that seems justified in light of the fact that radiologists are sued more often than other specialists, and mammographers are sued more often than any other subspecialists of radiology.

In many malpractice cases involving a missed imaging test, the image would not have made a difference in the patient's outcome. Suits brought against mammographers, for example, most commonly involve a woman under the age of fifty who had a clean mammogram shortly before being diagnosed with a malignant breast cancer. The patient or her family sues the radiologist for having failed to spot the tumor. But many breast tumors in young women are particularly aggressive, appearing so quickly that they can be invisible on a mammogram to even the most suspicious and careful mammographer, only to grow large enough to detect, sometimes even by feel, just a few months later.

In cases involving a head injury, it might seem as if it's better to be safe than sorry, but that's not always the case. Emergency doctors have clear rules to help them decide when they need to order a head CT scan. If they follow those rules, their chances of missing a brain bleed are next to nil. If the doctor suspects a brain injury, she is supposed to run the patient through a series of simple neurological tests, asking the patient, for example, to raise both eyebrows, turn his cheek against the doctor's hand, and touch his fingertips to his nose with his eyes closed. If the patient exhibits no outward neurological signs of brain injury, there's little reason to order a head scan, because the image will almost certainly come up clean. So why not order the scan, just to be sure? Because both doctors and patients think scans can't lie, and they may be falsely reassured by a clean scan that the patient is out of danger. But a brain bleed can develop slowly, and it won't show up immediately on a scan. The doctor sends the patient home. A few days later, the patient, thinking he's been given a clean bill of health, ignores the "thunderclap" headache that is a signal that he has begun to hemorrhage inside his skull.

Jeanne Lenzer, a former physician's assistant who is now an investigative medical reporter, tells the story of a patient she saw several years ago, an older man who walked into the emergency room with a deep gash in his forehead. The man, whom we'll call John Powers, had fallen from a ladder to a concrete floor, losing consciousness for a few minutes before waking up with his face covered with blood. His wife, Rita, brought him to the emergency room, where Lenzer stopped the bleeding from his cut, performed a neurological exam to make sure he was not in immediate danger of brain injury, and stitched up his wound. Before discharging him, she explained to Powers and his wife why she was not giving him a CT scan. She told the couple that the neurological exam was completely normal, and she was confident he wasn't bleeding in his brain, but that didn't mean he would not develop a bleed over the next few weeks. She gave them strict instructions to go to his primary care physician or come back to the emergency room if he began having any symptoms, like dizziness, disorientation, or a persistent headache.

Lenzer ran into the couple about a year later, when they came to the emergency room for another reason. She asked them how John was doing, and Rita replied that he had been fine—ever since his brain surgery. "I thought she was teasing me at first," says Lenzer. "When I realized they were serious, my heart stopped for a second." Lenzer suspected that Powers had gone on to develop a bleed, and that she was now in danger of being sued for malpractice for failing to order a CT scan of his head. She was only partly right. After returning home, Powers felt fine for a few days, until he developed a headache. Doing as Lenzer instructed, he called his doctor, who sent him for a scan, but it showed no evidence of bleeding. When the headache persisted, Powers returned to the emergency room for a third time. This time, a CT scan revealed a subdural hematoma—a significant pool of blood pressing on his brain. He was sent for immediate surgery. The couple thanked Lenzer for taking the time to explain why she was not ordering a scan and what they needed to watch for when they got home.

Most ER physicians know this is the right way to treat a patient with a normal neurological exam, and many are aware of the hazards of an unnecessary head CT, yet they order them anyway, they say, because juries in malpractice cases don't always pay attention to the medical evidence. In 2004, John and Robyn Sprague, of La Plata, Maryland, won a five-million-dollar judgment against their pediatrician and two doctors at a local hospital because they failed to order a head CT for the Spragues' infant son. In 1998, the Spragues brought their eleven-month-old son to the emergency room because his babysitter reported he had fallen backward from his high chair and hit his head. When the baby appeared perfectly normal neurologically, without so much as a bump on his head, the emergency physician and an on-call pediatrician agreed there was no reason to perform a head CT. The family went home with strict instructions to come back if the child's behavior changed. They did return, two weeks later, after the child had suffered a devastating head injury while in the care of the babysitter, who was

later charged with child abuse. The Spragues successfully sued their pediatrician, the hospital, and two other doctors for failing to order a CT the first
time they brought their son in, claiming that the image would have somehow shown the babysitter was abusing the boy.

Whether or not a CT might have uncovered evidence of abuse, cases like
the Spragues' send a collective chill down the spines of physicians. No matter how justified they might be in their clinical decision not to scan, they
often conclude that it is better to practice defensive medicine, to order an
unnecessary test, than to risk being hit with a lawsuit. Even when physicians win their cases, going through the ordeal of a malpractice suit leaves
many emotionally shaken and filled with distrust for their patients. Their
malpractice-insurance premiums may go up, and every time they renew
their licenses, they must register the fact that they have been sued and explain what happened. As one physician blogger responded to the Sprague
case, "What is the moral of the story? Order an expensive test and save
yourself the trouble."

The other reason physicians commonly offer for ordering so many unnecessary imaging tests is that patients demand them. Patients with back
pain ask for MRIs because a friend got one, or because they read about
MRIs in a story about a new surgical technique for back pain, or because a
radiology clinic was advertising MRIs. One freestanding clinic in the
Boston area ran radio ads during football games, urging New England Pa-
triots fans who had been "sidelined by an injury" to come in for a scan.
Parents want their children to get head CT scans for a bump on the head
and abdominal CTs for belly pain, perhaps because we all tend to believe
what the Air Force pilots thought during the first Gulf War: that photographs can't lie, that getting an image represents the surest path toward being safe rather than sorry.

Doctors say that when a patient demands a test, they often comply—even
when they know the test is not warranted. It's easier to acquiesce than to explain why a CT scan won't necessarily help diagnose appendicitis, or why
the doctor is certain that the patient's ankle is sprained, not broken, and
doesn't need to be X-rayed, or why an MRI won't change the fact that the
first remedy for mild back pain is ice, over-the-counter pain medication,

and normal activity. As one emergency physician who is a pediatric specialist tells me, he'd rather send a child to radiology than fight with the kid's
parents, who will only think he's incompetent because they know their child
needs a scan. "You can take fifteen or twenty minutes to explain why a head
CT for a tiny bump isn't a good idea," he says. "Or, you can get the CT and
be out of there in five minutes. They're happy because you did it. You're
happy because you didn't have to spend that time."

While doctors' fears of malpractice suits are real, and patients do make
demands for high-tech care, these two pressures can't be the whole explanation for the phenomenal number of unnecessary imaging scans being
performed each year. National Imaging Associates, a company that helps insurers decide how to pay for imaging services, estimates that at least two
thirds of MRIs contribute nothing to physicians' ability to diagnose their
patients accurately. In 2002, Blue Cross Blue Shield of Missouri calculated
that 20 to 30 percent of their claims for PET, CT, and MRI scans were for unnecessary tests. In states where malpractice laws make it less likely that doctors will be sued, there's only about a 15 percent difference in the amount
of unnecessary treatment doctors deliver. This suggests that only a fraction
of the useless scans being performed can be laid at the feet of defensive
medicine. No study ever conducted has shown that malpractice worries or
patient demand can account for any more than a tiny fraction of unnecessary care.

A far more important driver of excess imaging, in Stephen Baker's view,
is the fact that most doctors are as enamored of imaging as their patients
are, and for precisely the same reasons. "We have this slavish belief in technology," he says. Like the rest of us, doctors tend to place their trust in visual
information, perhaps because the eyes, as essayist Diane Ackerman puts it,
"are the monopolists of the senses." Human beings are by nature visual
creatures, and we perceive and appraise the world mainly through seeing it.

This faith in the visual is reinforced in medical school, where young
doctors quickly learn that it's better to know too much than too little. They
spend their first two years cramming their heads full of the minutiae of
symptoms, blood chemistry, anatomy, and drug interactions. As interns,
they're grilled mercilessly on their knowledge by residents and attendings,

who often demand clinical data about individual patients regardless of whether that information will actually affect diagnosis and treatment. The underlying message that's conveyed is that when it comes to tests, too many is a lesser sin than too few. One year, a colleague of Baker's at the University of Medicine and Dentistry conducted a survey of the surgical residents in the hospital, asking if they were ever corrected for ordering an unneeded radiological study. The young surgeons reported that they were routinely called on the carpet for not getting a study, but never for ordering a test they didn't need. The last thing a resident wants is for the attending to ask, "What did the MRI say?" and for the resident to have to answer, "I didn't order one."

All of which fuels an inflated belief in imaging technology's capacity to reduce ambiguity and doubt. "An image gives the illusion of a greater sense of certainty," says Baker. "But it's still an illusion; it's an article of faith that overpowers rational argument." Which helps explain why doctors don't follow the rules that exist to help them decide when they need to image and when they don't. These "decision trees" have been carefully constructed to help emergency doctors and radiologists decide when it is in a patient's best interests to order a test and when an image is not only unwarranted but potentially harmful. One set of rules, for example, which was designed to help physicians decide if they need a CT scan for a patient who might have a neck injury, could eliminate 12.6 percent of CT scans for neck trauma, or about one hundred thousand scans a year, without risking the possibility of leaving a patient untreated for a serious spinal injury. Yet doctors ignore these decision trees and persist in believing that malpractice-suit fears and patient demand are the entire explanation for their habit of giving patients what they know are unnecessary tests. Everything in their training told them that ordering images would protect them from making mistakes, or at least looking stupid when a resident or attending demanded the results of a test. Once they are out in practice, there are few incentives to discourage them from the habits they learned in medical school. But there's one additional impetus, one more reason for doctors to order images that aren't really needed, and that's the hospital's bottom line. Doctors are rarely discouraged by their hospitals or their radiology department chairs from ordering excessive tests, because imaging tests are a source of considerable profit.

A vast cultural delusion

A muggy July morning in Newark finds Baker in his crowded office, sitting at a small circular table with Dave Spencer, regional sales manager for General Electric, and Tim Lynch, the account manager who handles the University of Medicine and Dentistry's account for GE machines. Spencer and Lynch, both in their thirties, are dressed in the standard uniform of medical salesmen: dark suits, conservative ties, their white shirts still crisp, despite the withering heat outside. Spencer's blue eyes protrude slightly, giving him an expression of perpetual astonishment. Wearing a rumpled suit and a wonderfully loud tie decorated with a map of the world, Baker barely glances at the glossy brochure and colorful information sheets about GE machines that Spencer and Lynch have brought him. He already knows he wants to purchase GE's newest CT scanner. Unfortunately, he's a little short on capital funds; the state of New Jersey is staggering under huge budget deficits and is unable to provide much assistance to the hospital. Baker wants Spencer and Lynch to figure out a way for GE to lease his radiology department a two-million-dollar machine known as the LightSpeed VCT, for volume-computed tomography.

The LightSpeed VCT, which came out in 2005, has become a must-have piece of technology not just for the University of Medicine and Dentistry but for radiology departments all over the country. It's not hard to see why. The machine is a marvel of mechanical and electrical engineering. Inside its sleek, white, plastic husk are sixty-four X-ray sources and detectors, capable of taking two hundred separate X-ray images simultaneously from multiple points around the body in a single second. The LightSpeed is so fast that it can digitally capture an entire organ—the lungs, the heart, the liver—in less than five seconds. Yet the true genius of this machine lies in its dazzling software, which was borrowed in part from computer animation and can reconstruct the individual slices taken through an organ into a volume-computed, or three-dimensional, image.

To radiologists, 3-D is a kind of parlor trick, impressive but not terribly useful to them. They've grown accustomed to looking at multiple CT slices arranged in neat rows on a computer screen, mentally putting together the flat images into whole organs, bone, and blood vessels in order to spot a tumor, a blockage in the bowel, or bleeding in the brain. They don't need a computer to do that for them. Spencer acknowledges that "3-D development was invented for the nonradiologists." In fact, the LightSpeed VCT was created specifically for cardiologists, who had never had much use for CT scanning when it required looking at arteries and the heart slice by slice. Now, they can see a 3-D scan of the coronary arteries, which in the Light-Speed VCT's exquisitely colorized image look like a network of white tree roots encasing a crimson heart.

By the end of 2005, GE had sold nine hundred LightSpeed VCT scanners worldwide, at a cost of up to two million dollars each. Spencer, whose sales region includes much of New York State and New Jersey, earned commissions on nearly a hundred the first year the machine was out, most of them going to large academic medical centers. Now, everybody wants a sixty-four-slice scanner, he says. "This year, I've got rural, hundred-bed hospitals in upstate New York with no money trying to buy one." They want the new scanner partly because new means faster, and faster means greater throughput—more patients scanned per day. The higher the throughput, the more profit for a radiology department. They also want the scanner because it will appeal to ambitious cardiologists, who want to use the latest device and who will bring in more (profitable) business to the hospital that owns one. That's one of the reasons Baker is looking to buy the LightSpeed VCT. "If I don't get the technology, we can't get the research grants, and the hospital can't attract people to work here," he says. "It's like the growth of naval powers between 1870 and 1917; everybody needed another dreadnought. Now everybody needs the newest CT scanner."

The meeting concludes with instructions for the GE salesmen to find a deal that will let Baker spread the cost of the LightSpeed out over five years. Afterward, Baker slumps in his chair and rubs his face with both hands. Then he says, "The work I do to reduce utilization is at cross-purposes with the hospital." On the one hand, he wants the young doctors in his department to learn

how to use radiological images judiciously, so that an image adds to their ability to make sound clinical judgments, to improve care for their patients,
rather than detracting. He knows that if imaging machines were not so readily available, doctors would be less likely to use them so indiscriminately. (In
countries like England and Canada, where scanners are spread more thinly,
doctors make do with far fewer scans per patient.) On the other hand, as chief
of radiology he must continually purchase new imaging machines to bolster
the hospital's bottom line, knowing all the while that the availability of newer,
faster devices only encourages physicians to perform even more unnecessary
tests. "There is a certain amount of cognitive and moral dissonance here," he
says. "My success as a chair of the department of radiology depends on how
many toys I can get for the department. So I have to win turf battles, and get
more and more. That's what I do every day. Then I go home and think, 'What
the hell am I doing?' "

When it comes down to a fight between reducing overutilization of imaging tests and helping his hospital stay solvent, his hospital must win. Between
2003 and 2006, Baker spent twenty-five million dollars on new machines for
the radiology department. He lays out the economics for just one of those
machines, the PET scanner he bought for three million dollars three years ago.
A radiologist makes about two hundred dollars for reading a scan; the hospital is reimbursed between sixteen hundred and two thousand dollars. After
paying for the initial investment in the scanner; the maintenance fee, which
amounts to twenty thousand dollars a month; and a nurse and a technologist
to administer the radioactive drug and run the patient through the scanner,
the hospital makes an average profit of about a thousand dollars per scan.
"The more scans you do, the more money you make. If I do eight PET scans a
day, that's two million dollars a year, or a 35 percent profit margin," Baker
says. "But we don't use the word 'profit' in hospitals; it's called surplus."

Hospitals around the country are making the same calculations and con-
cluding that they all need newer, faster scanners. This strategy represents a
shift from the late 1980s through the '90s, when hospitals didn't vie for patients directly but rather for the business of managed care plans, which only
sent them patients if they slashed their prices. New technologies like high-
speed CT scanners were viewed as too expensive for the most part, and hos-

pitals refrained from investing in anything that did not promise to reduce the cost of care. By the late 1990s, however, a consumer backlash against managed care had forced insurers to loosen their grip on hospital reimbursements, and this "wholesale" strategy was no longer necessary. Hospitals reverted to more-traditional retail marketing, going after both patients and doctors by advertising their high-tech assets. They went on a buying spree for devices ranging from two-million-dollar CT scanners to million-dollar da Vinci surgical robots.

Today, hospitals in cities and towns across the country are engaged in a medical-technology arms race, buying up high-end machinery as fast as they can, even if it means duplicating a device that can be found in a hospital just down the road. In Minnesota's Twin Cities, for example, a region of three and a half million residents, five of the area's thirteen hospitals had already purchased sixty-four-slice scanners by 2006, from either GE or its rival manufacturers, Toyota and the German company Siemens. By 2005, the state of Ohio boasted more than 250 MRI units. That's more MRI machines than there were in all of Canada, and radiologists in Toledo sometimes joke that it's a wonder that cars don't swerve back and forth on the streets where many of the city's hospitals are located, owing to the strong magnetic fields that are created by MRI machines.

When hospitals buy faster machines, says Baker, it lowers the barrier for physicians to order yet another unnecessary test, setting up a vicious cycle. Why not send a patient off to get a scan—for bed control, to avoid a malpractice suit, because a patient demanded it? "They think to themselves, scans are fast, the machines are there, so why not use them?" he says. As doctors send more patients for scans, the hospital makes more money, but eventually the radiology department starts clogging up. Pretty soon, physicians are complaining that their patients have to wait too long to get their scans. The radiology department realizes there's enough demand that it can afford to buy another, even faster scanner, and soon the cycle starts all over again. You can think of it as a variation of supply-driven demand, or a version of Roemer's law: A purchased scanner is a scanner with a full schedule. It's also a little like widening roads to ease congestion. When the road is first improved, traffic eases and commutes get shorter. But then, more people move into an area because the commute isn't too bad, and eventually traffic is congested again until work starts anew to widen the road or build a new one.

Doctors in private practice have also figured out the economics of imaging tests, and more and more of them are investing in radiological equipment so they too can reap some of the potential profit. In 1993, according to a study published in the journal *Radiology*, radiologists received reimbursement for more than 210,000 imaging tests per hundred thousand Medicare beneficiaries. (Think about that number: If those images were spread evenly among all Medicare beneficiaries, each would get two images per year.) Doctors who weren't radiologists billed Medicare for another seventy-nine thousand scans per hundred thousand Medicare recipients, a little more than two thirds as many scans as radiologists. By 1999, the number of scans done by nonradiologists had gone up to more than one hundred thousand scans per hundred thousand Medicare beneficiaries, while the number of scans done by radiologists remained about the same. So the total number of scans done on people over sixty-five rose, along with the proportion of them being performed by nonradiologists. The reason for this increase among nonradiologists was managed care. With its ungenerous reimbursement rates, managed care indirectly drove many doctors in private practice to search for ways to bolster their falling incomes. As its grip on reimbursements tightened, the price of high-end equipment was simultaneously coming down, and the predictable result was that trade magazines for doctors began carrying articles bearing such titles as "Make Your Practice More Profitable." The authors provided information on where to purchase imaging equipment and predicted how much income physicians could expect from investing in it. Enterprising doctors in large group practices who have bought machines like CT scanners and MRIs outright, or cut deals with device makers to lease equipment, can collect anywhere from hundreds to thousands of dollars in fees for every scan done on an outpatient basis. Other doctors have invested in freestanding radiology clinics, taking a share of the profits based on the number of patients they refer to the clinic.

The problem here is that doctors who "self-refer," who send patients for procedures or tests in which they themselves have a financial stake, tend to order a lot more procedures and tests than doctors who don't self-refer. Studies have found that self-referral leads to as many as eight times more imaging tests than are requested by radiologists. Imaging from self-referring nonradiologists costs the nation about sixteen billion dollars a year. At this point, it almost goes without saying that many, if not most, of those images are entirely unnecessary.

New York Times reporter Gina Kolata wrote recently about her own experience with an orthopedist, who self-referred her for an MRI. Kolata, a runner, had been suffering from pain at the base of her third toe after a particularly long, hard run. After ignoring the pain for several weeks, she made an appointment with a local orthopedist. She waited nearly an hour to see the doctor, who never even touched her foot. Kolata wrote, "All I got was a cursory examination and an X-ray. When the X-ray showed normal bone, the orthopedist said I needed an MRI. His office said someone would call me when my insurer approved it. Then I could schedule it." Kolata went home, where she e-mailed a rheumatologist in Tulsa, Oklahoma, with whom she'd been corresponding. The rheumatologist told her the MRI wasn't necessary. He thought her problem was most likely an inflamed tendon, which could have easily been diagnosed with a hands-on examination. If the problem was as he suspected, a small dose of steroids injected into her foot should relieve the pain, and her injury would heal on its own. Kolata found another orthopedist, who gave her the injection: "The injection cured me. It also saved my insurer more than $1,000 for an MRI and subsequent doctors' appointments."

Another form of entrepreneurial imaging emerged in the mid-1990s, when hospitals and radiologists in private practice began offering CT scans directly to the public. For about $900, anybody off the street can get a whole-body CT scan, which proponents claim will protect against everything from heart disease to cancer. While most academic radiologists have been critical of the practice, by 2001 at least one hundred scanning centers had sprouted up around the country. Demand for their services was fueled in part by testimonials from celebrities like Oprah Winfrey, who actually underwent a whole-body scan on television. At one time, scan shops on the West Coast, like HealthView, in Newport Beach, the most popular center in the Los Angeles area, had ten-month waiting lists. Other entrepreneurial doctors load CT scanners into mobile units and send them on the road with a technologist. Like itinerant patent-medicine salesmen, who once traveled from town to town selling their potions and elixirs, CT technologists park their vans for a day or two, sell as many scans as they can, and then move on to the next small town. The results of the scans are read by a radiologist back at a central location and sent to patients by mail.

Scan centers advertise that "bad news can be good news, if you get it early enough" and that getting tested brings "peace of mind," but does it really? In most cases, a scan finds absolutely nothing wrong, and the customer does indeed walk away satisfied, thinking he's been given a clean bill of health. (He's also been given a big dose of radiation, but more about that later.) In a tiny percentage of people, a CT scan might actually do some good, uncovering a cancer of one sort or another that might possibly have caused the patient harm sometime down the road. But you have to scan a lot of people in order to find a single tumor that needs to be taken out. For instance, scanning twenty thousand men between the ages of forty and sixty will pick up on average only a single, solitary kidney cancer, and even then there's not much evidence to suggest that removing every kidney tumor that turns up in a CT scan will save anybody's life.

The real danger of whole-body scans is that when a scan turns up a lump, it's almost invariably an innocent, innocuous nothing, an "incidentaloma" in radiology-speak, that would never have caused symptoms had it never been found. Unfortunately, while incidentalomas are perfectly harmless when left alone, they can wreak havoc as soon as they are spotted by a radiologist. That's because radiologists often can't tell the difference between an incidentaloma and a potentially dangerous tumor just by looking at it, and that means that when a scan finds something positive, the patient has to be worked up, with more tests, biopsies, and sometimes even surgery. One study of twelve hundred whole-body scans found that 87 percent picked up an abnormal finding; 40 percent of those required follow-up tests. Only a tiny, tiny fraction, less than 1 percent, turned out to be a tumor.

In 2002, Dr. William Casarella, chairman of the radiology department at Emory University, underwent a virtual colonoscopy, a new way to screen for colon cancer using a CT scan instead of a colonoscope, an optical device that's inserted through the rectum and allows doctors to peer inside the colon. Casarella's colon was cancer free on the CT scan, but the image also captured other parts of his abdomen, revealing what looked like tumors on one kidney, a one-inch mass on his liver, and a scattering of lumps on his lungs.

Casarella underwent a contrast CT that showed the lumps on his kidney to be renal cysts, a common and entirely benign condition that affects half of all people over the age of fifty. After another contrast CT scan failed to identify the lump on his liver, he underwent a needle biopsy, which involved plunging a long needle into his abdomen so the doctor could extract a few cells from the lump. The pathologist couldn't tell whether the cells were benign or malignant. As for the lesions on his lungs, after a PET scan came out negative, which suggested they were probably not cancer, Casarella was left with two options: He could wait to see whether they grew bigger, or he could have them biopsied. Unfortunately, if the spots turned out to be malignant, surgery would not offer a cure, since the lesions were too large and too numerous.

Unwilling to go through life wondering if he had cancer, Casarella chose to undergo five hours of surgery, during which the surgeon collapsed one lung and cut out three wedge-shaped sections for a pathologist to examine. After his surgery, Casarella wrote about his experience in a letter to the editor of the journal *Radiology*, describing it in the terse, unemotional language of medicine, which nonetheless conveyed his sense of helplessness and the pain: "I woke up five hours later with a Foley catheter, a chest tube, a central venous catheter, a nasal oxygen catheter, an epidural catheter, an arterial catheter, subcutaneously administered heparin, a constant infusion of prophylactic antibiotics, and patient-controlled analgesia with intravenously-administered narcotics." After four days in the hospital, Casarella was allowed to go home, but it would be another two weeks before the agony was bearable and he could begin tapering off the narcotics. More than a month went by before he felt strong enough to return to work, and even then he was still in some pain. The bill for his surgery and hospitalization came to forty-seven thousand dollars. And the lung nodules that were removed? They turned out to be scars from an old histoplasmosis infection, a common fungal disease that is of no consequence in healthy people. The long-gone infection also explained the lump on his liver.

Beyond the dangers of workups for incidentalomas, unnecessary imaging tests pose the added risk of radiation. Over the past few years, many radiologists and emergency room physicians have grown increasingly concerned that one day we are going to wake up and discover that the millions of radiological tests patients undergo today will lead to thousands of cases of cancer tomorrow. With the exception of MRI and ultrasound, all imaging tests involve radiation—surprisingly high levels of radiation, in fact, depending upon what kind of scan it is. A whole-body CT scan, for instance, delivers a dose that's equivalent to about one tenth the radiation we are exposed to from natural sources—over the course of our entire lives. In other words, that's a lot of radiation all in one dose. The average head CT involves as much radiation as two hundred chest X-rays; performing angioplasty exposes a heart patient to the equivalent of more than one thousand chest X-rays. In big hospitals, CT scanning accounts for more than 10 percent of imaging exams that involve radiation, and two thirds of the radiation to which patients are exposed.

It's very clear that all this radiation is causing disease; the question is how much. Nobody knows the precise answer, but it's possible to come up with projections about the impact of medical radiation based on observations of survivors of the atomic bombs dropped on Japan. More than half of Hiroshima and Nagasaki survivors were exposed to relatively low doses of radiation; nonetheless, they went on to develop cardiovascular disease and several types of cancer, including leukemia, thyroid cancer, and breast and lung cancer. In a report by the prestigious National Academy of Sciences, issued in 2006, experts estimated that a sixty-year-old who undergoes an annual whole-body CT scan over the next fifteen years has a 1 in 220 risk of dying from cancer due to radiation exposure. The risk of dying in a car accident, by way of comparison, is nearly the same, 1 in 200. According to another estimate, out of about six hundred thousand children a year under the age of fifteen who receive a head or abdominal CT scan, five hundred could ultimately die in adulthood from cancer due to the radiation they received as youngsters.

Some radiologists have begun to worry that we are already seeing the ill effects of too much imaging in the skyrocketing rates of cancer of the thyroid, an organ that is located in the neck and is acutely vulnerable to radiation. The number of thyroid cancer cases per thousand people in the U.S. population has doubled since 1980, and it's now rising at a rate of 4.3 percent per year. Some of that, says Stephen Baker, may be that doctors have gotten better at detecting thyroid cancer or are becoming more vigilant, but he worries that at least part of the increase is a result of medical radiation.

Behold the human heart

There's no mention of radiation in the brilliantly conceived advertisements that began appearing on television shortly before the first LightSpeed VCT scanner rolled off the General Electric assembly line in Waukesha, Wisconsin, in early 2005. The first ad opened on a series of famous photographs—the black-and-white shot of a World War II sailor sweeping a pretty girl off her feet on V-Day; several of Eadweard Muybridge's time-lapse photos of a horse in full gallop; a colorized electron micrograph of a fly. Then a voice intoned, "Behold the human heart," as the LightSpeed's colorized rendering of a human heart appeared in living rooms across America. Behold, indeed—the machine's 3-D reconstruction of a human heart is undeniably, almost breathtakingly, beautiful, as detailed and delicately rendered as a da Vinci anatomical drawing. Since that first ad, GE has run several others on television for its CT scanners, all of them implying, if not stating directly, that CT scans can save lives by catching disease early.

In terms of inspiring patients to ask for a scan, GE and other manufacturers got an even bigger marketing boost from the news media. In September 2005, for instance, Time Magazine ran a photo of a sixty-four-slice 3-D reconstruction of a heart next to the cover line "How to Stop a Heart Attack Before It Happens." The story began by describing the case of Mike Fackelmann, a registered nurse at the Cleveland Clinic. Fackelmann "had no reason to think he had heart disease. Although his cholesterol was a touch on the high side, he had never experienced any chest pains and had just passed a stress test with flying colors." Even so, he agreed to serve as a guinea pig in a demonstration of the clinic's new sixty-four-slice scanner. The image revealed a partial blockage in one of his coronary arteries. Cardiologists at the clinic opened his artery with a stent a few days later, according to *Time*, "thereby preventing what could have been a heart attack." Yet as we learned in chapter 4, all the clinical evidence says that the stent Fackelmann was now carrying around in his chest likely would do no such thing, because stents don't prevent heart attacks. At best it could have relieved symptoms like chest pain and shortness of breath, neither of which was plaguing him.

Time's declaration that the sixty-four-slice scanner averted a potential heart attack converted many new enthusiasts of CT scanning. Within days of the magazine hitting newsstands hospitals and cardiologists around the country were taking calls from patients who wanted to get their hearts scanned too. "This has been huge," one cardiologist told me. More calls came in after another episode of *The Oprah Winfrey Show*. Oprah's guest was Mehmet Oz, a cardiothoracic surgeon at New York–Presbyterian Hospital, in Manhattan, who stood in front of a giant image of his host's heart and explained how the scan worked and why it was a good idea to get one. Meanwhile, the scientific evidence about the value of heart CT scans is inconclusive; some researchers believe that a small subset of patients with acute chest pain, who cannot be diagnosed by usual methods, will be helped by getting a cardiac CT scan.

No pushback

For more than a decade, the drug industry has successfully used direct-to-consumer advertising to boost sales of brand-name drugs, so perhaps it should come as no surprise that the device industry has finally caught on to this marketing tool. After all, it's their job to sell as many of their machines as they can, and stimulating patient demand for imaging tests is one way to do that. What is surprising is the blinding speed at which many new, medical technologies, not just imaging equipment, are adopted by hospitals and physicians, regardless of their true utility or costs.

One reason it's surprising that new machinery is adopted so quickly in medicine is that unlike technology in almost any other industry, new medical devices and equipment don't lower costs. In an industry like, say, steel, investing in expensive technology like automation ultimately brings down production costs by eliminating expensive labor. In health care, by contrast, technology generally drives costs upward. Health care economists say that's not a bad thing. They argue that medical technology like the LightSpeed VCT may be expensive in the short run, but it would be foolish to impede the flow of such devices into the marketplace, because they improve the practice of medicine. (Besides, new devices and drugs means new jobs for people in the device industry and health care, and new jobs are good for the economy.) The case for encouraging the flow of medical technology has been made time and again in scholarly papers, and it is an argument that carries enormous weight when it comes time for Congress to make decisions about what Medicare will and will not pay for.

Yet the view that all new medical technology is worth the price is often at odds with the evidence—and no more so than in the field of imaging. Payments for physician services by Medicare and Medicaid rose 31 percent between 1999 and 2004. During that same period, payments for imaging services grew more than 60 percent, twice as fast, largely because physicians ordered more images per patient and more expensive images. Payments for MRI, for example, grew 140 percent; CT payments went up 112 percent. Now, if the economists were right, the costs of all that imaging would be worth paying because it was actually helping patients. Yet studies of the effectiveness of imaging, including autopsy studies, have shown that the technology is improving care in only tiny increments, even as utilization and costs are rising at meteoric rates. A study performed for the Medicare Payment Advisory Commission, for example, found that patients suffering from heart attacks, hip fractures, and colon cancer did not benefit from more imaging tests.

To make matters worse, simply tracking the spiraling bills we're paying for all that imaging fails to capture its true cost. Many imaging tests lead to further testing and treatment, whose price isn't included when economists look at the amount we spend on CT and other imaging. Take the sixty-four-slice scanners that hospitals are snapping up as fast as they can. Far from replacing catheterization as a means of diagnosing heart attacks, as the manufacturers and some cardiologists are claiming, the new machines may in fact lead to more catheterization—and higher costs. "More angiograms will be done, not less," predicts cardiologist Eric Topol. Why? Because the 3-D scans are fast, painless, and easy to read, and because cardiologists are eager to use the latest gizmo. Just like doctors who order a belly CT even when they already know whether the patient has appendicitis, emergency physicians and cardiologists will undoubtedly order 3-D CT scans even for patients they are practically certain are at minimal risk of having a blockage in the coronary arteries or, on the other hand, are clearly suffering a heart attack. Ordering lots of 3-D scans for patients who are at minimal risk for heart disease is going to lead to lots of false positives, just as whole-body CT scans detect numerous incidentalomas. And like harmless incidentalomas that nonetheless must be worked up, harmless imperfections in coronary arteries discovered by 3-D scanners will lead to more cardiac workups, including unnecessary catheterizations, in order to confirm the diagnosis.

The issues surrounding imaging tests once again highlight one of the most pervasive problems in American medicine: the lack of a true market. In this case, there is no real "pushback" from the market against the rapid adoption of new, unproved technology. When Cordis, a manufacturer of cardiovascular stents, introduced the first drug-coated stent in June 2003, interventional cardiologists began using them without evidence that they represented an improvement over bare-metal stents. They just seemed like a good idea. Uptake was so widespread and so rapid that by 2006 over 90 percent of all stents placed in patients were coated. Clinical trials are now showing that the drug-coated stents increase the risk of a clot, which can cause a stroke, unless the patient takes drugs to prevent one. When GE develops a new scanner, hospitals and doctors are eager to get on the bandwagon. Hospitals want one in order to compete with other hospitals.

Doctors want to use new scanners because they're infatuated with the technology, which is readily available, and because they want to avoid malpractice suits and the wrath of patients who have been denied a test that dazzling GE ads and the media have led them to believe they need and deserve. On top of that, as we've seen, many physicians get paid more for doing more tests.

The multiple urges to image are so great that doctors ignore a mountain of data available in the medical journals telling them that many of the tests they are ordering are failing to help their patients. For instance, according to the American College of Radiology, patients with uncomplicated low-back pain (meaning there are no signs of serious disease, such as cancer) should not receive imaging studies. Not only is the image a waste of time and money, but it often leads to unnecessary back surgery. Yet the National Committee for Quality Assurance found that doctors often were unaware of, or ignored the academy's recommendation, giving nearly a quarter of patients with low-back pain in managed care plans an unnecessary image.

What about payers? Insurance is a competitive industry, and you would think that the market would create the right conditions for insurers to vie on the basis of providing the highest-quality care for the lowest price. In the case of imaging, high quality would undoubtedly mean fewer tests, not more. Insurers could deny payment for images that were contraindicated by a decision tool—say, for instance, a neck CT for a patient who clearly didn't need one. For insurers, however, providing quality doesn't pay, especially when it involves telling doctors—and patients—they can't have something they think they want. After the debacle of the 1990s, when patients and doctors rebelled against the restrictions imposed by managed care, insurers backed off from denying services or reimbursement, a retreat that triggered a return to rising health care costs and the current medical-technology arms race that is now helping spur the use of imaging tests. (You'll hear more about the demise of managed care in chapter 9.)

There are health care systems that are searching for ways to use imaging tests and other medical technologies more judiciously, to help doctors relearn the art of diagnosis—among them Kaiser Permanente, in California; Group Health, in Seattle; and the Veterans Health Administration. These systems pay their doctors a salary, removing one of the incentives that drive much of the unnecessary imaging we see in the rest of health care. They also strongly encourage their doctors to follow the decision tools for deciding when to image, and they measure the performances of their physicians and hospitals. All of them are HMOs, it turns out, or health maintenance organizations, but they work in a very different way from the managed care most patients have learned to hate. You'll hear more in future chapters about how we could apply the principles they've used so successfully in order to improve the quality of the rest of the system and bring down costs.

In the meantime, there's no denying that one of the greatest tragedies here is the way in which imaging has increased the distance between doctor and patient. Doctors worry they haven't covered all the bases unless they order an imaging test; patients worry they're being cheated when they don't get sent to radiology. Testing has replaced thinking on the doctor's part and feeling cared for on the patient's. What's lost in the process, says Stephen Baker, is the personal relationship, the trusting interaction that once formed the basis for healing. But when the patient views the doctor as a tool of the insurer, and the doctor views the patient increasingly through the narrow lens of a computer screen, it's difficult for either to see the other as a partner in the process of healing. "The personal interaction with patients has been discarded," says Baker, "and the hubris of all this has led us to use technology in ways that we don't really understand."

SEVEN The Persuaders

The desire to take medicine is perhaps the greatest feature which distinguishes man from animals.

—Sir **William Osler**

ON MARCH 14, 2001, twenty-year-old Justin Cheslek was found hanging from the balcony of his apartment. A sophomore at the University of Southern Mississippi, Justin had been a good student, a soccer player and an avid kayaker, and full of excitement on the phone to his parents just three weeks earlier, when he called to tell them about an independent study class he was taking in computer-network management. But like many college students, Justin was having trouble sleeping. On February 19, he went to the student health center, where the doctor gave him a thorough exam. She also questioned him to find out whether he was depressed and then prescribed Ambien to help him sleep. In Justin's file, the doctor noted, "No suicidal ideation," which meant he expressed no desire to kill himself. The boy returned to the clinic a few days later, complaining that the sleeping pills left him feeling groggy and "depressed." This time, the doctor diagnosed depression and gave him a sample package of Paxil, an antidepressant. Over the phone, Justin told his mother, Linda, that the drug made him feel "awful," wound up, jumpy, unable to sit still or concentrate. Linda, a pediatric nurse practitioner, assumed his symptoms would ease once the drug began to take effect. She gently suggested he give it a few days. At his one-week follow-up visit, Justin told the doctor he couldn't stand how he felt. She instructed him to stay on his current dose of Paxil rather than ramping up to the next, as planned. A week later, Justin was still feeling no better. The doctor told him to stop taking Paxil and handed him several samples of Effexor, a similar antidepressant.

The next day, Thursday, March 7, Justin took his first Effexor tablet. The following evening, while out with his girlfriend, he fell to the floor and suffered a seizure. He refused to go to the hospital, telling his girlfriend he just wanted to go home. On Sunday, Justin called his parents, telling his mother he still felt "really, really bad." She offered to make the two-and-a-half-hour drive to the university from their home in Vicksburg, Mississippi, but he demurred, saying he would be fine. On Monday, he called the school clinic, but it was spring break and his doctor was on vacation. So was the neurologist who had prescribed low doses of Elavil months before for his migraines. On Wednesday, Justin begged off going on a kayaking trip with his friends, saying he had suffered a seizure and was taking some medicine that made him feel strange. On Thursday, three weeks after Justin swallowed his first antidepressant, his roommate walked into their apartment to find his friend dead. Around Justin's neck was one of the straps he used for securing his kayak to the top of a car. Under his feet were his laptop computer, lying open, and his unfinished can of Coke.

In the months following Justin's death, his father, Gary Cheslek, a dentist in Vicksburg, agonized privately over what kind of terrible father he must have been, wondering to himself, how do you miss that your son is suicidal? Then a small article in the local paper piqued his interest. It concerned a patient who had suffered withdrawal symptoms coming off Paxil, one of the drugs Justin had taken. "Imagine my horror and relief the first time I typed 'Paxil and suicide' into a Web search engine and there was over 4,000 hits," he would eventually write in a letter to a plaintiff's lawyer. Linda Cheslek was not convinced that either Paxil or Effexor, the other antidepressant Justin had taken, had anything to do with their son's death. "I didn't believe Gary at first," she said later. "I thought he was reading junk science. I thought he was in denial. Because I'm a medical provider, I said, we have to look at medically based research." But even the scientific literature would not give them a clear sense of the true risks of the class of antidepressants known as selective serotonin reuptake inhibitors, or SSRIs. Only a handful of papers, half a dozen at most, reported an association between SSRIs and the condition known as akathisia: the extreme agitation, sense of unease, and feeling of wanting to jump out of one's skin that Justin described in the days before his death. At the time, there was virtually no published information about the frequency of akathisia as a side effect of antidepressants or its relationship to suicide. But after eighteen months of digging through the literature, Gary Cheslek felt he understood what had happened. "There was a reason for this tragedy," he wrote in the letter. "I did know my son. In and of himself he would not have done this."

In August 2003, Linda Cheslek received a "Dear Doctor" letter from Wyeth Pharmaceuticals, the maker of Effexor. In the letter, Wyeth warned health care professionals that clinical studies had found a heightened risk of hostility and suicidal thoughts in children and teenagers taking its drug. The company wrote, "You should be alert to signs of suicidal ideation in children and adolescent patients prescribed Effexor." Extreme agitation was one of those signs. In October 2004, a little more than three years after Justin died, the Food and Drug Administration issued a warning to health professionals and the public. Based on a review of data from more than four thousand children and adolescents, the FDA warned that SSRIs may double the risk of suicide in pediatric patients. A more-recent FDA study has found that SSRIs may trigger suicidality in patients as old as twenty-five.

There are many disturbing aspects to Justin Cheslek's case and others like it, not the least of which is the fact that nobody recognized his symptoms as potential side effects of the drugs he was taking. He came to the student clinic complaining not of depression but of sleeplessness, which can occasionally be brought on by Elavil, the drug that Justin was taking for migraine headaches. Instead of changing his headache medication or sending him back to the neurologist for reevaluation, the school doctor prescribed Ambien, a sleeping pill, which in rare cases can trigger depression, agitation, and suicide. When the Ambien left Justin feeling bleary and depressed, the doctor put him on an antidepressant, which can cause akathisia. Then she put him on another drug in the same class that has similar side effects.

Why wasn't the doctor alerted by Justin's agitation and worsening symptoms? Concerns that SSRIs might be dangerous for some patients had already surfaced by 1994, just four years after Prozac was approved. Researchers from the Yale Child Study Center published results from a clinical trial testing Prozac in forty-two children and adolescents who were suffering not from depression but from obsessive-compulsive disorder. (At that time, Prozac was not yet approved for any pediatric use, but it was already being widely prescribed to kids "off label," the term for the widely accepted practice of prescribing drugs to patients or for conditions not specifically approved by the FDA and not specifically listed on the drug's label.) Six of the children in the Yale study, who ranged in age from ten to seventeen, developed "intense self-injurious ideation and/or behavior," the researchers wrote. Some of the children experienced a state of agitation and extreme inner turmoil—akathisia.

The study wasn't proof that the drug could trigger suicidality or akathisia, but the details of one case, that of a twelve-year-old boy, now seem eerily prescient in light of the school shootings that would hit headlines later in the 1990s. Once he started taking Prozac, the child began having violent dreams of killing his classmates until he himself was shot. The nightmares seemed so real that, upon waking, the boy began refusing to attend school. He was taken off the drug and hospitalized until his violent thoughts subsided. Three weeks after his discharge, another physician, who was unaware of previous events, put him back on Prozac, and the boy once again became suicidal.

Yet few doctors in the United States knew about these findings, or that there was even a possibility that SSRIs might pose any danger at all to their patients. (In Germany and the United Kingdom, psychiatrists, many of whom were aware of the potential risk, were already using sedatives to reduce the anxiety SSRIs could provoke in some patients.) By 2001, drugmakers had submitted to the U.S. FDA a total of fifteen different pediatric studies of various SSRIs. Only one, Prozac, would eventually be approved for pediatric use. (Even now, the others have yet to be shown to be more effective than a placebo, or sugar pill, in patients under the age of twenty-one.*) Doctors had no idea so many trials had been conducted, and had failed to show a benefit, because the companies never published those studies. The industry also had internal documents and data suggesting the drugs could trigger agitation, along with suicidal thoughts and behavior, yet the published literature said SSRIs were "effective" in children and adolescents and "well-tolerated," medical-speak for safe.[†] Even Justin's mother, a trained health care provider, hadn't a clue that her son's agitation might be a devastating side effect that could provoke him to suicide, until she received the "Dear Doctor" letter from Wyeth. "The medical community thinks these drugs are safe and effective," she says. "They don't know what they're prescribing."

There's no way to know for certain if the drugs that Justin was taking caused him to commit suicide, or if he was hiding a profound depression from everybody around him—his family, his girlfriend, his friends. Even so, perhaps the most troubling aspect of this teenager's story is the fact that he was given three different, powerful psychoactive drugs to treat what began as mild insomnia, which may itself have simply been a side effect of another drug. He was suffering from a bout of sleeplessness, an affliction that has plagued generations of college students.

In 2002, doctors wrote nearly eleven million prescriptions for psychotropic drugs for kids between the ages of one and seventeen. Rates of pediatric prescriptions for the stimulant Ritalin, which is used to treat attention deficit hyperactivity disorder, have been going up dramatically, along with rates of

---

* For anyone who has found relief from depression by taking an SSRI, the fact that the drugs have proved no more effective than a sugar pill in clinical trials undoubtedly seems more than a little strange. The problem is the "placebo effect," the ability of placebos to make people feel better, a mysterious but common occurrence in medicine. In the case of depressed children and teenagers, the placebo effect is particularly strong: As many as half of kids in clinical trials get better on placebos. The other confounding factor here is the fact that not everybody responds in the same way to an SSRI. Studies in healthy volunteers, people who have no signs or symptoms of depression, have found that some people feel terrific, even better than well, on an antidepressant. Many feel little or nothing. For others, SSRIs can trigger akathisia and suicidal thoughts.

† Eli Lilly, the maker of Prozac, has data showing that 38 percent of people who take the drug become "activated," a term that includes varying degrees of agitation. But those data are considered "proprietary," and they have surfaced only once during a court case before a judge ordered them sealed.

pediatric prescriptions for antipsychotics, powerful drugs that were developed to treat such serious psychiatric conditions as schizophrenia, mania, and bipolar disorder. Psychiatric visits that included treatment of a child with an antipsychotic went from a little over 200,000 in 1993 to 1.2 million in 2002. More than 90 percent of those prescriptions (all of them off label) were for the atypical antipsychotics, newer versions of the drugs that may cause serious side effects, such as rapid weight gain, diabetes, and a movement disorder known as tardive dyskinesia. Among boys ages six to twelve, more than half of antidepressant prescriptions written are intended to treat so-called conduct disorders, like hyperactivity and attention deficit, behavior that might have been written off a generation ago as "boys will be boys," but that now is labeled as a disease and treated with a drug. In 2005, according to an analysis by Medco Health Solutions, a company that tracks prescriptions, about 1.6 million children and teenagers—280,000 of them under age ten—were given at least two psychiatric drugs in combination. More than 500,000 were prescribed at least three medications. More than 160,000 got at least four psychiatric drugs at the same time. Taking drugs has become so commonplace among children and teenagers that young people talk casually about needing to "adjust their meds" in response to a rough week at school or a bad breakup, and instead of snorting or smoking illegal substances at parties, they trade prescription pills.

Clearly, some kids benefit enormously from taking psychiatric medications. SSRIs, antipsychotics, and stimulants all have a place in treating mental illness, which can devastate children's lives and tear families apart. But it's hard to imagine that the incredible increase in psychiatric prescriptions for teenagers and children is due entirely to an epidemic of psychiatric disorders, that some combination of bad parenting, bad genes, and bad videos has created an entire nation of screwed-up kids. We're also in the midst of an epidemic of diagnoses, in which children who exhibit behavior that is even mildly out of the norm are labeled and treated, along with the kids who are truly mentally ill. The question is, why are we now so quick to diagnose mental illness?

The answer to that question turns out to have implications that go beyond just the number of children who take prescription drugs. When you look at

Americans of all ages, we consume about two hundred billion dollars' worth of prescription drugs each year, a figure that's expected to continue rising by more than 10 percent a year until at least 2010. We spend as much on drugs as we do buying retail goods online, and we take from 25 to 50 percent more prescription drugs per capita than citizens of Canada and European countries. The pharmaceutical industry argues that we're better off for it—that Americans benefit from its products by living longer, suffering fewer symptoms of disease, and spending fewer days in the hospital. There's reason to question this claim, yet we're nonetheless lucky to have many life-saving drugs: antivirals that have transformed HIV from a death sentence into a chronic infection, for instance; cyclosporine, which makes organ transplants possible; and insulin, which keeps diabetics alive. But the drugs that account for the meteoric rise in prescription rates are not for saving lives, for the most part. The pharmaceutical industry calls them "lifestyle" drugs, products that shield us from the slings and arrows of ordinary existence, or treat but don't cure serious conditions, or are intended to reduce the risk of disease but not treat the illness itself. Many of these drugs reduce suffering—asthma inhalers, for instance, and migraine medication. But we also pop pills to go to sleep and wake up, to feel more energetic and less jittery. We take stimulants to slim down. We give our children medications to help them act calmly, enhance their performance in school, and make them taller. We take drugs to reduce the chances we'll develop heart disease, stroke, and diabetes. There are prescription drugs for anxiety, baldness, hay fever, headaches, heartburn, and toenail fungus, to name just a tiny fraction of the conditions that are now commonly treated with lifestyle medications.

For every single prescription written, there must be a diagnosis, and over the past quarter century, the number of possible diagnoses that can be treated with a drug has exploded. Take all the new diseases listed in the *Diagnostic and Statistical Manual of Mental Disorders*, the psychiatric bible that gives doctors and clinical researchers a common set of criteria to describe and diagnose mental conditions. A slim little volume in 1980 that listed 226 diagnosable conditions, the manual had swelled to a weighty tome by 1994 and included 365 psychiatric disorders. As new conditions are added to the manual and the diagnostic criteria for those that already exist are expanded, the number of Americans who are diagnosed as mentally ill—and treated for it—continues to grow. For example, the redefinition of attention deficit hyperactivity disorder, or ADHD, in 1994 led to nearly double the number of children being diagnosed with that condition, and a corresponding rise in the number of prescriptions written for stimulants like Ritalin. During the 1990s, stimulant prescriptions tripled among preschoolers, some of them as young as six months old.

What lies behind this astronomical increase in the number of diseases we now must worry about? Sometimes, it's a drug company. Premenstrual dysphoric disorder, for instance, made its way into the psychiatric manual in 1999 largely as the result of behind-the-scenes efforts by Eli Lilly, the manufacturer of Serafem, a repackaged version of Prozac that the company wanted to market for premenstrual symptoms. The pharmaceutical industry has pushed new diagnostic categories in other medical arenas, and it has helped broaden the definitions of risk factors that can be treated with drugs. For instance, the criteria for who needs to be on a statin, or cholesterol-lowering drug, were redefined in 2001, more than doubling the number of Americans who could be put on drugs like Lipitor and Zocor from about thirteen million to thirty-six million. Many experts argue that these new guidelines are based on a faulty interpretation of the medical evidence and could actually prove harmful to many people who wind up taking the drugs. Critics also note that eight of the nine authors who crafted the revised guidelines were being paid by the companies that make statins.

Previous chapters have looked at the various ways that unseen economic factors push doctors and hospitals to provide unneeded medical care, and how these financial forces may put patients at risk for the complications that are inevitable in medicine as well as preventable errors. We've looked at how doctors may be misled by their own technology into thinking they have more power to see inside the body than they really do, and how the decisions that hospitals make about investing in everything from ICU beds to CT scanners can lead to unnecessary treatment. The subject of this chapter and the next is no less important. We'll now look at the drug industry's role (and to a lesser extent the device industry's) in persuading both patients and doctors that we're sicker than we really are, and that the path to wellness lies with medical intervention: with a pill, an operation, or a test. Today, direct-to-consumer ad campaigns routinely paint mild conditions as serious and normal variations in human characteristics as disease. Saturation advertising from the drug industry and slick "disease awareness" campaigns from patient advocacy groups, many of which are funded by pharmaceutical companies, make us fret constantly about illness and have helped turn us into a nation of the worried well.

Free speech

In his book *Generation Rx*, Greg Critser traces the beginning of direct-to-consumer drug advertising to a couple of young Madison Avenue hotshots named Joe Davis and William Castagnoli. In 1985, the two were hired by Merrell Dow to advertise its new antihistamine, a drug called Seldane. Merrell executives believed that Seldane was a huge advance because it didn't leave hay fever sufferers glazed with drowsiness the way existing drugs did. But Castagnoli and Davis faced three tall barriers to conveying that information to patients. To begin with, at that time pharmaceutical executives took great pride in the fact that they generally avoided advertising directly to consumers. They placed ads in the medical journals, and they sent sales reps, or "detail men" (and they were all men in those days), to doctors' offices, where they could calmly and rationally go over in detail the most appropriate uses of their companies' products. This antipathy for consumer advertising was on display in a remarkable set of letters sent by pharmaceutical executives to Representative John Dingell, who solicited their opinion on the subject in 1982. Charles Hagan, vice president and general counsel of American Home Products, wrote, "[Direct-to-consumer] advertising would make [patients] extraordinarily susceptible to product promises." The chairman of Abbott Laboratories wrote, "We believe direct advertising to the consumer introduces a very real possibility of causing harm to patients who may respond to advertisements by pressuring physicians to prescribe medications that may not be required." Charles Collins of Smith

Kline and French warned that "advertising would have the objective of driving patients into doctors' offices seeking prescriptions."

Number two on the list of Davis and Castagnoli's barriers to getting the word out about Seldane was the FDA regulation that required all drug ads, including those on radio and television, to include a "brief summary" of side effects and safety issues. While it was called a brief summary, the agency's list of what had to be included made it anything but short. Required information about drug interactions, side effects, and evidence for efficacy could be squeezed onto a single magazine page in very small type, but for TV or radio, spelling out safety issues could take a minute or more, making most drug ads for broadcast prohibitively expensive. Number three on the list was that people with allergy complaints tended to visit their doctors on average only once every three years. If the advertisers stuck to marketing only to physicians, it would take years before large numbers of allergy sufferers got a chance to try Seldane, no matter how good the drug might be at alleviating their symptoms.

What Davis and Castagnoli needed was to find a way to "drive patients to their doctors," which was, of course, the very thing drug company executives viewed with such disdain. But the two knew there was no other way to ensure Seldane a profit. Drug patent laws granted a company seventeen years of exclusive rights to develop and sell its product before the patent expired and generic drugs horned in on the market. (Today, drug patents have been extended to twenty years.) Three to six years of that patent were eaten up by testing the drug and getting it through the FDA approval process. If advertising only to doctors meant that a drug took another four or five years to reach its sales potential, that left less than a decade before the patent ran out and cheap generic competitors marched in. Davis and Castagnoli hit upon a solution that was sheer genius. They got around the FDA's brief-summary requirement by producing TV and radio spots that never named the drug. Instead, the ads touted the fact that "a new drug for allergies is out." In the spot, a young, attractive nurse wearing a little white hat came through a doorway and said, "The doctor will see you now." Allergy sufferers who wanted to know more could "go and see your doctor," said the voice-over. In a very low-key, public service announcement sort of way, the ad even hinted at Seldane's biggest selling point, no drowsiness, but since it never named the drug, it didn't have to include a long—and expensive—warning about its multiple other side effects. The ad closed with the tagline "Now you can put your hay fever to sleep while you stay awake!"

The Seldane campaign, launched in 1988, sent allergy patients scurrying to the doctor and Seldane sales through the roof. Drugmakers had never seen anything like it, and despite their reservations, they couldn't argue with Merrell Dow's profits. Other companies soon followed with their own brand-name-less ads, which television and radio networks were only too happy to run. Network executives saw the pharmaceutical industry as a vast, untapped source of ad revenue, while ad agencies viewed direct-to-consumer ads as their clients' best hope for extracting as much profit as possible from their drugs before their patents ran out. By the early 1990s, pharmaceutical executives, who only a few years before had been aghast at the idea of pushing their drugs on the public, had come around to the notion that patients might even benefit from advertising—that consumers had a right to know about drugs. They began pressuring the FDA to loosen its brief-summary requirement, arguing that far from helping consumers, the summary hurt them by overwhelming them with too much boring, scary, off-putting information, which could lead them to avoid going to the doctor or taking the medicine that was prescribed. Together with the advertising industry, drug companies also fought the FDA's restrictions on direct-to-consumer ads in the courts, by whittling away at legal distinctions between individual free speech and commercial speech. Companies claimed that their right to free speech was violated by restrictions on ads. A series of suits, culminating in a case heard before the Supreme Court in 1996, finally convinced the FDA that if pharmaceutical companies ever challenged its restrictions on direct-to-consumer advertising, the agency might well lose the case. In 1997, it issued a draft rule, finalized two years later, permitting companies to boil down the brief summary to a few seconds for broadcast advertisements, thus opening the gates to Zoloft cartoon ads during prime-time sitcoms and Ambien ads on the nightly news. That same year, Seldane was removed from the market, after it was found to cause fatal heart arrhythmias when taken with other drugs.

In 1995, the pharmaceutical industry spent a mere $595 million on direct-to-consumer advertising, virtually all of it on newspaper and magazine ads. By 1998, that figure had jumped to $1.17 billion. It doubled again, to $2.38 billion, by 2001, with more than 70 percent of the spending going toward television spots. By 2005, drug companies were spending $3 billion a year on ads aimed at consumers, and company executives had finally come around to their marketers' way of thinking: Consumer ads weren't vulgar; they didn't interfere with the doctor-patient relationship. They helped patients by informing them.

The disease mongers

Direct-to-consumer advertising is now so ubiquitous that you cannot walk past more than a few feet of airport hallway, watch network television for more than a few minutes, or turn more than a few pages of a popular magazine without seeing an ad for a drug. By 1999, one market researcher estimates, the average American saw nine drug ads on television a day. Not only have ads grown in number, but they have also become increasingly specialized, as ad agencies discover new ways to get consumers to think of drugs as the solution to a wider and wider array of ailments. Companies now use "reminder ads," which may simply name a drug and the disease it treats in order to urge viewers who have already been diagnosed with a condition to try that particular brand. "Disease-oriented" ads often list symptoms of an ailment, give a disease a new name, or make the disorder sound as serious as possible in an effort to scare consumers into going to the doctor for a test. Pfizer ran an ad in a popular magazine for its anticholesterol drug Lipitor that showed the tagged toe of a corpse above a headline urging women in their fifties to get their cholesterol checked. Of course, the ads glossed over the possibility that Lipitor itself might kill them. Then there are the so-called feel-good ads, which aren't intended to make patients feel better, but rather to encourage drug company employees, stockholders, and legislators to feel good about the beneficial work a company is doing. Merck's tagline for recent radio ads was "Merck, where patients come first," a theme the company undoubtedly wanted to emphasize in the face of hundreds of law-suits from patients who suffered heart attacks from its painkiller Vioxx.

Direct-to-consumer advertising has been a spectacular success, boosting sales and stock prices beyond the dreams of the early drug marketers. Every dollar the pharmaceutical industry spends on consumer ads generates $4.20 in increased sales. That's a better return on investment than that of the fast food industry, which spends about as much on advertising. Nearly one in three adults has talked about a specific drug to their doctor in response to a drug advertisement; one in eight walked out with a prescription for the drug they asked for. But perhaps what's most important about drug adver-tising is how sophisticated it has become, how each part of a marketing campaign fits neatly together with the others to mold the way we think not only about a drug but also about what it means to be healthy. As one doctor puts it, "Calling what drug companies do 'advertising' is like calling D-day a bunch of guys wading in the surf."

Consider the launch of Lunesta, a new sleep drug that was approved by the FDA in May 2005. The opening salvo for Lunesta's sixty-million-dollar direct-to-consumer ad campaign appeared, appropriately enough, during the sitcom *Desperate Housewives*. The ad, shot in dreamy black and white, opened on a bedroom curtain floating on a breeze. The camera panned to a young woman pacing the floor while her companion lay asleep in bed. Then, a computer-generated green luna moth, the only bit of color in the ad, flut-tered in the window. In the last ten seconds, the woman returned to bed to drift off to sleep, safe in the arms of Morpheus, while the female voice-over cooed, "Lunesta helps most people sleep all through the night." Print ads soon followed, featuring an image of the same green luna moth and the words "the first and only prescription sleep aid approved for long-term use."

A month and a half after Lunesta's debut, doctors were writing sixty thousand new prescriptions a week for the drug, and drug industry analysts were proclaiming the dawning of a new day for the sleeping pill market. The two existing sleep drugs, Ambien and Sonata, shared a two-billion-dollar-a-year market between them. Corey Davis, an analyst with JP Mor-gan, predicted in the *Wall Street Journal* that sleep drug sales could hit six billion dollars by 2008. Lunesta, said Davis, "could do for the insomnia market what Prozac did for depression." Meanwhile, the company's chief financial officer told investors, "It's a drug you can take again and again and again. The sky's the limit."

Lunesta's TV spots and print advertisements were only the most visible aspect of the company's marketing campaign—and in many ways they represented not the beginning of the drug's launch but its culmination. Following a script that has become standard operating procedure in pharmaceutical marketing, Lunesta's manufacturer, a small Massachusetts company called Sepracor, began selling the drug to the media long before it gained FDA approval. (It was also marketing Lunesta to doctors. At the American Psychiatric Association's annual meeting in May 2005, the company pulled out all the stops, erecting a fifteen-foot-tall luna moth out of gossamer chartreuse netting, the same stuff a child's Halloween fairy wings are made of. Physicians could mount a rotating dais between the wings to recline on chocolate-colored chaise longues, where they were given headsets that emitted the soothing sound of crickets before a ten-minute sales video began.) FDA rules don't permit companies to market a drug directly before it's approved. Instead, Sepracor and its Manhattan PR agency, the Zeno Group, began issuing press releases encouraging reporters to write not about the drug but about sleep, and the problems associated with not getting enough of it. In the twenty-four months leading up to Lunesta's May 2005 launch, more than a thousand stories about the science of sleep and the dangers of insomnia appeared in newspapers and magazines—compared with about six hundred in the previous two years. Reporters also received press releases from Duke University, which was contracted by Sepracor to conduct the clinical trials the company needed to gain FDA approval. Duke was under no FDA restrictions, so its releases named the drug, along with the university sleep researcher, Dr. Andrew Krystal, who led the studies. Krystal also served as a paid consultant and speaker for Sepracor.

Most of the resulting stories made Lunesta sound like the answer to an insomniac's prayers. "For Insomniacs, a Sleeping Pill for Every Night" was the headline in the *Los Angeles Times*. "Sleepless at Duke find cure," said the Raleigh-Durham (North Carolina) *News & Observer*. Several reporters quoted

Terri Bagley, a forty-three-year-old owner of a North Carolina cleaning business who had been paid to participate in the Duke trial and was offered to the press by Duke's public relations office. A chronic insomniac, Bagley raved about Lunesta, telling the *Washington Post* she was counting the days until the drug was approved and she could get a prescription.

Today, the marketing of a new pharmaceutical almost always involves help from the press, which can make the public see a new drug as a miracle cure even more effectively than the cleverest advertisement. Consumers tend to view information coming from the media and other seemingly independent sources as more reliable than company-sponsored ads, so the pharmaceutical industry routinely employs what's known as the "third-party strategy," the art of getting its message into the mouth of a more-credible source. The press is one of the best third parties around for publicizing new drugs, especially when reporters look no further than the press releases they receive from PR agencies like Zeno. In the view of Trudy Lieberman, a leading health care journalist, the press often plays a willing role in trumpeting new drugs. Reporters, she says, "share the American cultural belief in the inherent goodness of medicine and its corollary—that every new pill, every new treatment, works and should be treated as safe and effective until proven otherwise."

Sepracor and the Zeno Group were aided in their efforts to sell sleep to the press and the public by yet another third party, the National Sleep Foundation. Based in Washington, D.C., the foundation is run by Richard Gelula, a pleasant-looking man in his fifties with sandy hair and a sincere demeanor. One spring day, shortly before Lunesta's launch, when the cherry blossoms were blooming, Gelula explained the foundation's history and its mission. Dedicated to "improving public health and safety by achieving understanding of sleep and sleep disorders," the foundation was formed in 1991 by a group of sleep researchers, one of whom had lost a son who had fallen asleep at the wheel of his car. At that time, Gelula said, researchers were just beginning to piece together the biological and psychological importance of sleep. While most people were undoubtedly aware that getting a good night's sleep is important, the researchers believed that more and more Americans were ignoring the need for shut-eye. The foundation's leaders saw an opportunity to improve the nation's health by publicizing sleep's role in physical and mental well-being—and effectively turning sleep, or the lack of it, into a medical condition.

To do that, they began conducting an annual poll of American sleep habits, the results of which are released during National Sleep Awareness Week. The first poll, which was sent to reporters in June 1991 and managed to garner only five newspaper stories, found that 27 percent of Americans had occasional trouble sleeping and 9 percent suffered from chronic insomnia. Five years later, the survey was reporting that a whopping half of Americans had trouble sleeping, an increase that was probably not the result of an epidemic of sleeplessness sweeping the nation, but rather of skewed polling. Data from the National Institutes of Health suggest that the number of people suffering from occasional but recurring insomnia is closer to 21 percent. By the time Lunesta was launched, the National Sleep Foundation was saying that about half of adults suffered from frequent insomnia and that sleeplessness was "under-recognized, under-diagnosed, and as a result, under-treated." That year, the poll found that an incredible 75 percent of adult respondents' sleeping problems were so bad that they were interfering with their sex lives. That's a lot of sleepy, sex-deprived people. The problem seemed newsworthy to at least two dozen papers, which ran stories about the twin epidemics of insomnia and no sex that were gripping the nation.

The National Sleep Foundation has an obvious interest in inflating the number of people suffering from insomnia. The more widespread sleeplessness seems, the more seriously the press will take the foundation, and the more likely it is that the public will pay attention to its health message. Of course, inflating the prevalence of insomnia, and thus persuading as many people as possible that they might need treatment for it, also serves the foundation's corporate sponsors, the manufacturers of sleep drugs. Together, Sepracor; King Pharmaceuticals, which makes Sonata; and Sanofi-Aventis, the maker of Ambien, provide about a third of the sleep foundation's $3.6 million annual budget. In addition, Sepracor was a $250,000 platinum sponsor of the foundation's 2005 poll; another $300,000 grant from the company went toward a series of "Sleep Medicine

Alerts," brochures to educate doctors, who, according to Gelula, don't treat insomnia adequately because they "don't think sleeplessness is a sickness."

But is it? For some people, of course, chronic insomnia is a ruinous affliction. Night after night, they toss and turn; they try books, booze, hot baths, watching TV, anything to get to sleep. Many such people are truly impaired by their inability to do something that comes so naturally to most. For the chronic insomniac, oddly enough, sleeping drugs often don't work, or they stop working after a few weeks. Sleep experts say a more-effective method for true insomnia involves behavior conditioning, which can reset the chemicals in the brain that let us drift off. These chemicals can be controlled, with help from a sleep expert, by such seemingly simple activities as preparing for bed at a consistent time and turning down the lights an hour before bedtime. For those of us whose sleep problems crop up intermittently during stressful times at work or when we travel, the occasional sleeping pill can help. But that doesn't make sleeplessness a sickness. What both the National Sleep Foundation and its corporate sponsors did was conflate serious, chronic insomnia, which can be truly debilitating, with garden-variety trouble sleeping.

Australian journalist Ray Moynihan and Alan Cassels, a Canadian pharmaceutical policy researcher, point out that companies hook up with third parties like the National Sleep Foundation because these groups can help them sell their products, not by pushing a drug directly but by selling the sickness the drug can treat. Patient-advocacy groups, whether it's the National Sleep Foundation or the American Cancer Society, want people to take action on matters that affect their health, and one of the most common means they use to motivate people is to scare them, make them worry they have whatever condition it is that the group wants to stamp out. Getting people to worry about a disease also serves pharmaceutical companies, because it widens the potential market for their drugs. In their book, *Selling Sickness*, Moynihan and Cassels write, "With many medical conditions, there is great uncertainty about where to draw the line that separates the healthy from the sick. The boundaries that separate 'normal' and 'abnormal' are often highly elastic, they may differ from country to country, and they can change over time. Clearly, the wider you draw the boundaries that define a disease, the wider the pool of potential patients, and the bigger the market for those making drugs." Companies have found they can use patient-advocacy groups to widen their customer pool by making the well think they are sick and the mildly impaired think they have a serious condition that needs treatment.

In 1998, SmithKline, the maker of the antidepressant Paxil (the same drug that Justin Cheslek took shortly before hanging himself), took this idea a step further and created its own patient-advocacy group, a practice known as astroturfing, or putting together a fake grassroots organization. When Paxil was first approved by the FDA for depression, in 1993, its sales lagged far behind front-runners Prozac and Zoloft. With only so many depressed patients to go around, SmithKline needed a way to distinguish its drug from the pack. It decided to do this by positioning Paxil as a treatment for anxiety disorders, a "sort of latter-day Valium," as writer Brendan I. Koerner puts it. First, the company tried encouraging doctors to prescribe the drug off label for post-traumatic stress disorder by funding and publishing several clinical trials testing Paxil on people suffering from the condition. Unfortunately for SmithKline, however, the results of the trials failed to show the drug was effective, and the FDA refused to approve it for post-traumatic stress disorder. The company then turned to another condition, called social anxiety disorder, an extreme form of shyness that causes intense feelings of distress in social situations.

The only problem for SmithKline was that social anxiety disorder was a puny market, especially compared with depression. According to the *Diagnostic and Statistical Manual of Mental Disorders*, social anxiety is "extremely rare," afflicting between 1 to 2 percent of the population at most. That meant that SmithKline would have to concoct a market for its drug, by persuading millions of people they were suffering from what was, in fact, an uncommon disease. In 1998, a year before Paxil gained FDA approval for social anxiety, SmithKline's PR agency, Cohn and Wolfe, came up with a slogan, "Imagine Being Allergic to People," which it plastered on bus shelters around the country. Pictures of a dejected-looking young man toying with a teacup were displayed over the lines "You blush, sweat, shake—even find it hard to breathe. That's what social anxiety disorder feels like." The posters made no reference to Paxil. They did, however, bear the name of the Social Anxiety Disorder Coalition and its three member organizations, the American Psychiatric Association, the Anxiety Disorders Association of America, and Freedom from Fear, all of which made the posters seem more like public service announcements than advertisements. In reality, three of the psychiatric organizations listed on the posters receive significant funding from SmithKline and other drugmakers. The fourth, the Social Anxiety Disorder Coalition, existed only temporarily in the New York offices of Cohn and Wolfe, which fielded all media calls for a few months after the ad campaign began.

Cohn and Wolfe's strategy did not stop at posters. The firm put together a "matte release," a press release about social anxiety disorder made to look like a reported article, complete with a byline. Many smaller newspapers printed the article verbatim, never telling their readers they were looking at a press release. The company also issued a video news release and a radio news release, which some stations also ran as is. To help reporters "put a face on the disorder," as one of the firm's account executives would tell the trade journal PR News, Cohn and Wolfe offered up names of patients and academic researchers, anxiety experts for the press to call. Those experts were all paid consultants of SmithKline, a fact that was left out of the biographies that reporters saw. Cohn and Wolfe's press packets, which were sent under Social Anxiety Disorder Coalition letterhead, inflated the number of people afflicted with the condition, claiming that social anxiety "affects up to 13.3 percent of the population," or one in eight Americans, and is "the third most common psychiatric disorder in the United States, after depression and alcoholism." In reality, according to the Diagnostic and Statistical Manual of Mental Disorders, no more than four million people are sufficiently impaired or distressed by their condition to warrant treatment. Inflated or not, Cohn and Wolfe's press campaign paid off. In the two years preceding Paxil's approval, fewer than fifty stories on social anxiety disorder had appeared in the popular press. Hardly anybody even knew what social anxiety was. By the time the FDA had approved the drug for social anxiety, and SmithKline had unleashed its direct-to-consumer ad campaign, which could now link social anxiety to its cure, Paxil, hundreds of stories about the illness had cropped up in U.S. publications and on broadcast programs. Social anxiety was everywhere, in the *Washington Post*, the *New York Times*, and *Town and Country*, on *The Howard Stern Show* and *Good Morning America*, and huge numbers of Americans were now worrying they might have it. Patients began asking their doctors about Paxil in droves, having diagnosed themselves with social anxiety, and their doctors, most often primary care physicians with little specialized knowledge of psychiatry or the diagnostic criteria for true social anxiety disorder, complied by writing prescriptions. Paxil sales, most of which were for social anxiety disorder, hit three billion dollars in 2002, putting it ahead of Zoloft, the nation's number-two SSRI.

Some might reasonably argue that Cohn and Wolfe's marketing campaign was indeed a public service to people who did not realize that their debilitating shyness was actually a mental disorder, that help was available. It undoubtedly brought some social-phobes into a doctor's office for treatment. But marketing shouldn't be confused with education, and letting drug companies define who needs to take their products is like letting your local Lexus salesperson decide what kind of car you should buy, and how often you need a new one. In 2002, physicians wrote 30.4 million prescriptions for Paxil—far more than would be needed for the four million patients suffering from social anxiety disorder as estimated by the *Diagnostic and Statistical Manual*. The treatment would turn out to be worse than the disease for an unknown number of people who took the brightly colored tablets, which came in orange, pink, blue, or green, depending on the dose. By 2004, it appeared that all of the SSRIs could trigger dangerous side effects, and Paxil especially so. That year, New York's then–attorney general, Elliot Spitzer, sued GlaxoSmithKline (SmithKline merged with Glaxo in 2001) for concealing data on the drug's potential to cause suicide. Internal company documents that became public included a memo to company sales reps that instructed them specifically not to discuss the potential suicide risk with physicians. Other company research suggested that as many as one in four patients on Paxil suffer withdrawal symptoms if they abruptly stop taking the drug. As David Healy, a British psychiatrist who helped spark recent investigations into the potential dangers of SSRIs, puts it, "If you've got a very severe problem, and I treat you with a drug like Paxil, I may save your life, I

may save your marriage, I may save your career. But if you don't have [a severe problem], if you've got a very mild problem, then making you a psychiatric patient, and putting you on a pill, may pose more risks than leaving
you untreated."

Branded

Cohn and Wolfe's campaign was just one example of the technique that
emerged during the 1990s for selling drugs by selling sickness. Known as
"condition branding" in marketing circles, the sales technique has proved
itself time and time again as a potent means for getting people into their
doctors' offices. Where drug manufacturing was once all about searching
for cures, condition branding is all about "the creation of medical disorders
and dysfunctions," as marketing executive Vince Parry puts it in a 2003 issue of *Medical Marketing & Media*. "There are three principal strategies for fos-
tering a condition and aligning it with a product," Parry writes. Those
strategies are "elevating the importance of an existing condition; redefining
an existing condition to reduce stigma; building a new condition to build
recognition for an unmet market need." The genius of condition branding
is that it allows marketers to expand a market simply by redefining disease;
coming up with an entirely new disorder; or simply widening the definition of an old one, and then forging links in the minds of both physicians
and consumers between the new definition and a particular drug.

For all its genius, condition branding raises troubling issues surrounding
the pharmaceutical industry's shifting sense of responsibility to patients and
doctors. While many of the techniques drug companies use to market their
wares are no different from those used to sell other consumer products,
drugs are not like cars or iPods. They alter the body in profound ways, and
they all have side effects, some worse than others. In redefining diseases,
marketers have done more than sell product; they have blurred the definitions of wellness and health. They have changed the way consumers think
about themselves and transformed huge numbers of formerly healthy people into patients who view themselves as sick. The solutions to their illnesses have invariably rested with drugs, all of which have the power to

harm as well as heal. That potential for harm has inevitably been down-played in condition branding campaigns.

Take Viagra, which Parry helped launch in 1998. It was advertised as the answer to "erectile dysfunction," a problem hitherto known as impotence and not much discussed, even between sufferers and their doctors. Calling it erectile dysfunction, or ED, reduced the stigma of impotence, which was a good thing. The term became a password, as Parry puts it, allowing doctors and patients to open up a potentially embarrassing conversation. It also al-lowed a sober fellow like Bob Dole and a he-man like Mike Ditka to serve as spokesmen for Viagra and marketers to spread the word in ads that impo-tence was a real disease, not something to hide in the closet. The choice of the word "dysfunction," writes Parry, "refocused the condition from being associated with a lack of potency (i.e. virility) to the more enlightened con-cept of physical loss of function that could be simply reversed." All to the good.

What was tricky about condition branding erectile dysfunction was that while the marketing campaign allowed some men to get treated for their flagging sex lives, it undoubtedly caused others to suddenly begin worrying unnecessarily that they had a medical problem. Men can go limp for a host of nonmedical reasons—stage fright, too much alcohol, stress, grief, lack of sleep—but once impotence was condition branded, many men began to wonder if the occasional failure to perform meant it was time to go to the doctor and get a prescription, for a drug that is not without danger. In 2005, Pfizer was ordered by the FDA to put a warning on its Viagra labels that the drug can cause irreversible vision damage, and in rare cases, blindness.

Saying Viagra treated a disease also allowed advertisers to quietly appeal to the public's desire for self-improvement and -enhancement—while si-multaneously pretending the drug wasn't really about improving any-body's sex life. Viagra was for a *disease*, not for wild, all-night sex. In *Better than Well*, an insightful critique of America's search for perfection, philoso-pher Carl Elliott points out that this oblique approach to selling enhance-ment is necessary in a culture that craves the benefits of drugs while simultaneously fearing they are a crutch; sap initiative; erode the work ethic; and turn people into mindless addicts. Yet as Elliott writes, "Consumer capitalism works, at least in part, by presenting consumers with a vision of the good life. This vision of the good life suggests the ways in which a consumer's own life does not measure up, and which could be remedied by the consumer product. You could be hipper, sexier, not just liked but well-liked, if only you would buy what we are selling." (An interesting aside to this is the history of cosmetic surgery. The idea of self-improvement through surgery seemed vulgar and tasteless—until plastic surgeons began selling it as a way to improve self-image, as a utilitarian path toward personal and financial success.) In the case of Viagra, marketers had to reconcile these two opposing views of drugs in the American psyche by presenting impotence as a bona fide medical condition (which it is, of course, for some men) and the little blue pill as a treatment.

Once that was accomplished, subsequent marketing campaigns dropped the subterfuge and unabashedly promoted Viagra and newer drugs as sexual aids. Less than a decade after Viagra's launch, it's good-bye Bob Dole, hello TV ad for Levitra showing a good-looking couple in their forties, glancing sidelong at each other with suggestively raised eyebrows as a sultry voice-over narrates, "Remember that guy who used to be called 'Wild Thing'? The guy who wanted to spend the entire honeymoon indoors? . . . Yeah, that guy. He's back." As advertising executive Donnie Deutsch put it in 2005, " 'Erectile dysfunction' is old news. EQ—'erectile quality'—is now the name of the game."

Not only was Viagra a gigantic commercial success, hitting one billion dollars in sales in its first ten months on the market, but it also helped launch the age of Internet drug sales and pharmaceutically enhanced rave parties. College boys and even teenagers could buy "V" on the net, to take along with their "X," the street drug ecstasy (though one has to wonder what could possibly make teenage boys think they need erection enhancement). Along the way, Viagra opened the door to bolder, saucier drug advertising and gave a boost to the multi-billion-dollar porn industry, which now had a stable of studs who could sustain an erection whenever the camera needed one.

Generation Rx

Some doctors argue that direct-to-consumer advertising has benefited their patients, that it has helped bring the sick into their offices, where they can receive needed medical care. But for many other physicians, drug advertising has changed their relationship with patients for the worse, often in precisely the ways predicted by the pharmaceutical executives who were writing to Congress back in the 1980s. Patients now routinely diagnose themselves with conditions and come to their doctors demanding the brand-name drugs they see advertised. Many doctors don't even bother trying to dissuade their patients, even if another medication or treatment would serve them just as well or better. Doctors say that when they try to discuss another potential treatment or drug, some patients assume they are simply trying to save money for an insurer. Many physicians would like to see direct-to-consumer drug advertising banned, or at least more strictly regulated to present more balanced information. In a recent editorial, Dr. David Kessler, former commissioner of the FDA, worried that "consumers who make health decisions based on what they learn from television commercials ultimately take medicines they may not need, spend money on brand medicines that may be no better than alternatives, or avoid healthy behaviors because they falsely believe a medicine is all they need."

Thirty years ago, Henry Gadsden, the head of Merck, told Fortune magazine he wanted his company to be more like the chewing gum maker Wrigley. It was his dream to make drugs not just for the truly sick but also for the healthy, so that he could "sell to everyone." One has to wonder whether, if Gadsden were alive today, he would be gratified to see the manner in which his dream has been fulfilled, how condition branding and other drug-marketing techniques have turned healthy people into patients by transforming wide swaths of ordinary human existence—everything from baldness to wrinkles, grief, worry, sex, and even shyness—into ailments in need of medical treatment. In 1993, the average number of prescriptions filled per person per year was seven. By 2000, it was eleven, and four years later it was twelve. By 2002, the top 10 drug companies were enjoying profits that equaled those of the other 490 Fortune 500 companies combined. It's hard to imagine a better testament to the power of marketing, or as a recent forecast in *Reuters Business Insights* puts it, "the corporate creation of disease." One sign of how common prescription-drug taking has become: Some new homes are being outfitted with supersized medicine cabinets. Gone is that mirrored, rust-stained metal chest that hung over the bathroom sink. Now there are triple-wide and even floor-to-ceiling models, complete with defoggers, interior lighting, and rubber gaskets that prevent the door from going "click" when you close it. As more of life becomes medicalized by marketing, the industry moves closer to Gadsden's dream of selling to everyone.

And the culture of popping a pill for every complaint has had other, unexpected effects. Americans are among the heartiest people on the planet. Unlike previous generations, a vast majority of us live long, active lives, free from childhood disease, infected wounds, and fatal childbirth, the killers that were responsible for the majority of deaths until the middle of the last century. Yet we don't see ourselves as being exceptionally healthy—we think of ourselves as sick. We obsess over our latest cholesterol reading, bone density, body mass index. We scour the health sections of newspapers, wondering if we or our loved ones are exhibiting the symptoms of this or that rare or previously unheard-of ailment, like restless legs syndrome, sleep apnea, bruxism, panic attacks, micro-obesity, and metabolic syndrome, to name just a few of the conditions that have cropped up in the news in recent years. One survey found that many teenage girls are so frightened of getting breast cancer that they are now doing breast self-exams, even though the likelihood that a woman under the age of thirty will be diagnosed with breast cancer is about one in nineteen hundred, less than the chances of a person of any age dying from the flu.

Not all of the blame for our national obsession with illness can be laid at the feet of pharmaceutical marketers. Sometime in the late twentieth century, the medical profession and patient advocacy groups came to the conclusion that the best way to keep people healthy was to scare them into the doctor's office, where they could be screened for diseases they didn't even suspect they had. These days, it goes almost without saying that prevention is the path toward better health. "Prevention" has become the doctor's watchword, the mantra that lies behind the screening tests that are now a routine part of every yearly exam. Twenty years ago, the seemingly healthy middle-aged man who went for a physical would have his blood pressure checked, along with blood and urine tests. If he complained of chest pains, he might get on a treadmill for a stress test. A middle-aged woman would get the same tests, plus a Pap smear and possibly a mammogram. Today, the number of tests has exploded, and doctors no longer just treat the sick but instead go looking for disease among the well. A routine checkup for the average middle-aged American male will almost certainly include a cholesterol test, a colonoscopy, and a PSA, or prostate-specific antigen, test for prostate cancer. Women will be given many of the same tests, along with a DEXA scan for osteoporosis. Radiologists have recently begun setting up Doppler ultrasound booths in local malls, where you can have your carotid arteries checked for blockages. Then there's the CA-125 test for ovarian cancer, calcium screening for cardiovascular disease, and spiral CT scan for lung cancer. And that's only a partial list. As one doctor puts it, "If I did all the tests that are recommended, I would never have time to listen to my patients."

That's not to say that a few screening tests haven't proved to be effective at preventing serious illness, allowing doctors to catch disease and treat it before symptoms appear. Taking everybody's blood pressure is a good idea, because treating those with hypertension lowers their risk of a heart attack or stroke. But many other tests, which have their place if a patient has symptoms, have had the perverse effect of benefiting only a small minority when they are given routinely to apparently healthy people in the name of prevention—while exposing the majority to invasive, often dangerous treatment they don't necessarily need. This is especially true for the PSA test—a simple blood test that most Americans believe implicitly will help them avoid an untimely death.

On the surface, the logic of the PSA test seems unassailable. It can detect prostate tumors on average eleven years before a digital rectal exam, which involves the doctor sticking a finger into a man's rectum to feel the prostate directly. Catching cancer early, as we've all been told, leads to cures. But does it really? If early diagnosis of prostate cancer really worked, then the mortality rate, or prostate cancer deaths per one hundred thousand in the population, should go down, as more and more men are screened.* There has been a slight drop in the death rate from prostate cancer in recent years, but many cancer epidemiologists and doctors argue that there is little evidence that the PSA test is responsible. That's because tumors come in many types, only some of which are aggressive enough to threaten the patient's life. In the case of prostate cancer, the vast majority of tumors sit around for years, causing few, if any, symptoms, and autopsy studies have shown that far more men die with prostate cancer than of it. Even among men who have been diagnosed with the disease, more than 90 percent will live fifteen more years even if they are never treated. On the flip side, many dangerous prostate cancers can't be cured with current treatments, no matter how early they're caught. Unfortunately, radiologists and pathologists can't tell with much certainty how aggressive a particular tumor is going to be. In the face of this uncertainty, doctors feel they must err on the side of caution and treat practically every tiny prostate tumor they detect as if it were potentially deadly, in the hope of curing at least a few.

What all this means is that widespread screening for prostate cancer may be a lose-lose proposition: It has resulted in little or no drop in the mortality rate, while simultaneously leading to huge numbers of men suffering the side effects of unnecessary treatment. A study published in 2002 in the British journal BMJ compared PSA testing rates in the region around Seattle and in Connecticut between 1987 and 1997. Men in Seattle were five times more likely to get a PSA test than men in Connecticut—yet there was no significant difference in the death rate from prostate cancer between the two regions. (Actually, there was a difference in the mortality rate: Men in Seattle were slightly more likely to die of prostate cancer, perhaps because they underwent more surgery for it.) Men in Seattle were also five times more likely to undergo surgical removal of the prostate, the

* That's assuming no increase in incidence. There has been an increase in incidence since the introduction of PSA testing, but according to most experts, it does not appear to be due to more cancers, just more detection.

most common method of treating the disease. A prostatectomy is a delicate surgical procedure that often renders patients impotent, incontinent, or both, even in the hands of the most accomplished surgeon. In a study of patients at Harvard University hospitals, the majority of men were impotent a year after their surgery and still wearing adult diapers. A man who chooses not to be treated for his prostate cancer may also develop incontinence and impotence, but these symptoms don't usually appear for many years after diagnosis.

Today, debate over the PSA test rages on, and neither doctors nor patients know what the right course of action is. The evidence suggests that PSA testing is not saving any lives, and even if it is, the large numbers of men who are treated unnecessarily are paying a terrible price. They're the equivalent of civilian casualties in our war on cancer. A friend of mine describes the change in her father-in-law, who became a different person after undergoing a prostatectomy that left him permanently incontinent. He grew silent and morose, no longer willing to go out with friends or even leave his house, for fear of an accident. He died two years later of heart disease. Yet doctors and patient advocacy groups continue to push for widespread screening with the PSA test.

This is the power of magical thinking. We all want to believe that early diagnosis of cancer will protect us, that if we dutifully head to the doctor for our yearly screening tests, we can avoid disease and thwart even death. And yet, many of the screening tests we imagine will protect us— mammography, colonoscopy, and more recently, CT scans to screen for lung cancer—suffer from many of the same drawbacks as the PSA test. The only cancer screening test that has been shown unequivocally to decrease mortality is the venerable Pap smear for cervical cancer. Yet even that is not a fail-safe talisman for warding off premature death. Howard Brody, a primary care physician at the University of Texas Medical Branch, in Galveston, recalls a tragic case of a young woman who put her faith in the Pap test:

One of the saddest cases I ever took care of was a woman in her late thirties who died of cervical cancer. She'd had an abnormal Pap smear four or five years earlier.

A [biopsy] found some abnormal cells. Everybody thought we'd gotten it all. She had a normal Pap smear every year after that, year in, year out. Then one day, I reached in to do a pelvic exam, and I felt the cervix, and then I felt another cervix, and the other one was a cancer. She went through chemo, radiation, the whole nine yards. The whole time, she was just so pissed off, she died an angry woman. She left a husband and two children under the age of ten. I tried to get hospice; I tried to get her palliative care. But she was so angry, because she had done everything right in her mind. She went in to the doctor like clockwork; she never missed an appointment for her Pap. She thought, if I do what I am supposed to do, I will get my gold star from heaven; I will be protected. Then God violated the contract. It was bad enough that she died at age forty, but she was so angry, she wouldn't even say good-bye to her children.

Magical thinking is not the exclusive province of patients. Doctors, too, believe they can prevent disease by turning risk factors into conditions they must treat. Everything from high cholesterol to slightly elevated blood sugar, which aren't diseases in themselves but merely signs that a patient might be at risk for one, now warrants a prescription or treatment. We all assume that treating risk factors is based on good evidence, which has shown that early intervention will lower our chances of getting the disease, or dying from it. That's often not the case in the real world. Take below-average bone density among women in their forties and fifties, a condition that has been branded as "osteopenia," a precursor to osteoporosis that many doctors and patients believe has to be nipped in the bud with powerful drugs. Sometime between the ages of thirty and forty-five, women (and some men) begin to lose calcium in their bones, a natural process that may lead to osteoporosis, or truly brittle bones, by the time they are elderly. Brittle bones break more easily, and a hip fracture in a frail, elderly woman often leads to a host of complications that signal impending death. Fosamax, the best-selling antiosteoporosis drug on the market, works by attaching to bone cells and preventing calcium loss, and doctors prescribe it to younger women with osteopenia in the hopes of preventing fractures down the road. But there's not a single study to show that starting early makes any difference. In fact, one study of Fosamax found that women with osteopenia who took it suffered *more* fractures, not fewer. (The following chapter will discuss why doctors continue prescribing drugs even when the data say they probably shouldn't.)

An even more troubling aspect of preventive medicine involves the use of procedures whose potential for harm can outweigh any possible benefit. Take the carotid endarterectomy, a kind of Roto-Rooter surgery for the arteries that supply blood to the brain. In use since the 1950s, the procedure was performed on about 132,000 Americans in 2002. It's intended to avert strokes that are caused when a blood clot forms in one of the two carotid arteries in the neck and blocks the flow of blood when it reaches a narrower arterial branch in the brain. In 2002, carotid endarterectomy was the most common vascular surgery performed in the United States. According to the National Stroke Association's Web site, the procedure reduces the risk of stroke "by as much as 55 percent." But this figure is accurate only for a subset of patients, those whose arteries are significantly blocked and who have already experienced either a full-blown stroke or a transient ischemic attack, a kind of ministroke, or temporary loss of blood flow to part of the brain. Epidemiologists estimate that left untreated, three out of ten people who fall into this high-risk category will suffer a stroke within five years. Undergoing carotid endarterectomy reduces their risk to one in ten.

But for patients who have only moderately blocked carotid arteries, the surgery's benefit is offset by the 6 to 7 percent risk of stroke or death posed by the procedure itself. As for patients with only mild narrowings or who have never had a stroke, the procedure doesn't reduce the possibility of stroke—it increases it.

What's astonishing here is that two thirds of the carotid endarterectomies performed in this country are on elderly people who have no symptoms at all, or for whom the benefits of the surgery are offset by its risks. For whatever reason, because they don't know the scientific data, or ignore it because of financial incentives, or because they simply cannot believe that cleaning out the arteries won't do a patient good, vascular surgeons performed about eighty-eight thousand *unnecessary* carotid endarterectomies in 2002, thereby causing an unknown number of strokes. At an average cost of fifteen thousand dollars per procedure, that comes to more than a billion dollars the health care system could have put to better use.

Elder abuse

James Goodwin, a geriatrician at the University of Texas Medical Branch, argues that when it comes to aging patients, treating risk factors with invasive procedures like carotid endarterectomy borders on assault. In an eloquent and disturbing essay published in the *New England Journal of Medicine*, Goodwin writes about the medicalization of aging, the tendency for doctors and patients to see the inevitable breakdown of the body as a series of treatable diseases.

So little of what is done for old people seems aimed in any direct way at making the patient feel better. With medicalization, the role of physicians has become so expanded and technologized that we fail at our most important task—providing relief from suffering. Medical care of the elderly is particularly distorted by this new focus. Medicalization externalizes experience, whereas the major tasks of aging are internal. Every clinician has witnessed the medicalized 80-year-old obsessed with arthritis, Alzheimer's disease, and serum cholesterol levels. Contrast this patient with someone else in the same physical condition, who admits that her knees are bad and that she has trouble remembering things. Which patient is better off? Attention to some proto-illnesses arguably could benefit 80- and 90-year-olds: certainly osteoporosis, probably also high blood pressure. But 80-year-olds can ill afford the ceding of responsibility and loss of control inherent in medicalization. The challenges of very old age are spiritual, not medical. The appropriate role of the physician is as counselor or helper, not as scientific expert.

Goodwin goes on to tell the story of an older man who was in good health except for a hernia. When the man went to the hospital for surgery on his hernia, he was given a cardiac test, to see if his heart was in shape for the surgery. That test showed a slight abnormality, so he underwent catheterization. The catheterization showed a blockage in a coronary artery, and he was scheduled for bypass surgery. Before he could undergo bypass, he was given a test of his carotid arteries, which showed a slight blockage. He suffered a stroke during the carotid endarterectomy, which delayed his heart surgery for six months. A year later, the man was almost back to normal, writes Goodwin, "and his hernia (still unrepaired) was not bothering him as much, because of his decreased activity. Here is the scariest part of the story: he was grateful—thankful that his doctors had found the heart and carotid problems in time. Grateful also are the legions of older men who have undergone radical prostatectomy for prostate cancer discovered by PSA screening, grateful that their doctors found it in time." What the man with the hernia failed to realize was that the procedures performed on him, the catheterization, the bypass, the endarterectomy, probably did nothing to lengthen his life but instead led to a stroke that left him paralyzed for more than a year. But at least his hernia was no longer bothering him.

Our relentless search for wellness through medicine has created a kind of therapeutic imperative, the urge to treat every complaint, every deviation from the norm, as a medical condition. We've come to believe that if a test can be performed, it should be performed; if a treatment can be used to lengthen life, no matter how incrementally, it should be used, regardless of whether the intervention will improve the patient's sense of well-being, or is what the patient really wants. Families often tell doctors to "do everything possible" for their elderly and dying loved ones, often without realizing that "doing everything" won't necessarily stave off death for long but could make the patient's last few days or weeks more miserable than they might have been. Physicians, too, forget that their power to prolong life is limited, and that they are still able only "to cure, sometimes; to relieve, often; to comfort, always," in the words of a French proverb.

Diane Meier is a palliative care specialist at Mount Sinai Hospital, just off Central Park on Manhattan's Upper East Side. She is a tiny woman, with fragile-looking wrists and slender shoulders. Slight as she is, though, Meier is a fierce advocate for patients in her hospital who are dying or in pain. She and the doctors and nurses who work in her department try to ease symptoms for patients, and to keep the therapeutic imperative at bay by encouraging family members to think about what's best for dying patients, rather than focusing on prolonging life.

A former geriatrician, Meier switched to palliative care after being radicalized by a patient, an elderly Hispanic man who spoke barely any English, who was dying of lung cancer when she met him. Mr. S., as she calls him, had watched his wife succumb to lung cancer three years earlier. Then he too was diagnosed in the late stages of the disease, and he wanted no part of the side effects his wife suffered during her treatment. He declined chemotherapy, radiation, and surgery, saying he wanted to die at home, surrounded by his family. The hospital sent him home, but a few months later, Mr. S. was brought into the emergency room at Mount Sinai by his grown children, delirious and suffering seizures. The lung cancer had spread to his brain, where it was causing pressure to build inside his skull. The hospital admitted him to the neurology department, and the doctors stabilized his condition with drugs that reduced the swelling of his brain, but it was only a matter of days before the cancer killed him. Mr. S. went in and out of awareness, but his son, who was serving as his health care proxy, knew he did not want to be treated for his cancer.

When Meier entered the room, she found a frail, emaciated man who was unable to speak intelligibly but was nonetheless clearly agitated, thrashing around in his bed despite being pinned by his wrists and ankles in four-point restraints. A nasogastric feeding tube snaked into one nostril and down into his stomach, to provide nourishment, since he was refusing food. (In terms of pain, having this tube in their noses is the thing that repeat visitors to the emergency department dread the most.) Shaken, Meier went out to the nurses' station to find out what was going on. Mr. S. had terminal lung cancer, she was told. It had metastasized to his brain. Meier went looking for a neurologist who could give her the man's complete history. What she heard made her decide to spend the rest of her career finding ways to reduce suffering, especially among dying patients. "The lightbulb moment for me was when I got the neurology intern to explain to me why Mr. S. was in four-point restraints," she says. "The intern looked at me with enormous distress in his eyes and he said, 'He'll pull out the nasogastric tube. If I don't keep him in restraints, he'll die.' "

It might seem like a giant leap to go from the suicide of a young college student to the death of an elderly man riddled with cancer, yet Justin Cheslek and Mr. S. are linked to each other by the American belief that more is better when it comes to medicine. Twenty years ago, a kid like Justin might not have even gone to his college clinic for sleeplessness. And if he had, the doctor probably would have reassured him that a few nights spent tossing and turning were nothing to fret about, and that he should knock off drinking coffee and smoking cigarettes, which could keep him awake. Now, parents and doctors worry that every child who fidgets in class has ADHD, and that every teenager who can't sleep or hits a rough patch on the road to adulthood is clinically depressed and liable to take his own life. There are children who are impaired by ADHD, to be sure, and adolescents who suffer from debilitating and even suicidal depression. But by redefining "the boundaries that separate the healthy from the well," as Ray Moynihan and Alan Cassels put it, and by exaggerating the dangers of mild problems and the prevalence of rare conditions, drug marketing has helped persuade both physicians and patients that they must worry about the littlest sign of incipient illness—that getting treated as early as possible for disease will lead to a longer and healthier life.

By extending the notion of prevention to imply that we can stop illnesses in their tracks before they even begin, both practitioners and the health care system's recipients have come to perceive medicine as possessing even the power to deny death. Or as breast cancer specialist Susan Love once put it, "We like to think death is optional." We want doctors to do everything and try everything, and we think that failing to do so is tantamount to killing the patient. When you couple this attitude with what we learned in chapter 4—that the supply of medical resources can drive what kind of care patients receive, and how much of it—it's easy to see how we've arrived at a place where some hospitals can spend, on average, one hundred thousand dollars per Medicare recipient in the last two years of life. Mr. S., tied down to a bed in a hospital he didn't want to be in, serves as a vivid reminder of what happens to too many Americans as they near the end of life, and it happens not because doctors or families wish them harm but because everybody is stuck in a system where all the forces point in the same direction, toward more medicine, rather than compassionate, appropriate care.

Did Justin Cheslek die from taking Paxil, or Effexor, or a combination of the two, or none of the above? We'll never know for sure, because it's often impossible to lay blame for an individual act, especially one as unfathomable as suicide. Yet pinning down the exact cause of Justin's death may not be as important as a different sort of question: Was the risk of agitation and suicide worth taking for a teenager who may have been suffering from nothing more serious than a few sleepless nights in college? Justin's grieving family doesn't think so. In early 2007, six years after Justin's death, his father Gary was able to say, "The real tragedy in this is doctors don't let patients know what the odds are. If you read the list of side effects on this stuff, you would have to sit down and say, how damn bad do I have to feel to risk all that?" This is a question that wise doctors and patients should ask themselves every time they consider any medical intervention.

EIGHT Money, Drugs, and Lies

SOMETIME IN THE early weeks of 2001, the giant pharmaceutical house Merck realized it had a problem. Its flagship drug, the painkiller Vioxx, had been on the market for more than a year, and it had already reached blockbuster status, the term for drugs that sell more than a billion dollars annually. The company had recently published a massive study of Vioxx that showed the drug was safer than naproxen, a painkiller similar to ibuprofen, both of which can cause bleeds in the stomach and intestines, a rare but potentially deadly side effect. But buried in the fine print of the study was the finding that Vioxx increased the risk of heart attacks and strokes compared with the older drug. Now, outside researchers and doctors were beginning to dig into the data.

Merck's marketing department went into high gear. The company could have initiated a new clinical trial to investigate the magnitude of the cardiovascular risk Vioxx posed. Instead, the company quickly took steps to spin the results of its own trial, suggesting that Vioxx didn't so much *cause* heart attacks as naproxen was simply better at *preventing* them. Merck plowed millions of dollars into direct-to-consumer ads, including a television spot featuring Olympic ice-skating champion Dorothy Hamill, who told viewers her arthritis had gotten so bad that she nearly had to stop skating until her doctor prescribed Vioxx. In parallel campaigns to market the drug to doctors, code-named "Project Offense" and "XXceleration," the company instructed its sales representatives to emphasize Vioxx's protective effects against gastrointestinal bleeds and to tell doctors that this benefit outweighed any possible cardiac risks. Anticipating that physicians might be skeptical, the company distributed a training document titled "Dodge Ball Vioxx," which told reps to dodge sticky questions by handing doctors preprinted "cardiology cards" using discredited data from small, short-term studies, which claimed that Vioxx was actually eight to ten times *safer* than other painkillers. The company also held pep rallies for its reps, who were told to think of champions like Helen Keller and Martin Luther King Jr. and the odds they surmounted, if ever the reps should feel discouraged about selling Vioxx.

Sales skyrocketed. The company sold billions of dollars' worth of Vioxx over the four and a half years the drug was on the market, most of it after worries about the cardiovascular effects first surfaced. By the time new data forced Merck to pull its painkiller from the market, in 2004, doctors had written one hundred million prescriptions, for a drug that was no more effective than ibuprofen, offered slightly more protection against gastrointestinal bleeds, but doubled the risk of heart attacks and strokes. Food and Drug Administration safety expert David Graham estimates that as many as sixty thousand people died from taking Vioxx. That's more deaths than Americans sustained in the Vietnam War.

Throughout the current debate over prescription drugs, Vioxx has become the poster child for everything that's wrong with both the pharmaceutical industry and the agency that is supposed to regulate it. The FDA approved Vioxx knowing there was the possibility that the drug caused heart attacks. Once the company published its large study in 2000, which further substantiated the possible danger, agency higher-ups ignored FDA safety officers like Graham, who wanted Merck to launch a clinical trial aimed at pinning down the cardiovascular risk. Instead, the agency spent eighteen months wrangling with Merck over the wording of a warning to be placed on the drug's label. By the time the company complied, the warning was so watered down it had virtually no effect on prescription rates. In 2004, in testimony before Congress, Graham said, "I would argue that the FDA, as currently configured, is incapable of protecting America against another Vioxx . . . Simply put, the FDA and its Center for Drug Evaluation and Research are broken."

The pharmaceutical industry itself has come in for even harsher criticism. Marcia Angell, a physician and author of *The Truth about the Drug Companies: How They Deceive Us and What to Do about It*, charges that companies routinely misinform the public with their direct-to-consumer ads; buy the loyalty of doctors with favors and gifts; inflate the benefits of drugs while deliberately obscuring their risks; and charge far too much for their products. At $150 a month, Vioxx was ten times more expensive than older painkillers, which were just as effective for most patients at relieving pain in the clinical trials. The only reason to use Vioxx was that it was supposed to be safer, yet doctors prescribed it to millions of patients who were at little to no risk of getting a gastrointestinal bleed from older, cheaper drugs. Merck sent doctors to all-expenses-paid seminars in exotic locales to learn about the drug. Internal memos from Merck obtained by Congress show that company scientists knew about the potential cardiac risk as early as 1997 and deliberately excluded patients who were already suffering from heart disease from clinical trials in an effort to reduce the chances of seeing a cardiovascular event.

Other critics lay blame at the feet of doctors and insurance companies. In his essay "High Prices: How to Think about Prescription Drugs," *New Yorker* writer Malcolm Gladwell argues that doctors are professionals who ought to know the data before they prescribe a drug, and that insurance companies don't have to pay for drugs that aren't any more effective or safer than cheaper alternatives. If doctors write prescriptions for drugs, he writes, "and insurance companies pay for them, surely there is more than one culprit in the prescription-drug mess."

Of course, that's assuming that doctors and insurance companies know how safe and effective drugs really are. In the debate over prescription drug prices, drug safety, and oversight from the FDA, the assumption has been that everybody has access to the same data and that everybody, from drug safety officers to doctors to insurers, is equally capable of assessing the merits and dangers of a drug. That's not the case. In fact, maybe the real problem with prescription drugs, and indeed with medical technology in general, is not so much that they cost too much or that they're too dangerous or that they don't always work the way they're supposed to. Maybe the real problem is there's too little of the right kind of information.

Drug reps

Doctors have three main sources of information about medical products: sales representatives, other doctors, and medical journals. All three of those sources provide some good data, and a lot of misinformation. The drug industry spends about twenty-five billion dollars a year marketing drugs to doctors, and its sales reps are part of that strategy. According to one study, for every dollar spent on marketing a drug to doctors, a company reaps on average more than ten dollars in sales. At the front lines of this massive marketing campaign stands the drug company representative, or drug rep, usually a handsome young man or shapely young woman who has been recruited more for his or her good looks and outgoing personality than for any aptitude in science or medicine. Drug reps have been calling on doctors since the nineteenth century, but over the past two decades their numbers have increased dramatically, doubling between 1996 and 2001 to an army of ninety thousand, which makes about one rep for every nine doctors. As their numbers have increased, so has their influence on doctors' prescribing habits.

Kate Howard began working as a drug rep in 2003, after returning to the small town in the Midwest where she grew up in order to help her mother care for her eighty-year-old father. A petite woman with long dark hair and a voluptuous figure, Howard is charming, smart, and profanely funny, a chatterbox who can strike up a conversation with anyone. After getting a Ph.D. in archaeology, Howard wound up working as a sales rep for gin maker Charles Tanqueray. When she learned about a job opening for a drug rep back home, she figured selling drugs couldn't be all that different from selling booze. Her first few months were spent working for TAP Pharmaceutical Products, selling the antacid Prevacid and an atypical antipsychotic that was known to cause heart murmurs. Then she was recruited by Pfizer, the biggest drug company in the world. After a six-week training course, the newly minted Pfizer rep was given a company car, a base salary of fifty thousand dollars, and three drugs to cover, including Celebrex, the main competitor of Vioxx. (Howard asked that her real name not be used because she fears Pfizer might sue.)

By the time Howard began repping for Pfizer, Vioxx and Celebrex were in a head-to-head competition for market dominance. Within a year after Celebrex gained FDA approval, in 1998, the drug had hit a billion dollars in sales, which was faster than any drug in the history of pharmaceuticals. By 2000, the two drugs had rocketed to sales of four billion dollars between them. Pfizer employed a brigade of four thousand reps, whose job it was to hammer home the superiority of Celebrex over not just older painkillers like ibuprofen and aspirin but also, especially, Vioxx.

As a soldier in Pfizer's army, Howard's first order of business was to keep the supply closets in her doctors' offices stocked with free samples. Each year, drug companies give away an estimated twelve billion dollars' worth of free samples of brand-name drugs, which the industry likes to portray as an act of charity, a way of allowing doctors to treat the uninsured. But most doctors know that the real point of giving away free drug samples is the same reason grocery stores offer you free samples of cookies: to get you to try it and buy a whole box. (Or as one wag put it, the first bag of heroin is free.) Studies show that most free samples wind up being handed out not to the poor but to the insured, along with doctors' families and friends. Companies know that doctors tend to stick with prescribing a drug once they've given it to a patient as a sample—even if that particular drug isn't the best treatment for the patient or there's a cheaper or safer one that would do just as well. When there are several drugs available for the same condition, doctors are more likely to prescribe the brand they have in their supply closet.

In addition to supplying free samples, Howard was expected to visit her doctors regularly, to establish friendly relationships with them, and to talk up Pfizer's drugs. "The personal relationship with the doctor is everything," she says. "If the doctor likes you, then he will try your drug." Reps will go to great lengths to cultivate doctors, even sleeping with them upon rare occasion, as a competitor of Howard's was. But most reps rely on the other three Fs—food, flattery, and friendship—to move product. With a fifteen-thousand-dollar-a-month expense budget, Howard brought breakfast or lunch to at least one physician practice every day, while many of her evenings were spent at expensive restaurants, wining and dining doctors and nurses. "I was either making a reservation or carrying food around in the back of my car. I felt like a glorified caterer," she says. "And you did not want to be known as the pizza and Subway rep." The better the food Howard brought to doctors' offices, the greater her chances of buttonholing a physician when he or she came to the break room to grab a bite to eat. Along with food, she showered her doctors and their staffs with trinkets— pens, sticky notepads, paperweights, tissue dispensers, baseball caps, and stuffed animals for doctors' children, all emblazoned with the name of her drug.

Gifts are a critical selling tool for all drug reps. At medical meetings, reps hand out mountains of freebies—and doctors can be seen strolling among drug company booths carrying bags that overflow with passport holders, nifty CD carrying cases, giant beach towels, waterproof tote bags, automatic coffeemakers, elegant silver business card holders, and USB memory sticks. Some reps talk about offering doctors far more lavish gifts, including concert tickets, television sets for their waiting rooms, junkets to golf outings, wine tastings, and cigar parties. In an alarming yet funny essay in a recent issue of the *Atlantic Monthly*, philosopher Carl Elliott writes about Gene Carbona, a rep Elliott describes as being "in a class of his own." Elliott recounts the story of how Carbona worked a group practice of about fifty doctors in Tallahassee, Florida, that was struggling to make a profit. Carbona told the doctors they needed a practice management consultant, and he knew just the fellow for the job. He then paid a business consultant, who also happened to be a friend of his, $50,000 out of his expense account to help the doctors transform their office into an efficient and lucrative practice. Soon, the doctors were writing huge numbers of prescriptions for Carbona's drugs. When Elliott asked Carbona how he managed to increase prescriptions without making the doctors feel as if they had been bribed, Carbona told him that his consultant friend had done all the heavy lifting. The consultant never mentioned the drugs Carbona was pushing. Instead, he talked up Carbona himself. "Gene is putting his neck on the line for you guys," the consultant told the doctors. He emphasized what a great service Carbona was providing them, how valuable the consulting was, and how they were all going to make a lot more money. "Those guys went berserk for me," Carbona told Elliott. They wrote so many prescriptions for his drugs that in one year Carbona earned a $140,000 bonus.

Most patients would probably find it at least a little unsettling to think that any kind of gift, whether it's a pen or a fancy dinner or free business consulting, could influence their doctors' decisions about which drugs to prescribe. After all, a physician's first duty is to his patient, and he's supposed to write prescriptions on the basis of medical evidence, not which drug rep gave him the coolest insulated coffee mug. The medical community has debated for years whether or not drug reps and the gifts they bear have any effect on the prescribing habits of doctors. A majority of doctors believe that the gifts and favors they receive have little or no effect on their prescribing habits, and they find it deeply insulting for anyone to suggest that they do. If you were to ask your own doctor if she prescribed a particular drug for you because she likes the free sticky notepads the rep brings each week, she would likely swear on the Hippocratic oath that she based her decision on sound medical science. And her belief in her own incorruptibility would likely be sincere.

But the research says otherwise. At least sixteen studies have found that drugs that are most heavily marketed to physicians are the ones most likely to be prescribed. The more time doctors spend with drug reps, and the more free gifts, drug samples, and food they accept, the more likely they are to prescribe the brand-name drugs that the reps are pushing. Physicians who have the most contact with reps prescribe the most "irrationally," which means they give patients expensive, brand-name drugs when there are cheaper and often better, safer alternatives—or when no drug at all would have been the best choice. At least two studies have found that doctors who take gifts are far less likely to believe that their prescribing habits can be influenced than doctors who shun drug reps.

The relationship between doctors and drug reps begins on the first day of medical school, when students find presents in their mailboxes, usually a useful item, a reference book, a stethoscope, something that makes them feel they are truly on their way to becoming doctors. As the student makes his way through medical school and then his internship and residency, he gratefully eats the food that drug reps provide at grand rounds. He sees the trinkets that reps bring to his instructors, he knows about the trips senior doctors take, and he watches them head off to fancy dinners, all courtesy of the industry. By the time doctors go into practice, many of them view presents and favors from reps as an entitlement, a little payback for the sleepless nights and low wages they put up with during their training. In a recent survey of more than one thousand third-year medical students, more than 80 percent reported they felt entitled to gifts (68 percent reported they did not believe gifts would influence their prescribing decisions). Some doctors feel that reps are truly their friends—which isn't surprising, given how amiable and engaging most reps can be. For their part, many drug reps believe they are doing God's work selling pharmaceuticals. While he was stocking a doctor's supply closet, one young rep told me he was inspired to quit his job selling copiers and join a drug company because "if you sell copiers, you're just selling a machine. It's not the same as saving lives."

At a deeper level, however, reps are trading on the psychology of reciprocity, the ingrained sense, shared by most human beings, that those who receive favors should repay them. The gifts aren't attached to an explicit quid pro quo, says Michael Oldani, a former drug rep turned academic. Now a professor of anthropology at the University of Wisconsin-Whitewater, Oldani worked for Pfizer for nine years, until 1998, when he suffered a crisis of conscience. He entered graduate school in anthropology at Princeton and wrote his dissertation on the anthropology of selling pharmaceuticals. His thesis is a gold mine of insight into the game of give-and-take in which doctors and reps engage. Often the gift itself is not what's important to the doctor; it's what the gift symbolizes, Oldani told me. "The gifting shifts the doctor's sense of obligation ever so slightly from the patient's best interests to those of the rep." All of this happens at a subliminal level. In an essay titled "All Gifts Large and Small," a group of bioethicists at the University of Pennsylvania point to the power of reciprocity in the case of the Hare Krishna movement. Hare Krishnas hung out in crowded airports in order to thrust trinkets, most often a flower or a pamphlet, into the hands of passersby with the words "This is our gift to you." Recipients often tried unsuccessfully to refuse the gift, or threw it in the nearest trash can. And yet, write the authors, "they were frequently so compelled to make a donation that the Hare Krishnas became quite wealthy." In the same way, when a drug rep repeatedly gives a physician presents, no matter how small or insignificant they might be, eventually the doctor feels compelled to reciprocate with the one thing the rep really wants: more prescriptions.

"Drug whores"

Gift giving is nothing new in the drug business. As the son of a family practitioner in Clover, South Carolina, Carl Elliott grew up surrounded by trinkets from drug reps. "I think I was eight years old before I figured out that not all Frisbees come with the word 'Merck' written on them," he says. Like his father and elder brother, Elliott attended medical school. He never went into practice, however, choosing instead to go on to a Ph.D. in philosophy. Now a professor at the University of Minnesota, Elliott has recently turned his attention to the ethics of gift giving in the pharmaceutical business. He points out that while the gifts have always been there, they have assumed greater importance over the past two decades, as drug companies have transformed themselves into marketing powerhouses. Once driven by research and development, the industry underwent a shift in focus that came about, in Elliott's view, as a result of key regulatory changes. In 1992, under pressure from the industry, Congress passed the Prescription Drug User Fee Act, or PDUFA. Known around Washington as "Padoofa," the act permits companies to pay fees to the FDA in order to speed up drug approval— creating in the process the absurd situation in which the agency is now partially funded directly by the industry it is supposed to regulate. At the same time, drug companies expanded their influence in Washington, donating heavily to congressional war chests and creating the largest, and probably the most powerful, lobbying group in the country.

Once the FDA opened the door in 1997 to less-regulated direct-to-consumer advertising, says Elliott, "companies began hitting for the fences." They concentrated their efforts on potential blockbuster drugs for chronic illnesses that could be taken by millions of patients. A new antibiotic might save lives, but a new lifestyle drug—Prozac for depression, Claritin for allergies, or a drug like Lipitor that treats a risk factor like high cholesterol—could be taken every day by huge populations, sometimes for years on end. Companies stepped up their marketing not only to consumers but also to doctors, and sales reps found themselves in a gift-giving arms race, trying to outdo one another in an effort to get doctors to write more and more prescriptions. Kathleen Slattery-Moschkau is a former rep who carried the bag for nine years for Bristol-Myers Squibb and Johnson & Johnson before quitting to write and direct *Side Effects*, an independent film about a fictional drug rep. She recalls that the pressure on reps to hit their quotas was intense. "If Pfizer was having a dinner at a really nice restaurant, you had to come up with [Green Bay] Packers tickets—and a bus to the game," she says. As reps upped the gift-giving ante, doctors began feeling entitled to increasingly luxurious favors. In an online chat room, one rep reported that a doctor asked him for money to build a music room in the doctor's house; another said she was asked to cater a doctor's daughter's wedding. An "unrestricted grant" from Gene Carbona paid for a doctor's swimming pool.

But the most profound change in the pharmaceutical industry was the new emphasis on "me-too" versions of existing drugs. No sooner would one company come up with a blockbuster than other companies would follow with competing versions. First there was Mevacor, then Prevachol, Zochor, and Lipitor. We have seven different versions of SSRIs, along with multiple me-too pills for erectile dysfunction and allergies. But there's a catch to this strategy: In order for a manufacturer to boost a second, not to mention a third, fourth, or fifth, me-too drug into blockbuster status, it has to sell the living daylights out of its drug. There are only three ways to do this: capture market share, increase the total market for the class, or create an entirely new market. Taking market share away from existing me-toos can be tough, since by definition one me-too is chemically similar to every other in its class, and they may share similar safety and efficacy profiles. Reps have to work especially hard to convince doctors that their company's drug is a cut above the rest—that, say, Celebrex is better than Vioxx. Sometimes it's easier to expand the total market for a class of drugs by condition branding that persuades doctors and patients that more people suffer from the disease the drugs treat than anyone ever suspected. Companies create entirely new markets for me-too drugs by selling a new sickness, like social anxiety disorder. No matter which strategy a company chooses, one of the most effective means of marketing a drug to doctors is getting other doctors to do it for you.

Kate Howard recalls enlisting a doctor to help her push Celebrex, a local orthopedist who was a "high-writer," or a physician who writes more prescriptions than average for the drug. As a high-writer, it was clear he already liked the drug. Sitting in the orthopedist's office one day, Howard and her partner suggested that he come aboard the company as a paid speaker. "My partner started to talk about the money angle," says Howard. " 'I realize you and your wife want to have a summer home. You can get your summer home so much faster if you just give us a couple of nights of your time, to give lectures . . . We'll pay you fifteen hundred dollars per speech. We will work the training around your vacation time. You can bring your family.' All he had to do was talk to a group of doctors and tell them he likes Celebrex." Within a few weeks, the orthopedist was jetting off to a speaker-training session at a luxury hotel, courtesy of Pfizer. When he returned, Howard began organizing extravagant dinners, at which the doctor would serve as the featured guest and speaker. "You go to all your orthopods in the area, and you say, 'Dr. So-and-So is going to talk about knee pain postsurgery,' " Howard says. She and her partner were careful not to make the dinner sound like a drug sales pitch to the other physicians they were inviting. "You don't say he's going to talk about Celebrex. You tell them he's talking about postsurgery knee pain."

After a dozen or so of these dinners, Howard found she could no longer stand her job. She began to feel she was bribing doctors with gifts and expensive food and misleading them about the drugs she was touting. She'd lasted only nine months as a drug rep.

For companies, the payoff for recruiting doctor-speakers can be spectacular. After one dinner Howard arranged, one of the doctors in attendance began handing out 25 percent more prescriptions for Celebrex, going from about 100 prescriptions a month on average to 125. At a dollar a pill, 25 more prescriptions a month translated into thousands of dollars in increased

annual revenue for Pfizer—after a single event that cost the company fifteen hundred dollars for the speaker's fee and another two thousand for
the dinner.

The drug industry has a term for such physician partners: They're
called thought leaders, or sometimes KOLs, for key opinion leaders. Like
patient advocacy groups, thought leaders are recruited to serve as third-
party, or covert, marketers, salespeople who will be seen as both authoritative and objective. Thought leaders are also critical to the medical device
industry, which has been known to pay prominent orthopedic surgeons as
much as four hundred thousand dollars a year to tout a particular brand
of artificial hip or knee. Some thought leaders, like Howard's orthopedist,
come from private practice, but most are academics, hired by the industry
to serve as consultants, sit on advisory boards, or join company speakers'
bureaus. Thought leaders can be paid fees ranging from a few hundred
dollars to several thousand dollars per day for consulting or speaking. A
few academic thought leaders earn hundreds of thousands of dollars a
year by working for multiple companies.* Among drug reps the unofficial
name for thought leaders who work for multiple companies is "drug
whores."

Companies court their thought leaders with great care. The last thing
they want is for the thought leader to figure out that her opinion is being
bought, or for her colleagues to think she's a shill. Drug reps are often the
ones who make the first contact with a new recruit, flattering her by saying
how widely respected she is by her peers and how much the drug company
values the opinions and counsel of doctors like her. Ever so slowly, the
thought leader's company contacts introduce the idea that she should help
them get the word out about their company's drug. A recent issue of *Pharmaceutical Marketing* included a guide for drug marketers on how to recruit
and train thought leaders to ensure "your product champions communicate
effectively on your behalf." Thought leaders aren't supposed to sell directly
but rather to create buzz, talking up a drug in casual conversation or while

---

* One psychiatrist from Brown University earned $556,000 in 1998 from his various financial relation-
ships with drugmakers, according to a report in the *Boston Globe*.

delivering lectures about the condition it's intended to treat. The guide suggests that marketers avoid using the same thought leaders too often: "If you front the same people at your symposia, or to write publications etc., they will inevitably be seen as being in your pocket."

Carl Elliott tells the story of how his brother Hal was lured, ever so gradually, into becoming a paid spokesman for a company that makes an antidepressant. First a company representative approached Hal Elliott, a respected psychiatrist at Wake Forest University, suggesting he speak about depression to a community group. The honorarium was a thousand dollars. He thought, why not? "It seemed almost a public service," Carl Elliott writes. Soon, the psychiatrist found himself speaking to clinicians at local hospitals. Then the company reps were urging him to talk less about disease and more about antidepressants. Elliott tried to ignore their suggestions. "The company began giving him PowerPoint slides, which he also ignored," writes his brother. "Then the reps began telling him, 'You're medical school faculty; we could get you on the national circuit. That's where the real money is.' . . . Eventually the reps asked him to lecture about a new version of their antidepressant drug." That's when Hal Elliott pulled the plug on his short career as a thought leader.

Plenty of other academics don't pull the plug, deciding instead that they can maintain their academic and intellectual integrity and still take the money. Today, a third of academic clinicians have financial ties to either the drug or the device industry, though nobody (except the companies themselves) has any idea how much money actually changes hands. Some, though not all, of them really are thought leaders—chairs of departments, winners of prestigious prizes. The more illustrious the thought leader is in his field, the more indispensable he is to his industrial sponsor's marketing efforts. Academic thought leaders defend their financial conflicts of interest, arguing that their opinions aren't for sale, that their integrity can't be bought. They say their time is worth money, and it's only fair they should be paid for their work as consultants and speakers for drug companies. They carefully weigh the scientific evidence before accepting a check for a lecture, where they express opinions they already held before being hired to speak.

That's doubtless true for some academic thought leaders, but the central problem is not so much whether an individual academic can be bought. Some can and some can't—and some are undoubtedly swayed by the money without even realizing it. The larger problem is that academics who are willing to endorse a particular drug are given a platform by their sponsors for disseminating their enthusiasm. Thought leaders put their names, for a fee, on medical articles ghostwritten by companies, lending an air of authority and veracity to the publication—even when they had nothing to do with the gathering, analysis, or write-up of the data. They serve as paid speakers at medical meetings and at grand rounds in hospitals; as white-coated spokespeople in promotional films aimed at other physicians; and as lecturers at continuing-medical-education courses, which doctors are required to attend each year in order to maintain their medical licensure. As of 2003, drug companies were providing more than half of the nearly two billion dollars spent on continuing medical education, gaining the industry a great deal of control over what doctors know and don't know about drugs and how to use them. By contrast, academics who are critical of a drug or device have to work harder to get their views disseminated. They don't have companies flying them around the country to tell other physicians about their concerns.

Another crucial role played by thought leaders involves the marketing of off-label, or unapproved, uses of drugs. Companies and their reps are strictly forbidden by the FDA to promote drugs for conditions not specifically approved—and listed on the drug's label. Doctors, on the other hand, are given wide latitude when it comes to prescribing off label. (And rightly so, for the most part. Nobody would fault a pediatrician for giving steroids to an asthmatic child, even though steroids, like most medications, have never received specific pediatric approval from the FDA.) Thought leaders help drug companies get around the no-off-label-marketing rules by doing the promotion for them. A doctor's decision to prescribe off label can be influenced by the recommendation of other doctors or by scientific articles in the medical literature, which the physician may or may not be able to interpret. Companies use thought leaders to reach doctors from both directions. They pay them to write positive editorials, for instance, or to talk up an unapproved use for a drug at a continuing-medical-education course.

The power of this under-the-table marketing can be seen in the tragedy of fen-phen, the wildly popular but potentially deadly off-label combination of two different diet drugs, fenfluramine and phentermine, that was removed from the market in 1997. At least forty-five thousand people, according to the manufacturer's own estimates, were harmed by the drug, which may cause pulmonary hypertension—high blood pressure in the lungs that can lead to damage to the heart valves and death. Estimates of how many patients were actually killed by fen-phen are hotly disputed to this day, and it's not even absolutely certain the drug was at fault. One of those whose death may have been caused by the drug was Mary Linnen, a young Boston woman whose story is told in detail in *Dispensing with the Truth*, writer Alicia Mundy's devastating chronicle of the fen-phen saga. Linnen's doctor prescribed the drug in 1996 so she could fit into her wedding dress. After being on fen-phen for twenty-three days, Linnen became dizzy and short of breath. She stopped taking the pills, and her symptoms improved for a time. But over the next few months, the young woman developed pulmonary hypertension, a condition that is rare in one so young. The disease damaged her heart so severely that she spent the last few months of her life hooked to an external pump with a tube leading into her chest. She could not risk walking down the street, lying on her side, or making love with her new husband. If an alarm sounded because the pump had failed, she had two minutes to repair it or call an ambulance. Mary Linnen died of heart failure in 1997, at age thirty.

The cruel joke here is that fen-phen was never particularly effective. The results of small-scale studies, which suggested early on that the combo drug worked spectacularly well at helping people lose weight, didn't pan out in larger, more-careful clinical trials. When Wyeth Pharmaceuticals, which manufactured two different versions of fenfluramine, conducted its own trials, they showed only a 3 percent difference between fen-phen and a placebo. Patients who took the drug lost on average about 5 percent of their body weight; patients who took a sugar pill lost 2 percent.

So how did Wyeth manage to turn fen-phen into a blockbuster diet pill, which some seven million people had taken by the time the drug was pulled from the market, in 1997? The company's fifty-four-million-dollar marketing campaign included generous grants to professional medical societies like the American Diabetes Association and the American Society of Bariatric Physicians, who went on to endorse fen-phen. The company sponsored all-expenses-paid seminars for community physicians, where they could hear about the drug from Wyeth's paid thought leaders. It dispatched Louis Lasagna, a famed clinical researcher and writer of essays on bioethics, to downplay the dangers of Wyeth's drug Redux, its new version of fenfluramine, when an FDA committee was considering whether or not to approve the drug in 1996. According to Mundy, George Blackburn, a Harvard researcher and chairman of the Committee on Nutrition for the Massachusetts Medical Society, was instrumental in getting the state of Massachusetts to lift a ban on fen-phen after cases of pulmonary hypertension surfaced.

But perhaps the most significant moment in the fen-phen saga occurred when a group of researchers in Europe and Canada published a study of ninety-five patients with pulmonary hypertension in the *New England Journal of Medicine* that linked the disease to diet pills. The study wasn't proof that the diet pill caused the condition, but Redux had just been approved, and news that it might cause pulmonary hypertension could have been bad for sales. Prominent obesity researchers JoAnn Manson, of Harvard, and Gerald Faich, from the University of Pennsylvania, argued in an editorial that the benefits of weight loss for the obese justified any potential risks from the drug. The editorial failed to mention to readers that the writers had financial ties to fen-phen's manufacturers. In a subsequent editorial, *New England Journal* editors Marcia Angell and Jerome Kassirer bemoaned the authors' failure to disclose their financial relationships, noting that Manson and Faich's conclusion, that fen-phen's benefits outweighed the risks, was just the sort of practical summary the journal wanted—if only the experts offering it had not had a conflict of interest. The fact that the authors were paid consultants, they wrote, "raises troubling questions." Later, Manson and Faich chalked up the omission to a "series of unfortunate misunderstandings" with their editors. Misunderstandings or not, one of the most important observations to be drawn from the story of fen-phen is the degree to which the drug industry has been able to penetrate the single most important source of medical information for both doctors and the public: the journals.

Lake Wobegon science

When doctors are in medical school, they're taught that good medicine is based on good science, and that the place to find the best medical science is in the top medical journals. Each year, tens of thousands of articles are published in hundreds of medical journals, only a few dozen of which rank in the top tier, the must-read category. Publishing in them is highly competitive, and each article must be peer-reviewed, or vetted by experts for accuracy and credibility. The journals that are most familiar to the public, the *New England Journal of Medicine*, the *Journal of the American Medical Association*, the *Annals of Internal Medicine*, are also the publications that physicians consider the authoritative sources, their most cherished repositories of medical knowledge.

Imagine Dr. John Abramson's dismay when he first discovered that a paper published in the esteemed *New England Journal* was wrong, and worse yet, when he began investigating more deeply and found that the authors had obscured information that might have prevented doctors from writing thousands of prescriptions for a potentially dangerous drug. In 2001, Abramson was still a family practitioner in a small town forty-five minutes north of Boston. A man of medium build, with dark, curly hair and a serious yet kind demeanor, Abramson considered himself an exceptionally well-informed doctor, a conscientious and discerning reader of the medical journals. One day, while eating his lunch in his office in between seeing patients, he came across a drug therapy article that changed the way he thought about himself and about medicine.

The article discussed research that had been published previously on the painkillers Vioxx and Celebrex. The authors of the paper, both of whom Abramson would subsequently notice had financial ties to the drugs' manufacturers, reviewed the data on the drugs, including Merck's huge trial of Vioxx, known as the Vioxx Gastrointestinal Outcomes Research, or VIGOR, trial. The authors opined that both drugs could protect patients against gastrointestinal bleeds better than older painkillers like ibuprofen. Then, almost as an aside, they noted that patients taking Vioxx in the VIGOR trial were more likely to suffer a heart attack, stroke, or death from a cardiovascular event than those taking naproxen, the drug that's similar to ibuprofen. They dismissed this finding, however, saying it may have been a statistical fluke, nothing more than "the play of chance," because the total number of cardiovascular events was small. But when Abramson looked carefully at the numbers, it looked like more than chance at work. The number of cases of serious gastrointestinal bleeding that Vioxx was supposed to prevent was actually smaller than the number of people who developed a heart attack, blood clot, or stroke. Abramson began digging around, eventually uncovering on an FDA Web site the original data Merck had submitted to the agency from the VIGOR trial.

The data Merck had submitted for Vioxx told a different story from what had been presented to physicians in the *New England Journal* article Abramson had read. The authors had played down the likelihood of a cardiovascular event, yet when Abramson began recalculating the odds, he found the risk was quite serious. "That's when the lightbulb really went on," Abramson told me recently. "If I as a family doctor gave Vioxx instead of naproxen to a hundred patients, there would be two and a half extra serious adverse events in the following year—serious as in hospitalization, permanent disability, or death—and I would have caused them." Abramson had already been sifting through other papers in the journals and finding similar problems—papers presenting results of drug research that glossed over risks or accentuated benefits. But the most unnerving discovery of all was the Vioxx research. After doing his calculations, says Abramson, he found himself almost incapable of writing a prescription. What if he gave a patient a drug that killed her? If he couldn't trust what was in the journals, how was he supposed to know what to prescribe? In 2002, Abramson closed his practice in order to research and write the book *Overdo$ed America*.

The discrepancies that Abramson found between what the data said and what the authors of the Vioxx and Celebrex article concluded are by no means an isolated instance. Rather, they represent a single example of the kind of thing that routinely afflicts the medical journals: complex findings, which are reported by academics with conflicts of interest, who portray the results in a way that obscures risks and plays up benefits. The authors of the drug therapy article tell readers right on page 436 that naproxen is just about as effective at reducing pain as the expensive new drug. That much is plain. The paper doesn't hide the fact that there were double the cardiovascular events in the group taking Vioxx. What's wrong with this article is the interpretation of the data. It buries the information about cardiac effects in a complicated discussion of why they probably aren't real, but rather due to "the play of chance." In the paper presenting the actual results from the VIGOR trial, the abstract at the top focuses on the benefits of the drug, while failing to emphasize in simple, clear terms the potential risks. The conclusion section ought to point out that the patients in the trial didn't reflect the general population of people for whom the drug would likely be prescribed. Later it would turn out that Merck failed to include three heart attacks that occurred during the VIGOR trial when the data were published in the *New England Journal*. Most doctors had no idea; they took the abstracts and conclusions of these articles at face value, because that's all most of them read, never digging far enough, as Abramson did, to get at the truth.

This situation has only gotten worse in recent years. Thirty years ago, a vast majority of scientific studies involving human subjects was funded by the federal government. Today, the pharmaceutical industry underwrites at least 80 percent of this clinical research, a shift that has given the industry unprecedented leverage over what shows up in the medical journals. At least eleven large studies, involving thousands of journal articles, have shown that industry-sponsored research tends to produce conclusions that favor the sponsor's product. A dozen other studies have found that when academic researchers have financial conflicts of interest with the industry, when they serve as paid thought leaders, they also tend to produce research results that shine a rosy light on their benefactors' products. In the view of Richard Horton, a British physician and editor of the prestigious medical journal the *Lancet*, "Journals have devolved into information-laundering operations for the pharmaceutical industry."

There is a long list of ways in which companies have been known to launder clinical research. In a hilarious spoof in the British journal BMJ titled

"HARLOT plc: An Amalgamation of the World's Two Oldest Professions," respected British clinical researchers David Sackett and Andrew Oxman list at least thirteen different methods for making drugs (and devices) look better than they really are. Their imaginary corporation, HARLOT plc (for How to Achieve Positive Results Without Actually Lying to Overcome the Truth), offers to help "the manufacturers of dodgy drugs and devices" increase market share by cooking the data. Among their list of services, Sackett and Oxman offer to compare the sponsor's drug to a placebo, rather than to an established therapy, a common method companies use to make their drugs look as effective as possible. (In the case of Vioxx, however, adding a group of patients on placebo to the VIGOR trial would have quickly shown that the drug increased the cardiovascular risk.) The authors suggest treating a side effect of a drug and then claiming the side effect rate was low. They offer to " 'accentuate the positive' . . . by reporting only favourable subgroup analyses," or using data only from those patients who did well on the product. "We 'eliminate the negative' by omitting or burying all unfavourable results where nobody can ever find and report them. After all, what they (patients, clinicians, regulators, and the public) don't know can't hurt you. We have a contact in the Wieliczka salt mine who can guarantee burial of negative results 200 metres underground . . . Our SAFE (Say Anything For a Euro) panel of experts is ready, at the drop of a banknote, to appear on television, chummy up to reporters, or write favourable commentaries in leading clinical journals."

What's not so funny about Sackett and Oxman's send-up of clinical trials is that the medical journals are filled with articles that appear to have adopted their methods. Here's just one example. In a survey published in 2006 in the *American Journal of Psychiatry*, a group of researchers from the United States and Germany looked at the results of nearly three dozen published papers on the atypical antipsychotics, powerful drugs used to suppress disordered thinking and behavior in patients with schizophrenia and other serious mental conditions. The studies they looked at were a particular type of clinical trial known as a head-to-head trial, which compares the efficacy and safety of one drug with those of another. Companies commonly use positive results from head-to-head trials to encourage doctors to prescribe their drug rather than a competitor's. When the authors of the

Journal of Psychiatry survey looked at the trials, they found a curious thing: In five trials that were paid for by Eli Lilly, its drug, Zyprexa, came out looking superior to Risperdal, a drug made by the company Janssen. But when Janssen sponsored its own trials, Risperdal was the winner three out of four times. When it was Pfizer funding the studies, its drug, Geodon, was best. In fact, this tendency for the sponsor's drug to come out on top held true for 90 percent of the more than thirty trials in the survey.

Now, it's pretty obvious that all atypicals can't possibly be superior to all other atypicals, unless the drugs were tested in some fantasyland like an M.C. Escher print or radio host Garrison Keillor's fictional Lake Wobegon, where all children are above average. How, then, could the head-to-head trials of these drugs come up with such impossible results? When the authors of the Journal of Psychiatry survey looked closely, they found that many of the trials had been designed in such a way as to favor the sponsor's drug.

All of this might be laughable if not for the stakes involved, for payers, who have been shelling out $10.7 billion a year worldwide for atypical antipsychotics, and especially for patients who take these drugs, which are prescribed—mostly off label—for conditions ranging from dementia and Alzheimer's in the elderly to oppositional behavior in children as young as four years of age. When the drugs first came along, a decade ago, manufacturers touted them as being more effective and safer than conventional antipsychotics. But in 2006, a study sponsored not by manufacturers but by the National Institute of Mental Health found that the atypicals are no more effective than conventional antipsychotics and may cause just as many side effects. In fact, the study found that some of the the atypicals may cause high rates of stroke, sudden cardiac arrest, rapid weight gain, and diabetes, side effects that a leading psychiatrist and former champion of the drugs calls "staggering in their magnitude and extent." This pattern repeats what happened with the SSRIs, which were widely used until publicly funded studies finally showed that they are not as safe and effective as doctors and patients had been led to believe.

It turns out, companies have known for years about the atypicals' possible side effects. In late 2006, a scandal erupted when a plaintiff's lawyer from Alaska sent internal company documents obtained during a court case against Eli Lilly, the maker of Zyprexa, to a reporter at the *New York Times*. The newspaper reported that the documents, which included e-mail, marketing material, sales projections, and scientific reports, showed that the company had hidden information about the drug's potential to cause severe side effects. The company told sales representatives to downplay its own published data showing that a third of patients gained an average of twenty-two pounds or more on the drug within a year. Some gained as much as a hundred pounds. In a March 2002 e-mail message, for instance, a Lilly manager recommended against giving psychiatrists guidance about how to treat diabetes, because that might make them reconsider prescribing the drug: "Although M.D.'s like objective, educational materials, having our reps provide some with diabetes [information] would further build its association to Zyprexa." The documents rocketed around the Internet and were subsequently published on several Web sites. Lilly sought and obtained a court injunction, ordering anybody who had a copy of its documents to return them promptly or risk being sued. But trying to get all of them back was a little like trying to stuff toothpaste back into the tube. As of January 15, 2007, the documents sat defiantly available on Swedish servers, under a domain registered on Christmas Island, a tiny, coconut-tree-studded chunk of volcanic rock in the Indian Ocean.

Information, please

It's tempting to lay the blame for all of this—the distortions in the medical literature, the co-opting of academic thought leaders, the wooing of physicians with lavish dinners, free samples, and trips to exotic locales—on either the pharmaceutical industry or the FDA, the agency that is supposed to regulate it. Marcia Angell and other critics charge that the FDA's record on ensuring the public's safety is poor. The agency has approved dangerous drugs far too quickly and then failed to monitor them once they hit the market. Meanwhile, say critics, the drug industry is designing biased clinical trials, recruiting compliant academics to run them, controlling the analysis and write-up of the results, and then using freebies to help peddle its slanted results to gullible doctors. The industry has also engaged in the immoral, though not necessarily illegal, practice of deliberately hiding potentially deadly side effects of drugs like Vioxx and Prozac and then paying academics to mislead their fellow physicians.

But there's plenty of blame to go around beyond the drug companies and the FDA. For all of its faults, the pharmaceutical industry has been doing what it is supposed to do, which is come up with new drugs and make money for stockholders. The rules for drug companies are set up such that their fiduciary responsibility lies with shareholders, not with doctors and patients—despite advertising slogans like Merck's "Where patients come first." No drug company is going to take it upon itself to quit marketing aggressively, for the simple reason that it would be slaughtered on Wall Street when profits fell. The FDA could be doing a much better job of holding companies to a higher standard of evidence before it approves their drugs. It has the regulatory powers allowing it to require companies to conduct postmarketing studies in the event that safety officers suspect there's a potential problem with a drug, as they did with Vioxx. Yet the agency rarely forces the industry to follow through, even when it does ask for additional studies. When it comes to covert marketing and poorly conducted and interpreted research, though, the agency does not have much control over academic researchers and doctors in private practice, the people in the best position to put a stop to influence peddling in medicine. After all, doctors don't have to accept free samples and gifts, and it's up to their professional societies, not the FDA, to set codes of ethical conduct. Physicians don't have to attend continuing-medicine-education courses that are underwritten by industry, and they don't have to let all those cute drug reps in the door. There's no reason for academics to serve as paid advocates for drugs, and stopping the practice is more a job for their institutions than for the FDA. And nobody is forcing editors to publish the thousands of poorly designed, biased, or badly interpreted articles that appear on an annual basis in their medical journals.

Why have they all continued to do it, despite overwhelming evidence that ignoring the problem is harming patients? Partly because, as Carl Elliott so delicately puts it, "change is in nobody's financial interest." But they also do it because the harm can only be seen in the aggregate, while the responsibility for it is diffuse. The individual doctor can't imagine that his prescribing habits are being influenced by something as insignificant as a free meal. The academic can't see anything wrong with taking a speaking fee from a pharmaceutical company, as long as he already agrees with everything his corporate sponsor wants him to say. The researcher may think there's nothing amiss when she lets a drug company design the study she conducts, or control the data she's allowed to publish, because the company has deep enough pockets to hire the best clinical trial designers and the finest statisticians. She also knows that if she objects to their rules, she may not get any more funding. The journal editors pretend that they can publish industry-funded trials and editorials written by academics with conflicts of interest because peer review will catch any improprieties. Besides, they say, if they refused to print papers and editorials written by academics with conflicts of interest, they wouldn't have anything to publish. Only when all the pieces are put together is it possible for the public to see that companies have commandeered the very machinery of medical information.

There are signs that the cozy relationship between the industry and physicians has begun to cool ever so slightly. Half a dozen books have come out in the past five years, many of them written by physicians who are critical of the industry's influence over medical research. At the same time, two physician organizations, No Free Lunch and the American Medical Student Association, have adopted platforms that encourage doctors to eschew gifts and free samples, to avoid drug reps, and to seek out more objective information about drugs.* Leana Wen, past president of the American Medical Student Association, says medical students are becoming increasingly aware of the need to wean themselves from industry influence. "In 2002, our PharmFree campaign was first launched at our annual convention," she

---

* Their campaigns have proved to be a tough slog. In 2005, No Free Lunch was barred by the American College of Physicians from renting a ten-by-ten-foot space in the exhibit hall at the college's annual meeting (where Pfizer, the maker of Celebrex, occupied a twenty-five-hundred-square-foot booth, and Sepracor, the maker of Lunesta, took up ten thousand square feet). When No Free Lunch members tried to distribute a brochure to attending physicians, they were ordered to stop, and the College of Physicians rushed to assure its exhibitors that the college had nothing to do with No Free Lunch. There was a delicious irony here: The brochure No Free Lunch wanted to distribute contained the American College of Physicians' own ethical guidelines, which instruct member physicians to decline industry gifts, no matter how small.

says. "I was at a seminar with Bob Goodman, founder of No Free Lunch. He gave a talk about pharmaceutical company influence. There was stony silence at the end of his presentation. No applause. Then the audience bombarded him with angry comments, like 'I want my pizza' and 'You have no right to tell me what I can't do.'" At the 2005 convention, says Wen, Marcia Angell spoke about the same issue and received a standing ovation.

Academic medical centers are also becoming increasingly aware of the need to reduce industry influence on both research and prescribing practices. In 2006, after the *San Jose Mercury News* published an embarrassing exposé of conflicts of interest among Stanford University medical school faculty, the school banned drug reps, free food, and gifts from its hospital. Several medical centers, including Kaiser hospitals, Yale, and the University of Virginia, had already barred drug reps from their facilities and forbidden their physicians to accept gifts. In response, the drug industry is already shifting some of its marketing effort away from drug reps. In early 2007, Pfizer announced it was cutting ten thousand jobs worldwide, including a 10 percent reduction in its sales force.

Concerned doctors have taken it upon themselves to help their colleagues learn to read the medical literature more critically. The Cochrane Collaboration, for instance, performs meta-analyses, or studies of studies, to provide physicians with the most valid data. InfoPOEMs is an online subscription service that sifts through the medical literature and then translates the valid studies into simple, clear language. Founded in the 1990s by three family practitioners and a pharmacologist, InfoPOEMs, for Patient Oriented Evidence That Matters, sorts through more than two thousand articles published each month in a hundred medical journals, looking for the few articles that could make a real difference in patient care. The research team, all of whom are experts in dissecting clinical trials, pick apart each article to make sure the results are credible. Only about one in forty studies makes the cut. Qualifying articles are then summarized and posted on the InfoPOEMs Web site and sent to doctors who subscribe to daily e-mail alerts. For example, one recent alert informed subscribers of the results of a large study looking at vitamin E supplements, which showed that contrary to widespread belief, they don't help patients with heart disease. They do, however, slightly increase the risk of death.

When doctors pay more attention to the Cochrane Collaboration and to InfoPOEMs than to drug reps, and when they learn to read the literature more critically, they will undoubtedly do a better job of treating their patients. And the journal editors will raise the quality of the papers they publish by tightening the rules for who can write them. But as valuable as the efforts of the InfoPOEMs team may be, along with those of Michael Stuart and Sheri Strite's courses for doctors discussed in chapter 5, and groups like No Free Lunch, they can't fix the problem on their own. Putting medicine on more scientific footing, and ensuring that patients aren't harmed unnecessarily by useless or dangerous procedures and products, is going to take a multipronged campaign. There's growing awareness among medical professional societies that conflict of interest is a real problem that isn't going to go away if they ignore it. The press is (finally) investigating the myriad ways in which medicine's financial ties to the pharmaceutical industry are harming patients and distorting medical science. Many doctors don't want to have to change their ways—a doctor at a recent medical meeting stood up in the back of the room where a speaker was discussing the issue of gifts to doctors and said, "I like getting pens and sticky notepads and free lunches. Don't ruin it for me!" But as the public grows increasingly aware of the insidious effects of those gifts, it will be more and more embarrassing for doctors to take them. At the same time, academic medical centers are recognizing that they need to scrutinize more closely the relationships between their clinical researchers and the industry. Even if reform can only come slowly, now that the issue is out in the open it won't go away.

That still leaves the question of how to get research that we need done. In giving the industry increasing responsibility over the years for funding clinical studies, says John Abramson, we have granted it the power to leverage the direction that medical research takes. "The primary mission of medical research has been transformed," he says. "It used to be all about gathering information to improve health. Now, clinical research is aimed at gathering information that will maximize return on investment."

Given that drug and device companies are in business to sell products, not to increase medical knowledge, it's not surprising that they don't want to pay for research that might hurt the bottom line. For doctors, patients, and payers, however, this creates two problems. The first is that by allowing drug and device companies to become their principal source of information, doctors have been lulled, as we've seen, into prescribing and using billions of dollars' worth of products without demanding unbiased evidence that they are actually improving health. (Many people mistakenly believe that the FDA requires companies to produce such evidence before gaining approval to market their products. It doesn't. In the case of most new devices, the agency only asks that they be substantially equivalent to an existing device; for most drugs, companies must show only that their products are as safe as and more effective than a placebo.)

The second problem is that letting industry dictate what research gets performed has meant there is often little relationship between what we pay for devices and drugs and what they are actually worth. Together, the drug and device industries took in more than three hundred billion dollars in 2006, roughly 15 percent of our total health care spending. Implantable devices, defibrillators, artificial knees, cardiac stents, and other bionic body parts amounted to thirty-six billion dollars. Spending on drugs and devices is the fastest-growing sector of health care costs. Outlays for drugs doubled between 1995 and 2003, owing in part to more prescriptions but also to rising prices, which went up 7.2 percent, nearly three times the inflation rate. Of course, many of those drugs and devices helped patients enormously. I have a friend in her forties with two young children who would not be here today if not for the pacemaker implanted in her twenties that keeps her heart ticking. She's just one of millions of Americans whose lives would be shorter or more painful if not for a device or a drug. But what's not so clear is whether we're paying the right price for all those medical products. Was the five billion dollars we spent on Vioxx and Celebrex in 2004 really necessary, considering the fact that one drug was pulled from the market for killing people and the other one is no better than over-the-counter ibuprofen? Is a three-thousand-dollar drug-coated cardiac stent nearly three times better than an eight-hundred-dollar bare-metal stent? Recent research says maybe not.

When you factor in the harm caused by the overuse of drugs, devices, and procedures, it starts to seem completely crazy that we don't have a better system for assessing the clinical value of medical technologies, the degree to which they actually improve the lives of patients. Ray Elliott, the chairman of Zimmer Holdings, the world's largest manufacturer of knee and hip replacements, told investors at a Bank of America conference in 2005: "There's a lot of bell-and-whistle stuff in this industry over the last five or six years where you got pretty good money for stuff that was pretty fluffy."

We can't control costs or improve the quality of health care without better evidence for what works and what doesn't, and it is unreasonable to expect companies to produce the research that's necessary to give us that evidence. Getting medicine that's based on reality, rather than potential return on investment, requires a new source of funding for clinical research. We collectively, as taxpayers and health insurance purchasers, have to find ways to fill the gaping holes in the science of medicine. If we want better health care at the best price, we need valid and clinically useful information about devices and the wide array of medical practices that have never been put to any kind of real test.

David Eddy, a heart surgeon turned mathematician turned health care economist and a leader in the evidence-based medicine movement, estimates that as little as 15 percent of what doctors do is backed up by valid evidence. What's the best treatment for chronic sinusitis? Surgery? Antibiotics? Nobody really knows. How well do fertility treatments really work? (Probably not as well as fertility clinics advertise.) What's the most effective way to bring down skyrocketing rates of diabetes? New drugs? Screening people for high blood sugar? Sending patients to weight-loss clinics? Does fetal monitoring reduce the risk of a bad outcome during childbirth, or just increase the chances of a Caesarean section? Does screening for prostate cancer with the PSA test save lives? If prostate cancer is found, which treatment is best? (There are four kinds of surgeries, several types of implantable radioactive seeds, and multiple external radiation regimens to choose from.) These are just a few of the questions that can only be answered if we stop leaving the job of funding clinical research to the pharmaceutical industry.

NINE The Doctor Isn't In

THERE WAS A time when Gordon Peabody thought that being a doctor was the greatest job in the world. As a pediatrician just starting out in Spokane, Washington, in the 1970s, he had colleagues he liked and respected and a full practice of wonderful parents and patients. He didn't mind going to the emergency room if one of his patients was injured, or staying up all night in the hospital with an asthmatic child. In fact, he relished it; it felt good to help someone, to make a difference in a child's life. He would come home from the hospital in the morning, wash up, and head for the office, where he would see ten or twelve patients in the morning and the same number after lunch. He felt proud when the parents of his patients stopped him on the street or in a store to thank him for caring for their children. Most of his patients were insured; some were on Medicaid, and a few had no insurance at all, but he and the two other pediatricians in the practice felt a duty to care for their share of the poor. They could afford it, because their insured patients provided a decent living. It was a good life.

All that began to change sometime in the 1980s. Peabody can't put his finger on an exact date, but one day he began to realize that he didn't feel like he was doing his patients any good, and that practicing medicine was no longer rewarding. His colleagues felt the same way. They stood around over coffee in the hospital or at medical meetings, complaining that they could no longer practice medicine the way they wanted to, the way they had been taught. They were buried in paperwork and were being forced to hire more office help to deal with the increasingly confusing welter of rules and roadblocks that insurers threw up before they would pay. The primary care doctors—the pediatricians, general internists, and family practitioners—weren't permitted to send a patient to a specialist as they saw fit. Now, they had to get permission from the insurance company—from some clerk who sometimes had nothing more than a high school education. They had to refer their patients to specialists who appeared on a list of insurance companies' "in-network" doctors, whatever that meant—all they knew was they were sending their patients to doctors they had never met and therefore couldn't entirely trust. To top it off, long-standing patients, people they had nursed through ailments and divorces and car accidents, were no longer allowed to see them. In their place came patients who had picked the doctor's name from a list, who felt no obligation to show up for appointments, who distrusted the doctor if he happened to suggest that the drug or test the patient had learned about from a friend might not be necessary. The doctors were seeing their expenses go up and their incomes go down; meanwhile, insurance company executives were raking in the profits. The name of their problem was managed care.

It wasn't supposed to be that way. When the managed care revolution was launched in the 1980s, insurers proclaimed an end to the era of the high-priced specialist and the rebirth of primary care. Patients, they said, would learn to be responsible consumers, and managed care would reduce their ever-increasing out-of-pocket expenses. Primary care doctors, the thinkers of medicine, would be restored to their former place of power and authority as the physicians in charge, the quarterbacks of good care, the doctors who saw the whole patient, not just her parts. Best of all, managed care would rein in both unnecessary care and out-of-control health care costs.

But it didn't work out as planned. Gordon Peabody was an ordinary doctor in private practice, not unlike thousands of other primary care physicians across the country who saw their livelihoods change with the advent of managed care. Like many young college graduates in the late 1960s, Peabody went into medicine because he was smart, he did well in school, and he wanted to do something important with his life. He wanted to make a difference. He didn't go into medicine to make a lot of money. "I thought anybody who made fifty thousand dollars a year and who had a hundred-thousand-dollar house was rich," he says. He was drafted before medical school, and once he got out of residency, he did his time in the air force before starting his practice. Once he began practicing, he turned out to be a good doctor, intelligent, hardworking, and kind.

But managed care drove him out of medicine, as it did countless other primary care physicians, and he agreed to tell his story as a way of explaining why dedicated doctors would decide to abandon their profession and their patients. He asked that his name and details of his life be changed because he still lives in the town where he practiced, and he still sees former colleagues, doctors who in his opinion forgot the part of the Hippocratic oath that bound them to put their patients' needs above their own. His story is important because it illuminates many of the changes managed care brought to American medicine—most of them for the worse. Embraced by employers and patients as a way to control double-digit increases in health insurance premiums, managed care did manage to rein costs in for a time. By the late 1990s, however, managed care was paradoxically encouraging doctors to provide unnecessary care, while simultaneously driving a wedge between patients and their physicians. But managed care's most devastating legacy is that it has damaged primary care, the backbone of the nation's health care system.

Gordon Peabody grew up in Pennsylvania, just outside of Philadelphia, the son of a legal secretary and a clothing salesman. He attended medical school at Cornell University with no financial help from his parents, scraping by on odd jobs, scholarships, and loans. He graduated in 1967 owing thirty-five thousand dollars. When Johns Hopkins offered him a two-year residency in pediatrics, he turned it down because the salary was twelve hundred dollars a year, not enough to cover expenses and pay back his loans. His residency at the University of Virginia paid four times that. He and his wife, a schoolteacher, lived in a seventy-dollar-a-month, one-bedroom walk-up apartment. The apartment was so small, Peabody recalls, "you could sit in the living room and watch TV and stir the spaghetti at the same time." After completing his residency, he entered the air force, which sent him to Mountain Home, Idaho, where he served as a base pediatrician. In 1973, the Peabodys moved with their infant son to Spokane, just east of Seattle, to join a pediatric practice with two other physicians. Peabody was told he could expect to earn about fifteen thousand dollars his first year— the equivalent of seventy thousand dollars today.

Peabody loved being in practice. At that time, the local hospital had no pediatric intensive care unit, so Peabody cared for the sickest children himself, the ones who ended up in the hospital with asthma or seizures or uncontrolled juvenile diabetes. "I would stay up four to six hours, stabilizing a kid," he says. "There was an increased stress level, and increased malpractice risk, but it was very rewarding. It's the complexity that's interesting." He remembers one case, an anorexic teenage girl who was hospitalized for weeks, strapped down and fed intravenously. "She was so terribly ill. I would spend every day with her, before rounds, after rounds. I told her, 'I'm not going to let you kill yourself. I'm going to dance at your wedding.'" Once she was released from the hospital, says Peabody, "I took her on eating dates. Her mother would drop her off, and we would go out, and her goal was to eat two french fries." As promised, he danced at her wedding. Recently, she called Peabody with questions about her pregnancy.

Spokane was growing when Peabody went into practice, and the pediatric group's business thrived. By the mid-1980s his group included seven doctors and four nurse practitioners. Together they cared for twenty-five thousand children. They took their share of Medicaid patients and children who were uninsured. Medicaid paid lower fees than private insurance, but the practice could absorb the difference. Before managed care came along, primary care doctors did well. Not as well as specialists, of course, but Peabody was making about two hundred thousand dollars a year by the time he was in his late forties.

At first, the doctors in his practice were only dimly aware of managed care, because the vast majority of their patients continued to be covered under traditional fee-for-service plans. With this form of insurance, also known as an indemnity plan, employers paid most of the premium, and the

insurer reimbursed patients for 80 percent of the doctor's fee—for practically anything the doctor ordered. There seemed to be no limit to what
insurers would pay. By 1980, there were nearly 400,000 physicians in practice, or about 163 doctors per 100,000 in the population. That was up from
260,000 physicians in 1965, the legacy of medical school expansion that
had been underwritten by the federal government in the '60s to reverse a
perceived doctor shortage. The idea of putting more doctors into practice
was partly to ensure a supply of physicians, but also to keep their fees low.
Instead, more doctors meant fewer patients per doctor, which led them to
increase their fees and deliver more care per patient: more office visits,
more tests, more surgeries. The rising number of doctors also led to increasing specialization. Now there were surgeons who only did gall blad-
ders, orthopedists who focused on backs. The more of these procedures
doctors did, the more they were paid by insurers—who simply passed their
rising costs on to employers.

By the early 1980s, employers were in a panic. Fee-for-service plans were
an important part of the benefits package companies used to retain workers,
but with the economy sagging and the price of health insurance premiums
rising at double-digit rates, employers began putting pressure on insurers
to get a grip on costs. Insurers had long known that the only health plans
whose costs weren't going through the roof were the traditional health
maintenance organizations, the true HMOs like Kaiser Permanente, in California and much of the West, and Group Health Cooperative of Puget Sound,
in Seattle. In these so-called staff-model HMOs, doctors worked in groups
comprising several specialties; their salaries were paid by integrated insurance plans, which also ran the HMOs' hospitals. Patients paid a yearly premium, just like with indemnity plans, but unlike traditional insurance
companies, HMOs did not give their doctors and hospitals free rein to decide what patients needed. Instead, HMOs set yearly budgets for their clinics and hospitals. Within those budgets, the doctors set priorities for how
best to maintain the health of the population of patients for whom they
were responsible. They tended to practice more conservatively than doctors
in fee-for-service plans, and HMOs were generally less likely to embrace a
new technology, like faster CT scanners, or a new surgical procedure, until

it had been shown to benefit patients. HMOs also monitored the performance of individual doctors and groups, as well as the satisfaction of their patients.

At staff-model HMOs, insurers knew, higher quality care was being delivered at much lower cost than in traditional indemnity plans. Patients in HMOs spent fewer days in the hospital, on average, than patients covered under fee-for-service plans, and they made fewer visits to specialists. When researchers scrutinized the quality of care HMO patients received, they found it "at least comparable to care in other health care facilities, if not superior."

Yet traditional HMOs had never been able to expand much beyond northern California; Seattle; and Rochester, Minnesota, home to the Mayo Clinic, largely because of opposition from the American Medical Association. The AMA considered prepaid, staff-model HMOs another threat, like Medicare, to the autonomy and income of its members. In the 1930s, physicians who joined prepaid group practices were often denied membership in local medical societies. The societies also strong-armed hospitals (at the behest of the AMA) into blackballing physicians belonging to salaried group practices. In one instance in the '40s, a doctor who worked in Washington, D.C., for a branch of Seattle's Group Health took a patient to a hospital for surgery and he and his patient were barred from the operating room. The AMA's antipathy toward HMOs not only prevented many doctors from joining them but also seeped outward to patients, who believed the AMA's propaganda portraying HMOs as badly run and interested only in denying patients care to save money. By 1970, there were only thirty-three HMOs in the entire country, serving a scant three million people.

A little more than a decade later, with stagflation in full bloom and employers clamoring for relief from mounting health care costs, private insurers felt emboldened to exert some measure of control over physicians and hospitals. The old fee-for-service way, they said, rewarded greedy doctors, who padded their incomes by giving patients unneeded tests and procedures and putting them in the hospital unnecessarily. Their version of HMOs, dubbed managed care, would impose discipline on medical providers. Now, doctors would no longer be paid for every office visit and every procedure they performed. They would be paid to "manage" their patients' care. Quality medicine, said the insurers, is cost-effective medicine. In cost-effective medicine, doctors would neither withhold needed care nor deliver care that was unnecessary. At least, that was the slogan.

Like most doctors, Peabody and his partners were only to happy to oblige when patients began coming in and asking them to sign up with their managed care providers. Peabody didn't want to lose patients, and signing up was easy. All he had to do was send in a form to the insurer, and he would be included in the company's list of preferred providers. Of course, the word "provider" seemed a little strange, as if he were a merchant, not a doctor, but he signed the contract because he wanted to keep his patients and their parents happy. As more people left fee-for-service and enrolled in managed care, Peabody noticed he was getting calls out of the blue from parents who said he was their childrens' new doctor. The old way meant that he got new patients based on his reputation. Another physician or a current parent recommended him, and the new family came in already primed to trust him as a competent and caring pediatrician. The new way meant parents found his name in "the book," the directory of in-network providers they got from their employers. From their perspective, he was no better or worse than the next guy on the list.

Pretty soon, Peabody and his partners noticed something else: more and more paperwork. Managed care companies began sending them notices, instructing them on how to manage their office and care for their patients. They were told to put a sticky note on the records of patients who needed to be tested for allergies. They received the vaccine schedule for children from infancy to adolescence and instructions on how to spot scoliosis, or curvature of the spine, a strep infection, meningitis. It was as if managed care thought they had never attended medical school. Managed care companies sent them lists indicating which labs they could use for blood tests, which specialists were acceptable for referrals, and which hospitals their patients could be admitted to. And each company had its own list. The office began to fill up with three-ring binders to accommodate all the paper. They had to hire first one administrative assistant, then another, to handle it all.

Over the course of a decade, overhead costs went from 30 percent of their income to sixty.

Peabody worried every time he referred a patient to one of the specialists on the managed care company lists, or sent blood samples to their designated laboratories. What if the lab made a mistake? What if the specialist was a jerk with kids, or worse, incompetent? In the old days, he sent patients to doctors he trusted. Now, he was sending them into the great unknown. On top of it all, making a referral or admitting a patient to the hospital required a telephone call to the insurer to get permission. It was 1-800-MOTHER-MAY-I medicine. If he wasn't on the phone himself, one of the office assistants the practice had been forced to hire was begging an insurer to approve a prescription or a test. As more of his patients enrolled in managed care, Peabody began to see that this new insurance was not even remotely like fee-for-service.

It also wasn't anything like the true HMOs, with their prepaid plans and salaries, that it was supposed to be modeled on. In fact, it was less about managing care and more about managing money. Managed care companies borrowed the cost-control policies from the true HMOs, while ignoring the need for doctors who were committed to a new way of practicing medicine. Companies began squeezing price concessions out of hospitals and pressuring physicians to accept lower and lower fees by threatening to take away their patients. Doctors, notes Guy Clifton, a Texas neurosurgeon, "were overwhelmed by a cartel of large insurance companies, all determined to find the level at which doctors and hospitals refused to work, and then to pay just over that." The balance of power, which had been firmly fixed in the hands of doctors for most of the past century, was shifting. As more and more patients enrolled in managed care, doctors like Gordon Peabody were forced to accept the terms it was offering. "I could see the writing on the wall in 1989," he says. "I didn't want any part of it, but I didn't have any choice."

Double booked

In the early days of the managed care revolution, patients didn't notice much difference between the old fee-for-service and the new way, except for the price. Most employers offered a choice between traditional fee-for-service; one of the new, so-called HMOs; and a PPO, or preferred provider organization, doctors who had agreed to work for lower fees. The employee's share of the premium was lower for HMOs and PPOs than for fee-for-service, and so were his out-of-pocket expenses. Under the old indemnity plans, the patient had to pay 20 percent or more; under managed care, there was at most a five-or ten-dollar co-pay for an office visit. If you didn't like managed care, you could always go back to fee-for-service. But then employers began dropping the more-expensive fee-for-service option and offering only managed care plans. When that happened, patients began to discover they were expected to jump through hoops that had never been part of going to the doctor before. Under fee-for-service, they went to the doctor of their choice whenever they wanted, and the insurer paid for whatever the doctor ordered. If you had a skin problem, you went to the dermatologist; a sore knee, the orthopedist. Now, you had to go to your primary care physician to get a referral slip before going to a specialist. There was an 800 number to call before undergoing an expensive procedure. New mothers discovered they were allowed only twenty-four hours in the hospital after giving birth. If the physician you had been seeing for years wasn't on the in-network list provided by your employer's managed care provider, well, too bad; you would just have to get naked in front of a new doctor. When your employer switched to yet another plan the following year, you had to look for a doctor all over again.

Peabody began to feel as if there were a revolving door at the entrance to his office. Patients disappeared when their parents' employers switched insurers and he was no longer one of the in-network doctors on their plans. In their place came patients whose parents had picked his name out of the book. The number of no-shows started to rise. What did they care if they missed an appointment? They didn't know him from Adam. Peabody desperately wanted to tell the chronic no-shows to find another doctor, he says, "but of course, they would report you to the plan if you did." That could mean losing the end-of-the-year bonus the plans dangled in front of doctors to get them to toe the line, to keep costs down while somehow simultaneously managing to keep patients happy.

With each passing month, Peabody could see his practice changing. In 1985, nearly nineteen million Americans were enrolled in a managed care plan or a traditional HMO. By 1990, that number had leaped to 36.5 million. Five years later, a majority of Americans with employer-based health care coverage were enrolled in managed care. Each plan imposed a slightly different set of rules. Some PPOs simply pushed doctors to accept reduced fees for office visits, procedures, and surgeries by threatening to stop sending them patients. Other plans paid a capitated, or flat, fee per patient, a system that loosely mirrored the budgets that constrained traditional HMOs. Under a capitated plan, if the primary care physician sent a patient to a specialist or ordered a test, the cost would be deducted from the primary care doctor's "account," a pool of money he would receive at the end of the year. Capitation worked best for everybody, Peabody and his partners were told, if they thought twice before sending patients off to specialists willy-nilly or ordering expensive tests. All of which was a good idea in theory, given the unnecessary care that was rife in the system. But capitation turned primary care doctors into mini–insurance companies, forcing them to assume the risk associated with the possibility that some of their patients could wind up being very sick and very expensive, which meant the doctor would lose money. If they had patients who never got sick, of course, they would make money, but doctors had no way of knowing what kind of patients managed care would send them. Unlike real HMOs, individual doctors couldn't risk-adjust, or set their fees according to how sick they expected patients would be over the course of a year. Some doctors made money by denying patients care even when they needed it, while others lost their shirts with capitation. One Chicago family physician joined a capitated plan and was handed four patients who subsequently received back surgery, costing him fifteen thousand dollars out of his own pocket after the end-of-the-year pot of money was used up.

Managed care had other carrots and sticks to use to force doctors to comply with its cost-cutting measures. Companies offered bonuses, but only if doctors refrained from ordering what the plans considered to be too many tests or procedures. They punished primary care doctors who sent their patients to expensive specialists or prescribed high-priced drugs by "deselecting" them, or dropping them from the in-network lists. Sometimes the plans based their decisions about what constituted too many tests and unnecessary drugs on good science. They tried to get doctors to refrain from ordering an MRI for uncomplicated back pain, or sending a patient with a suspected ulcer to a gastroenterologist without trying to treat him first with drugs. But doctors didn't know that they were overtreating their patients, or that by sending them off to a specialist unnecessarily, they were being wasteful. All they knew was that when they were deselected, they could wake up one morning to discover that they suddenly had dozens fewer patients. For some doctors, that simply meant lost income. For others, like Peabody, it also meant saying good-bye to patients he had cared for—and cared about—for many years.

Wall Street only added to physicians' misery when it began to view health care as a moneymaking opportunity. Once Medicare began insuring the elderly, there was a steady stream of money flowing through the system, and little likelihood of a downturn. Disease and sickness were not going to go away anytime soon, and as the population aged, demand for health care was only going to keep rising. At the same time, health care was highly fragmented, with hundreds of different businesses: hospitals, doctors, HMOs, medical device companies, assisted living centers, pharmacies, testing facilities, and insurance companies. There was little coordination between all the moving parts and huge inefficiencies in the system. Wall Street began to envision a new business model for medicine, one that would put money into investors' pockets. Remaking this sector offered what *Investment Dealers' Digest* called a "once-in-a-lifetime opportunity for creative investment bankers."

That opportunity took many forms. Nonprofit hospitals were snapped up by for-profit conglomerations that were underwritten by investors. New managed care companies emerged to compete with older insurers like Aetna and Blue Cross. Wall Street was soon bankrolling an entirely new type of corporation called a physician practice management company, or PPM. The idea behind PPMs was that they would bring good management to doctors' offices, which were, after all, small, and often poorly run, businesses. PPMs promised to provide economies of scale by pooling administrative duties and billing for multiple physicians. You treat the patient, PPMs said to doctors, and leave the business side of medicine to us. Physicians were only too ready to sign up. A few small group practices and solo practitioners sold their businesses outright to PPMs in exchange for a salary and stock options. Other doctors agreed to pay PPMs a percentage of their revenue, often as much as 15 percent, in exchange for new equipment and administrative services. By 1998, 10 percent of the nation's nearly seven hundred thousand physicians were affiliated with a PPM. PPMs, crowed Wall Street pundits, were "the brave new world of health care."

In the end, PPMs proved to be an empty promise. They made a few Wall Street entrepreneurs rich, but they failed to add value either to patient care or to doctors' incomes. One of the first PPMs to rise and then fall was MedPartners, which went public in 1995. Within two years, the company was affiliated with thirteen thousand physicians across thirty-seven states and had grown to be a $6-billion-a-year business. With money rolling in from investors and the company's physicians, CEO Larry House built himself a twenty-one-bedroom, twenty-two-bathroom mansion with a guitar-shaped driveway and Italian white marble floors. But physicians who accepted stock in MedPartners as part of their payment didn't do as well. The value of their stock plummeted in 1998, when auditors discovered that the $54.4 million profit the company had posted in the first quarter of that year was actually an $840.8 million loss. By the fourth quarter, losses had reached $1.2 billion, and MedPartners declared bankruptcy, leaving the doctors who had joined the company with nothing but their medical diplomas. As insurers continued to reduce physicians' fees, doctors found themselves being squeezed by both managed care and the PPMs, which continued to demand their pound of flesh from the physicians' shrinking reimbursements. Family practitioner Steven Myers, who worked for a clinic owned by a PPM in Pittsfield, Massachusetts, estimated that in 2000, the last year he practiced in the PPM, he cleared only $15,000.

Meanwhile, managed care companies continued to extract price concessions from physicians. With each new contract, they offered less and less per patient in capitated plans, first it would be $15 a patient per month, then $12, then $9. Then $6. PPO plans also dropped their reimbursement payment rates for everything from office visits to procedures. In 1995, aver-age income for primary care doctors was about $135,000 a year. Specialists made almost twice that amount on average, while some specialties, like in-vasive cardiology and orthopedics, were averaging more than $300,000 an-nually. By 2005, physician incomes across the board had fallen by 5 percent, but primary care incomes had tumbled the furthest. The average primary care doctor was making $161,000, a 10 percent loss over ten years after adjusting for inflation.

Primary care doctors felt as if they'd fallen down the rabbit hole. Like Al-ice and the Red Queen, they were running as fast as they could just to stay in the same place. Many responded to their declining incomes by "bulking up," or increasing the number of patients in their practice. That meant they had to either find more hours in a day or see more patients per hour. In the early years of his practice, Peabody would see at most two dozen patients a day. Now, under managed care, he needed to see thirty or forty. Some physi-cians were jamming in as many as thirty patients in a morning session and another thirty in the afternoon. It wasn't so much that managed care com-panies were telling doctors they had to see more patients per hour; it was a matter of economics. Doctors needed the extra patients if they wanted to maintain their incomes. To many in the business world, more patients per hour seemed like a good thing. It meant that doctors were working harder; they were more productive. But this change in the way doctors practiced primary care helped shred the already increasingly fragile relationship be-tween physician and patient. On top of seeing more patients, the doctors in Peabody's practice began double booking appointments to make up for all the no-shows, the way airlines oversell seats. "Then one day everybody would show up," says Peabody, "and all your patients are mad at you. Then they would report that to the health plan."

Horror stories

Eventually the press caught wind of the frustration among doctors and patients, and by the late 1980s, the managed care horror stories began appearing, tales of patients being refused care by heartless insurers. When a Michigan mother of two in her early thirties complained to her primary care physician of vaginal bleeding and pain, the doctor referred her to a gynecologist. The bleeding and pain persisted, so she asked to see the gynecologist again, but, she claimed, the doctor refused, saying she was not sick enough. The woman took herself to the emergency room, where she was diagnosed with advanced cervical cancer. When the woman brought suit, her managed care company said it could not be held responsible for the behavior of the two doctors. Mary Jane and John Bohnen's son, Daniel, was accidentally shot in the face with shotgun pellets. A few minutes before Mary Jane was to take Daniel to the hospital to have his right eye repaired, she got a phone call from their insurer. The managed care company wanted Daniel to get a second opinion from one of its medical consultants before the surgery. Even though Daniel's surgeon had warned that any delay could cost the eight-year-old his sight, his mother did as she was asked. The medical consultant quickly confirmed that Daniel needed surgery, but by the time he went to the hospital, it was too late. Without admitting guilt, the company settled the malpractice suit brought by the Bohnens for $1.2 million.

The subtext of such stories carried a powerful message of good versus evil, of greed crushing hope. Every story had a victim, vulnerable and sick, who was denied care by a villainous, unfeeling corporation. Only occasionally did a doctor appear as the hero. These kinds of stories proved irresistible to the media. From 1980 to 1990, only 137 news articles were written about HMOs and managed care. Over the next decade, the number of stories swelled to 2,659, the vast majority of them tales of care denied. Readers were particularly outraged by stories of managed care "drive-through deliveries," the practice of sending women and their babies home within twenty-four hours of birth. Managed care companies based this coverage decision on sound scientific research, which had been conducted by Kaiser Permanente. Most mothers and their newborns, said the research, could safely go home within a day, sometimes even within twelve hours after birth. The secret to Kaiser's success was excellent prenatal care; follow-up visits by nurses to the family's home; and communication between doctor and patient about the decision. When managed care mandated no more than twenty-four-hour stays, it too provided nursing follow-up at home and allowed doctors to argue with a reviewer if they thought the mother or baby needed to be in the hospital longer. But many doctors hesitated to ask for more time for their patients, for fear they would be dropped from the insurer's list of physicians if they argued about the twenty-four-hour stay too often.

Soon there were stories in the media about mothers and babies suffering harm from being sent home too early. New Jersey residents Steve and Michelle Bauman delivered heartbreaking testimony before Congress in 1995 after their infant daughter, Michelina, died from a strep infection two days after she was born. Had mother and baby not been discharged only twenty-eight hours after the birth, said the couple, "her symptoms would have surfaced and professional trained staff would have taken the proper steps, so that we could have planned a christening instead of a funeral."

Maybe their baby would have been saved by spending another day in the hospital, and maybe not, but the facts took a backseat to the power of the story, the idea that ordinary Americans were being screwed by the big, bad insurance business. Even feature films joined the bash-fest. In the 2002 film John Q, Denzel Washington played a father whose employer-provided HMO refused to cover a heart transplant for his dying son. Audiences cheered and stomped their feet when the father held an entire emergency room hostage at gunpoint until doctors agreed to perform the operation. Moviegoers exploded in applause when Helen Hunt's plucky heroine in 1997's *As Good as It Gets* called the bureaucrats controlling the care of her asthmatic son "fucking HMO bastard pieces of shit."

These films and others like them tapped into a deep well of resentment over what was happening to medicine. Patients hated having to switch doctors all the time. They disliked being forced to go to their primary care doctors to get a referral to a specialist. Half the time, they didn't even like their primary care doctor, a person whose name they had chosen off a list and whom they had known only since the last time their employer had changed managed care plans. They were fed up with not being able to get appointments, having to wait because doctors had double booked, and getting the bum's rush after only a few minutes with the doctor. By the mid-1990s, the economy was picking up, labor was getting tight, and employers began listening to their employees' complaints. Big companies told managed care to ease back on some of its most onerous restrictions. By 1995, some plans had loosened their restrictions on referrals, tests, and prescriptions. Many abandoned capitation entirely and retreated to PPOs, simply keeping a lid on doctors' fees.

That year, Peabody and his partners sold their pediatric practice to a larger, multispecialty group of doctors. Physicians all over the country were banding together into group practices in the hope that they could exert more leverage on insurers when it came time to sign managed care contracts. Peabody agreed to stay on with the new practice for five years, with a salary guarantee for the first three. The group paid its doctors according to a complex formula based on their specialty and productivity. Pediatricians and family practice doctors were at the bottom of the salary heap, and cardiologists and radiologists were at the top, with other specialists ranged in between. The more patients a doctor saw over the course of a year, the more the group earned as a whole from PPO and fee-for-service plans and the higher the individual physician's pay. A few of their patients were still in capitated plans, which meant the group was paid a flat fee for each of those patients. In addition to seeing patients, Peabody agreed to serve as the group's utilization reviewer, a post that was sometimes required by managed care. Large practices often assigned utilization reviewers to monitor what their doctors were doing, in an effort to police themselves, to keep their use of referrals, tests, and procedures low enough that they could avoid being punished by managed care companies.

Being the utilization reviewer of a large group was an eye-opener for Peabody. He began to see what insurers were up against in their efforts to control costs. "Even if the plan was capitated, the specialists weren't," he says. "They couldn't control themselves. This one ear, nose, and throat guy would take the tonsils out of anybody. But nobody wanted to criticize him. You couldn't say anything to the back surgeon, even though he was doing unnecessary surgery. Nobody wanted to be utilization reviewer because it meant you had to talk to your peers. These doctors did not want to be told what to do. It was worse than telling your three-year-old what to do." Utilization review was an idea managed care had borrowed from traditional HMOs, which routinely monitored the performance of individual doctors, groups of doctors, and entire hospitals. Traditional HMO doctors were accustomed to being reviewed, and most of the time, they welcomed the chance to learn how to practice medicine better. Doctors on the outside, however, saw utilization reviews as just one more burden imposed by managed care.

Peabody began to see doctors making decisions that were based not on what was best for the patient but on what kind of plan the patient was in. If a diabetic was in a PPO, for instance, which paid a fee for every office visit, the doctor would tell him to come back every few weeks in order to have his blood sugar monitored more closely. (The less a diabetic's blood sugar fluctuates, the more slowly he will develop the downstream effects of the disease, including heart disease, kidney damage, and blindness.) But if the patient was in a capitated plan, he might be told not to come back for months.

At the same time that managed care began to abandon capitation and loosen some of its restrictions, patients seemed to become even more demanding. They had seen the stories about patients who were refused needed care. They knew their doctors were all in cahoots with the insurance companies, just trying to save money. They came in angry, distrustful, and ready to complain if they didn't get the referrals they wanted, and the prescriptions for brand-name drugs—which were now being advertised on television. Peabody tried to practice medicine the way he had always done. He patiently explained to parents that their child's sore throat was caused by a virus and the antibiotics they wanted wouldn't make him get better any faster. When a kid came in with a sore back, he would tell her parents that a referral to an orthopedist wasn't necessary; she just needed to put fewer books in her backpack. But all that explaining took time, and time was the one thing he didn't have if he was going to see five patients an hour.

Primary care doctors found themselves in a catch-22. On the one hand, with managed care squeezing their fees, they had to see more patients in order to make any money. One the other hand, more patients meant shorter visits, and shorter visits meant less time to perform the delicate questioning that was often necessary to coax a patient out, to get him to describe symptoms that would lead to a correct diagnosis. Shorter visits meant having to rush through explaining to patients what was wrong with them and what they needed to do to get better. As late as 1993, the average visit with a family practitioner lasted twenty minutes. Seven years later, patients could expect on average only seven to ten minutes, scarcely enough time to discuss much of anything. Like how to use an inhaler properly. Or why it was important for a patient with high blood pressure to keep taking her medicine despite feeling better. Even when Peabody did take time to discuss things, parents didn't always believe him. They didn't want to hear that a trip to the neurologist wasn't necessary for a child who was having occasional headaches, or that earaches nearly always clear up on their own without antibiotics. They came in with their printouts from the Internet, ready to do battle if he tried to deny them care.

Many primary care physicians decided the fights weren't worth the effort. As soon as managed care relaxed some of its restrictions on referrals and prescriptions, many doctors began handing them out as fast as they could write them. Primary care doctors were no longer diagnosticians or healers, says Peabody; they were dispensers of referrals and prescriptions. One pediatrician in Peabody's practice started each day with a stack of referral slips in one hand and her prescription pad in the other. "She could get through more patients in a day than any other doctor in the practice," he says. Soon, Peabody made the bitter discovery that other physicians in the group were using him as an excuse, in his role as utilization reviewer, when they needed to say no to patients who wanted unnecessary treatment or referrals. "The doctor would say, 'Sure, you want to go to the dermatologist for a pimple, and your six-year-old hasn't even hit puberty? Sure, I'll send you. But I don't think Dr. Peabody will approve it.' Then the parent would decide Dr. Peabody was an SOB," he recalls. Patients began to complain to their managed care companies about Peabody, who had always received high marks in the past from his own patients. Now, he was being cast in the role of the bad guy, as Dr. No. At the end of the year, the medical director of the group told him he would not be getting a bonus; his ratings were too low. Peabody told him to find a new utilization reviewer.

Doctors had other ways of getting around managed care's low reimbursements. Many physicians turned up the volume of discretionary procedures and tests, or "ancillary services," in order to produce extra income. Primary care doctors invested in laboratories that performed blood work, and inexpensive machinery, like X-ray and EKG machines, and then self-referred patients to get additional tests that would result in extra income. An EKG machine, which is used to measure heart rhythms, cost as little as a thousand dollars and would bring in about twenty-four dollars every time the doctor used it on a patient. Specialists earned considerably more on their ancillary services. An endoscopy, which involves slipping a flexible scope down a patient's throat, earned ear, nose, and throat specialists an extra three hundred dollars. Dermatologists turned to cosmetic procedures like Botox injections and chemical peels. Ophthalmologists began specializing in surgical procedures, like eyelid tucks. Between 2000 and 2005, the number of elective procedures performed by physicians around the country rose dramatically, most of them paid for by insurance. Among Medicare recipients, colonoscopies went up 40 percent; angioplasties, 34 percent; and cardiovascular stress tests, 45 percent. As physicians (and hospitals) figured out ways to regain lost income, the savings that had been wrung out of the system by managed care in the early nineties evaporated. By 1999, a vast majority of people who were insured by their employers were enrolled in managed care plans, the so-called solution to America's health care crisis, yet health care costs were once again rising at double-digit rates.

Despite the fact that managed care's grip had loosened, Peabody found himself feeling angry all the time. Angry at his colleagues. Angry with the people he still had to do battle with every day at insurance companies, most of whom were clerks, who were arguing with him over whether or not a sick child, his patient, needed to go to the hospital or take an expensive drug or undergo a test. He was angry at parents who failed to show up for appointments. He found himself resenting the mothers who came in with their printouts from the Internet wanting to talk endlessly about some disease their child did not have. After a ten-hour day of rushing from patient to patient, he would come home for dinner exhausted and still have calls to make. He was having trouble sleeping at night; he felt frustrated and tired all the time. He didn't feel like he was practicing good medicine. One day in 1999, his wife looked at him and said, "You're not happy. You don't have to do this anymore. We'll be fine." When Peabody's contract with his multispecialty group expired the following year, he decided to retire early. He was not yet sixty years old.

Losing doctors

In the end, managed care reneged on all of its promises to doctors, to patients, and to employers. It didn't return the primary care doctor to his former place as the quarterback of medicine, the person who saw the whole patient, not just his parts. Instead, primary care doctors found themselves cast in the role of "gatekeeper," a term they came to loathe once they discovered that it boiled down to denying care and access to specialists.

By keeping a tight lid on physicians' fees, managed care paradoxically drove costs up, largely because its executives failed to predict the obvious: The minute doctors sensed their incomes going down, they began to behave less like professionals and more like pieceworkers in a shirt factory. If a garment worker is paid a dollar a shirt and makes ten shirts a day, what does she do if her boss reduces her pay to ninety cents a shirt? She makes one more shirt a day. Doctors responded in a similar fashion when their fees were cut; they increased the volume of care. They began providing more ancillary services, more discretionary, and often-useless, procedures like endoscopies, stress tests, and MRIs. They bought laboratories and sent patients for extra lab tests. For primary care physicians, the main way to increase income was to bump up the number of patients seen per hour. In doing that, however, they no longer had time to explain why an antibiotic wouldn't cure a sore throat caused by a virus, or why it would be a better idea to go home and ice a sore knee than to see an orthopedist. To get through their appointments, they often resorted to handing out the prescriptions to expensive brand-name drugs and the referrals to specialists that their patients demanded, rather than use up precious minutes educating patients. All those referrals and prescriptions just drove up costs even more.

Indeed, managed care's biggest mistake may have been its failure to translate the methods of the traditional HMO, including the practice of paying doctors a salary. In a fee-for-service world, doctors are rewarded financially for providing more care, regardless of whether it helps the patient. In the early days of managed care, doctors were rewarded for withholding care. But in the traditional HMO, which managed care was supposed to be modeled after, doctors are salaried and there are financial incentives for neither. In missing this central point and applying only certain aspects of traditional HMOs, like utilization reviews—but without a cooperative environment among doctors—managed care made the same mistake that many companies have made in the past: It borrowed selectively from a successful organization without bothering to understand how all of its various parts interacted. For example, companies looked to General Electric's spectacular success in buying other companies and making GE not only bigger but also more profitable. But when they tried to copy GE's success, they often failed to adopt several key aspects of CEO Jack Welch's management ethos. Welch believed in a corporate culture of accountability and in cultivating new leaders from the lower ranks. These values came to be known as "the GE way," and Welch required intensive training for managers in each new firm that GE bought, in order to indoctrinate them. But when other CEOs tried to emulate the GE way, they forgot about creating a common corporate culture. In the same way, managed care companies forgot to import the culture of traditional HMOs when they instituted their cost-saving methods. "Doctors never bought into the managed care revolution," says Robert Blendon, a health care policy analyst with Harvard's John F. Kennedy School of Government. "It was a top-down phenomenon that was driven by employers who were desperate to control their costs. Doctors didn't think to themselves, this is the way medicine should be, so they had no obligation to defend the health plans to patients."

In neglecting to get buy-in from doctors, managed care ultimately helped damage primary care, a shift in medicine that could prove disastrous for

America's health and our pocketbooks in the coming decades. In a recent report, the American College of Physicians warned of an impending collapse of the nation's primary care system, which is losing doctors faster than medical schools can replace them. In 1949, 59 percent of doctors were in primary care. While the absolute number of primary care doctors rose over the years, by 1970 they made up only 43 percent of practicing physicians; by 1995 they had fallen to 37 percent. Ten years later, 21 percent of primary care physicians who had entered medicine in the early 1990s had left their practices, many undoubtedly driven out, like Gordon Peabody, by the frustrations of managed care. Many went back for additional training in order to pursue more-lucrative second careers as specialists. Anesthesiology has proved particularly attractive as a second-career specialty because it offers high pay and regular hours. Some primary care doctors fled to Wall Street to work as biotech and medical stock analysts; others took jobs as medical directors with insurance companies.

When medical students look ahead toward the day when they will enter practice, the picture for primary care must look bleak indeed. In 2004, 15 percent of family practice physicians earned less than $100,000 a year. That's still about double what the average American makes, and many patients undoubtedly have little sympathy for doctors who cry poor mouth. On the other hand, the average American doesn't spend four years in postgraduate education and emerge $120,000 in debt before getting his first paying job. Medical students are keenly aware that the average family practitioner will make far, far less than the average specialist; 20 percent of invasive cardiologists, 25 percent of neurosurgeons, and 14 percent of orthopedists have incomes over $600,000.

Given those numbers, it should come as no surprise that the percentage of medical graduates choosing family medicine has declined precipitously, from 14 percent in 2000 to 8 percent in 2005. As one medical graduate puts it, "To quote Tupac Shakur, 'Fuck the fame, just give me the money.' " Since 1998, the number of family practice residency positions that go empty has risen by more than 50 percent. Today, for every ten family practice residency positions, fewer than five are filled. Primary care physicians express higher levels of dissatisfaction with their jobs than any other doctors.

Medical students also can't help perceiving the decline in respect that primary care commands within the pecking order of academic medicine. Thirty years ago, those who went into internal medicine were drawn from the top of their classes. Primary care physicians really were considered the thinkers back then, the diagnosticians of medicine, and they were held in high esteem, though they never made as much money as the specialists. Specialists had to command a deep well of knowledge about their particular corner of the body, but primary care doctors, along with emergency room physicians, were expected to master broad swaths of information. They also had to possess the qualities that both physicians and patients once valued, including compassion, the ability to listen, and the intelligence to look at a constellation of symptoms and test results and then put their finger on the right diagnosis.

In today's world of increasing specialization and dependence on technology, primary care is often viewed in academic medical centers as a dying art, little more than triage, a perception that is reinforced by the politics of academic medicine, where money and prestige are tightly linked. As specialists earn more and more in comparison with their colleagues in primary care, they often acquire an inflated view of their contribution to patients' health. "Primary care is dead," an academic specialist recently told me in a conspiratorial whisper. "Nurse practitioners can do it a lot cheaper."

Maybe. But it could also be that primary care is precisely what people really want as well as need. Americans will usually pay for what they value, at least if they have the means, and, in the view of Dr. Lisa Sanders, a recent trend suggests that what many Americans want is a return to the days of Marcus Welby. Doctors are now turning to "boutique practices," charging patients an up-front fee of as much as ten thousand dollars a year in return for being available to the patient whenever the patient wants. Others are carrying their black bags on house calls once again. Only now, their bags are bigger and sometimes contain such technology as portable EKG machines.

And there's more to primary care than simply treating minor illnesses and figuring out which specialist to send patients off to when something is seriously wrong. A doctor, writes Bernard Lown, winner of the Nobel Peace Prize and developer of the defibrillator, "must rely on the art of a human understanding to amplify the insights provided by science." Francis Peabody,

a physician from the early twentieth century famously wrote, "One of the essential qualities of the clinician is interest in humanity, for the secret of the
care of the patient is in caring for the patient." A vast body of research supports this notion that medicine is still very much an art, and that caring for
patients involves more than simply applying the right technology. Two ingredients are necessary for keeping patients healthy and helping them recover
when they are sick. One is a long-standing, trusting relationship with a primary care doctor. In the 1960s, Kerr White, an expert in public health at Johns
Hopkins, argued that what the country needed was not more specialists but
doctors who were specifically trained to keep people healthy. White—the
man who a few years later would send Jack Wennberg to Vermont—knew
from his epidemiological work that while specialists were necessary, the overall health of the nation depended upon doctors with a broad understanding
of many conditions as well as the importance of personal attention in diagnosing and treating most illnesses. White showed in paper after paper that in-
timate and long-term relationships between doctors and patients often
mattered more than specialized training or new technology. Partly this was
due to the placebo effect. The comforting presence of a familiar doctor, and
the laying on of hands or the writing of a prescription, could (and still does)
do wonders for many patients. But Kerr also discovered that patients were
more likely to modify their behavior, to quit smoking, take their medicine
properly, and begin exercising, on the advice of a trusted and caring doctor.

The second ingredient in maintaining health is making sure patients are
given the correct diagnosis and the right treatment. Research has shown that
the ability to diagnose turns on a doctor's skill at establishing a bond with
her patient, to coax the patient into revealing the nature of his illness. Debra
Roter, a professor at the Johns Hopkins Bloomberg School of Public Health,
and Judith Hall, a social psychologist at Northeastern University, have analyzed thousands of hours of videotape and direct observation of physicians
and patients to define the qualities that all good diagnosticians possess. Doctors have to like their patients in order to treat them well, or at the very least
be able to empathize with them. Patients are often filled with anxiety and
fear, or they may feel embarrassed about their illness or symptoms. The best
doctors listen to both the patient's words and his body language. When a

doctor responds to a patient's unspoken feelings, she is doing more than providing comfort; she's creating emotional space, a quiet moment that allows the patient to talk more freely about his symptoms and help the doctor come to the right diagnosis.

Cyndra Mogayzel was a gifted diagnostician, one of those doctors who could get even the most reticent patient to talk. A delicate-featured woman, with alabaster skin and light blue eyes, Mogayzel grew up in a small town in Montana, the first person in her family to go to college. She was also in the top 10 percent of her class in medical school, where she had already developed a reputation for having an intuitive ability to diagnose. Mogayzel no longer practices medicine in part because she suffers from serious asthma and can't afford to be exposed to germs that could trigger it. But she also knows she could no longer afford to spend the kind of time she believes is necessary for good primary care.

Over coffee one morning in Annapolis, Maryland, near the school our children attend, Mogayzel talks to me about her first practice, which she opened in Tacoma, Washington, in 1992, while her husband was finishing his residency at the University of Washington, in Seattle. "I had a 100 percent inner-city Medicaid practice. I had Laotians, Hmong, Russian immigrants. At one point, I had the state of Washington calling me asking how I was keeping all my asthma patients out of the hospital. How I was able to get a 92 percent immunization rate," she says. One half of her secret was a team that included her receptionist and a nurse. As for the other half of her success, she says, "the moms trusted us. We took care of their kids. I had five translators that I called in. We found courtesy vans for my patients so they could get to my office. If they missed a scheduled immunization, my receptionist tracked them down. If a homeless asthmatic kid needed a nebulizer, we found a way to get it to the homeless shelter."

As Mogayzel gained a reputation for being able to handle tough cases, other doctors began dumping their "hysterical" mothers on her. "A quote 'hysterical mother' is one of three things," she says. "One, her kid is really sick, and nobody is listening to her. If you think something is wrong with your kid, and nobody is listening, nothing makes you crazier. Two, her kid isn't sick, and nobody has bothered to take the time to explain to her what's going on and why she doesn't need to worry. Or three, she is stressed for some other reason—divorce, domestic violence, financial problems—and you need to know what's going on in order to properly care for and protect the child."

The key to helping mothers and their children, says Mogayzel, is taking the time to listen. She recalls a case involving one of her "hysterical" mothers and the woman's fifteen-year-old daughter, who was suffering from irregular menstrual periods. The mother landed on Mogayzel's doorstep after she had taken her daughter to half a dozen other physicians, including an endocrinologist. All of them had dismissed the mother's fears, telling her that irregular periods were not uncommon in adolescent girls. But the more they tried to quiet the mother's fears, the more adamant she became. She knew something was wrong. When mother and daughter came to Mogayzel, she sat them down in her office and asked an open-ended question: "Tell me about your daughter."

The girl began menstruating at age eleven, and her periods were quite regular for the first two years. But then, said the mother, they began to vary wildly, not only in how often they came but also in how long they lasted and how much she bled. That was the clue that Mogayzel needed, the fact that the girl's periods had started out being regular and then changed. She ordered a full set of tests to look at the girl's hormones. When the results came back, they showed abnormally high levels of prolactin, a hormone involved in milk production. Mogayzel suspected a pituitary tumor, which was confirmed with a head CT. The girl underwent brain surgery to remove the tumor. Afterward, the neurosurgeon called Mogayzel. "He said that was the smallest tumor he had ever resected, and he wanted to know how I caught it so early," says Mogayzel. "I did it by listening to the mother. Nobody had ever bothered to take the time to get a complete history."

The vast majority of Americans whose insurance is covered by their employers continue to be enrolled in some form of managed care. Most plans have abandoned capitation, though not all, and primary care physicians continue to be squeezed financially, even as their numbers dwindle. Meanwhile, the number of specialists continues to rise. In the years to come, increasing numbers of specialists coupled with the destruction of primary care will, if left unchecked, almost certainly lead to higher health care costs—and worse health, for all the reasons that have been discussed in this book. But also because primary care, it turns out, forms the foundation of high-quality health care. While the family practitioner's status in the medical hierarchy has fallen in the past two decades, along with his income, his importance to the health of nations has never changed. Building on Kerr White's work, studies continue to consistently show that having more primary care physicians per capita results in lower rates of hospitalizations and healthier patients. People who have well-established, long-term relationships with a doctor who is a generalist have lower overall health care costs than those who don't have a primary care physician. Regions of the country where the ratio of primary care physicians to specialists is higher have lower health care costs.

Today, political debate about health care is focused for the most part on the problem of how to cover the forty-seven million Americans who are uninsured. Many of us have come to realize that as health care costs rise, more and more of us are losing coverage through our employers. It's not just the poor who are uninsured anymore but also the middle-class workers who are laid off temporarily or whose employers can no longer cover enough of the premium to make insurance affordable. As many as sixty million Americans go without health insurance at some point during the course of a year. Today, more than one third of the uninsured—seventeen million of the nearly forty-seven million—have family incomes of forty thousand dollars or more, according to the Employee Benefit Research Institute, a nonpartisan organization. More than two thirds of the uninsured are in households with at least one full-time worker.

While the plight of the uninsured is very real, in many ways the focus on them reflects another, unspoken fear—that the system won't take care of any of us when we fall ill, regardless of our insurance status. In one recent *Consumer Reports* poll, 40 percent of patients surveyed said they got more

information from the Internet about diseases and treatments than from
their doctors. Patients reported that they didn't understand about half of the
instructions they received during visits. They complained that doctors failed
to mention the side effects of medication they prescribed and didn't return
lab test results promptly. One in five respondents said that when they or a
family member was seriously ill, they had trouble getting needed care. Patients also resent time spent waiting to see the doctor, and they continue to
worry that their doctors are simply saving money for the insurer when they
try to dissuade them from getting a prescription for a brand-name drug or
a referral to a specialist. And we still think that better treatment is the same
as more treatment.

What all of this says is that what we need is a health care system that we
can trust will actually care for us when we are ill and help us stay healthy
when we're not. We don't really want unnecessary treatment, but after more
than a decade of managed care, we've concluded that our doctors and insurers are in business to deprive us, so we have to demand everything we
can possibly get. Though we can't articulate it, sometimes what we really
need is not a doctor who delivers more care but one who seems to care
more—and has the time to make sure we understand what we need in order to be well.

Getting to a health care system that works better than the one we have requires reframing the problem, and acknowledging that American medicine
is filled with paradoxes. Jack Wennberg spent thirty years trying to persuade
his peers that geography matters, that the care a person receives depends
less on what kind of care he needs and more on where he happens to live.
An even more difficult fact to digest is that too many specialists means
worse care. While you wouldn't want your primary care physician doing
brain surgery on you, the more specialists involved in your health, the more
likely it is that you will suffer from a medical error, that you will be given
care you don't need and be harmed by it. Unlike in most industries, where
demand determines supply, in medicine the supply of everything from hospital beds to doctors determines whether or not you will be hospitalized or
undergo surgery, and how much we all will pay for it. Things we think will
make diagnosis easier, like the ability to use CT scanning to peer into the

body, can cloud the picture. In other industries, new technology brings costs down; in medicine, it usually increases them, regardless of whether it improves our health. And the final paradox: While managed care was a colossal failure in so many respects—it has driven good doctors like Gordon Peabody out of medicine, destroyed the trust between doctor and patient, and led to spiraling health care costs—in one way, it may be the best thing to happen to American medicine. It's a little like the joke about how many psychiatrists it takes to change a lightbulb: just one, but the lightbulb has to want to change. Managed care has made many Americans realize that they want a change too. With what we've learned in the preceding chapters, it's now possible to envision a health care system that actually delivers what it's supposed to deliver, which is better health.

TEN Less Is More

IMAGINE, FOR A MOMENT, that you have not yet been born. You have no idea what your lot in life will be, whether you'll be born to a wealthy family or a poor one; whether you will enjoy good health or constant sickness; whether you'll be successful in life or wind up a homeless alcoholic. Now consider what kind of health care system you will want, not knowing ahead of time what sort of health care you will soon enjoy. This thought experiment is what philosopher Norman Daniels, author of *Just Health Care*, calls "the veil of ignorance," and it's a useful tool for thinking about how we would create an equitable and more-functional system if we had the luxury of starting from scratch.

Looking out from our unbiased vantage point, it's a pretty good bet that we wouldn't want a system like the one we have now. For one thing, we might wind up being among the forty-seven million uninsured. It's an accident of political history that a little less than half of the health care insurance in this country is covered by our employers, those who are willing or able to pay for it. (The government picks up the tab for the rest through Medicare, Medicaid, or a military agency.) A rational system would cover everybody, not only because it's the right thing to do, morally (and because it's what we would hope for if we didn't know whether we would have insurance), but also because the uninsured help distort our current system, pushing hospitals to shift costs to insured patients in order to cover their losses from the uninsured. (Think back to chapter 3, which discussed how hospitals invest in their refuges of profit, the departments that make money, and overtreat patients in those departments—at the expense of departments that are also needed to improve the health of their patients. The uninsured contribute to this to some degree.)

We would also want a system that used the best, most valid evidence available, employed doctors who knew how to interpret medical science correctly, and rewarded them for using evidence whenever they could. It would make valid evidence readily accessible to doctors, patients, and payers. Where evidence was lacking, as it is in so many areas of medicine, we would want an institution prepared to fund and direct the necessary research. We wouldn't leave clinical research to the drug industry, which has a vested interest in the outcome. Our doctors would make clear to us that they really didn't know if the PSA test would reduce our chances of dying prematurely, and that they had no idea if spinal fusion would ease the pain in our backs. Then they could help us weigh the various trade-offs before we decided to undergo a test, surgery, or treatment.

If we know anything about our current, dysfunctional system, we would also want health care that's more coordinated. When we're sick, we need all of the people in hospitals who take care of us, every specialist, nurse, and pharmacist, along with our primary care physician, to work together. Lack of cooperation in the current system is one of the major causes of medical error, and it encourages overtreatment. We would want our doctors to work as a team not only when we were hit with acute disease or injury but also when we had a chronic condition that required constant monitoring for many years. And while we're asking, we should wish for a system that doesn't consume such a large percentage of gross domestic product. That means we need hospitals to be efficient; they should deliver the best care they can for the lowest cost.

Believe it or not, such systems already exist in the United States. You've heard of some of them, the Mayo Clinic, Kaiser Permanente, and Group Health of Puget Sound, to name just three that are widely known. But maybe you don't know about one of the best: the Veterans Health Administration. That's right, the health care system that is run by the U.S. Department of Veterans Affairs. The same agency whose reputation had sunk so low during the 1990s that conservative opponents to the Clinton administration's plan for health care reform had only to point to the VA system and say the words "socialized medicine" to scare Americans into sticking with the status quo. Back then, the VHA's bad reputation was well deserved. Underfunded, overbedded, and poorly administered, it was a model of waste and inefficiency. Workers were dispirited and patients neglected. In 1992, three decomposing bodies were discovered on the grounds of a veterans' medical center in Salem, Virginia. Two of the bodies were of men who had wandered off a few months earlier. The other was of an eighty-four-year-old patient who had been missing since 1977. Movies like Coming Home (1978) and Born on the Fourth of July (1989) had immortalized VHA hospitals as crumbling, rat-infested sinkholes of shabby treatment and substandard care. By the mid-1990s, Congress was considering shutting the whole system down.

The Veterans Health Administration of today, however, outpaces most of the rest of American health care on nearly every measure of quality. In 2003, the New England Journal of Medicine published a study that compared veterans' health facilities with fee-for-service Medicare. Between 1997 and 1999, the VHA outperformed Medicare on all eleven measures of quality. In 2000, it bested Medicare on twelve measures. The VHA's prescription accuracy rate is 99.997 percent, compared with the 92 to 97 percent rate in the rest of the country.

Outside observers come up with equally surprising results. The nonprofit National Committee for Quality Assurance ranks health care plans on seventeen performance measures. It looks at how well doctors manage blood pressure and whether they use care that's proved helpful to patients, like being sure to measure something called glycosylated hemoglobin in the blood of diabetics at least once a year. This test tells doctors how well a diabetic has maintained his blood sugar over the previous two months. Left uncontrolled, high blood sugar can lead to complications like blindness. In every single category, the VHA outperforms even the best-ranked hospitals in America. According to a RAND Corporation study, the VHA system delivers two thirds of the care recommended by medical professional societies, which might not sound all that great until you remember that another RAND study found that outside of the VHA system, providers manage to deliver, on average, only about 50 percent of recommended care.

Veterans themselves sing their health system's praises. That may come as a surprise if you were reading the news in early 2007, when newspapers reported on the poor conditions at the Walter Reed Army Medical Center. These stories sometimes confused the army's medical system with the VHA; they're separate. Veterans complained about access and difficulties establishing eligibility to be cared for by the VHA system because the Bush administration withdrew the promise of benefits to vets who made over twenty-five thousand dollars or whose illness was not directly service related. Yet these complaints were about access, not the quality of the care received by veterans who are enrolled in the system. Those who get their care from the VHA consistently report high levels of satisfaction. "I couldn't be happier," says Raymond B. Roemer, a World War II veteran who spent eleven months in a German POW camp. A successful businessman in Buffalo, New York, Roemer can afford to be treated in any hospital he wants, but the VHA is where he prefers to go. He says, "My friends in the POW group I belong to all feel the same."

The VHA manages such high levels of satisfaction and quality while taking care of a population that is older and sicker than the rest of the country. As a group, the vets enrolled in the VHA system are fatter, poorer, and more prone to mental illness than the general population. They have more chronic disease, including Alzheimer's, cancer, congestive heart failure, and cirrhosis of the liver. One in five veterans has diabetes, compared with one in fourteen in the general population. They're more likely to be homeless and to be substance abusers. More than a third of the veterans enrolled in the VHA system smoke. Yet in 2002, the VHA's cost per enrollee was just $2,910, down from $3,720 in 1999. The bill for the rest of the country that year came to $4,576 per capita. And the people who work at the VHA are an exceptionally motivated bunch. They feel honored to care for men and women who served their country. On a recent visit to a VHA hospital, I had nurses coming up to me in the halls to tell me they wouldn't want to work anywhere else, even though the pay is often better on the outside. One nurse said, "I thank God I get to work here." Kathleen Jones, an emergency physician, said, "It's like a little utopia."

If the words "utopia" and "Veterans Health Administration" being used in the same sentence sounds strange, that's not surprising. We've been told enough times by various groups—the American Medical Association, for instance, the private insurance industry, and conservative believers in the power of the free market—that government-run medicine is inferior. The fact that it's actually better in many ways than the health care the rest of us receive violates everything we think we know. It's a government-run health care system—socialized medicine—that doesn't have long lines; doesn't ration care; isn't filled with lazy, poorly trained doctors; and costs less per capita than our private system. The VHA even costs less per capita for its over-sixty-five patients than Medicare. The story of how the VHA turned itself around offers clues to the qualities we should be asking for from all of our hospitals and doctors, as well as lessons in how to get the system we want.

Overhauled

The VHA's transformation began in 1994, when a man named Kenneth W. Kizer became undersecretary for health, effectively the CEO of the VHA system. The system had hit rock bottom. Facilities were worn and dirty. It was losing patients, as veterans of World War I and the Korean War began passing away. As aging veterans moved from the Rust Belt to the Sun Belt, VA hospitals in places like Pittsburgh and Detroit were left empty, while hospitals in Tampa and Tucson were being overwhelmed. At the same time, there were calls in Washington, D.C., to shut the system down. "They should . . . put out to pasture the sacred cow known as Veterans Affairs," wrote William Safire in the New York Times. In October 1996, President Bill Clinton signed a bill opening the VA health system to any veteran, regardless of his income or whether his condition was service related. A former emergency physician with a degree in public health, Kizer knew he had to perform major surgery on the VHA quickly, or it would be dead.

His first step was to decentralize management. Kizer and his top managers carved the country into twelve regions, giving each region its own budget, authority, and performance goals. The regions were left to reorganize their own hospitals, and they were rewarded for hitting performance measures that were set by Washington and are even today continually being ratcheted upward as the system gets better. Kizer also began getting rid of unused hospital beds, even shutting down entire hospital wings. In their place, he opened a series of satellite primary clinics and hired primary care physicians, transforming the VHA from an acute care, hospital-based system to one centered on preventive care. Since 1997, the VHA has opened 500 clinics nationwide and doubled the number of veterans who are seen by a primary care physician on a regular basis. The goal is for every veteran to have access to a primary care doctor, either a VHA staff physician or, if the veteran lives in a rural area where there are too few other vets to keep a staff doctor busy, a physician who has a contract with the VA. Kizer helped pay for all of his changes by bargaining hard with drug and medical suppliers and cutting a deal with the Office of Management and Budget that allowed him to plow any money he saved back into the VA health system.

Kizer's efforts were aided by a computerized medical-records system now known as VistA. VistA was developed in secret by VA doctors and other workers in the 1970s and '80s, often in violation of government policy that restricted them from tinkering with government computers. It is actually a collection of nearly twenty thousand different programs, each tailored painstakingly over the years to the specifications of nurses, pharmacists, and doctors, the people who must use it. Today, a veteran can walk into a VHA clinic or hospital anywhere in the country, and his medical records are instantly available to any provider who needs to see them. This proved crucial in the aftermath of Hurricane Katrina, when paper records for thousands of patients in Louisiana hospitals were lost. Louisiana veterans who fled to other states were able to go to a local VHA facility, and the doctors there could access their records without missing a beat.

But VistA does more than simply make it possible for vets to move around the country more easily. It also provides the data that has allowed the VHA to measure its own performance. VistA has helped reduce error and infection rates, while also improving the coordination of care. It has helped doctors cut down on both overtreatment and undertreatment and aided researchers in developing medical protocols for the best way to care for patients with specific conditions based on hard data.

To see VistA in action and learn more about how the VHA manages to provide such good care, I decided to visit one of the system's flagship hospitals, in Palo Alto, California. This was once one of the disaster areas of the VHA. It ran the psychiatric clinic just up the road, in Menlo Park, that served as the location for Ken Kesey's *One Flew over the Cuckoo's Nest*. It was overbuilt and filled with empty beds. Veterans came only for emergencies. The day I visit, a group of vets smoke and chat quietly in the sun outside the entrance to the main building, a five-story brick structure just a few miles from Stanford University. One man is in a wheelchair, the lower half of his right leg missing. Inside, the hospital seems much like any other, with slightly worn chairs in the lobby and the smells of breakfast wafting from the cafeteria. Patients dressed in hospital gowns sit on benches located in an interior courtyard.

You only begin to see what's different about a VHA hospital once you are upstairs, on the wards. The first thing you notice is the doctors and nurses striding down the halls pushing chrome carts that carry wireless laptops. Every nurse and every doctor has instant access to patient records here. Up in the intensive care unit, chief nurse Shirley Paulson sits down in front of a desktop computer to show me a medical record used for patients in the unit. Paulson pushes a key and a brightly colored record appears on the computer screen. The patient has just undergone surgery, and he is on a ventilator. "When I come on a shift, I can find out instantly how the patients are doing and what's been happening," says Paulson. She shows me how the record is organized, where test results are displayed, the location of notes left by a surgeon and a pulmonologist.

This computerized record stands in stark contrast to what you typically see in other hospitals, where nurses and doctors spend minutes at a time flipping back and forth through pages and pages of paper charts just to find out the results of a test, or if it has even been performed. Paper records not only waste time but also lead to duplication of effort. An estimated 18 percent of tests and radiological scans are repeated simply because they can't be located or can't be transmitted from one doctor to another in a timely fashion. Interns and residents who work in paper systems can be seen rushing from floor to floor of a hospital in order to retrieve X-rays from radiology or test results from pathology, or to locate a doctor because nobody can read her notes.

Paulson tells me that VistA also helps reduce drug errors. In the old days, she says, nurses kept track of which patients needed which drugs and at what dose on three-by-five cards or sheets of paper, which they kept stashed in their coat pockets. Today, VistA keeps track for them. She motions toward a nurse who has been sitting near her dozing patient. The nurse's computer is beeping; it's time for another dose of a drug. The nurse goes to the man's side and says quietly, "I'm going to scan your ID band." The patient's eyes flutter open, and he lifts his left hand, shakily, from the bed. Using a handheld bar code scanner like the ones you see in the grocery store, the nurse scans his ID bracelet, which has a bar code printed on it. She then walks to a cart located in the hallway, opens a drawer containing the drug she needs, and scans the bar code on one bottle and then another. She looks back at her computer screen. Only then does she inject the medicine into her patient's IV line.

In the rest of the U.S. health care system, adverse drug events injure or kill as many as four hundred thousand patients a year. Estimates suggest that there is on average about one drug error per day per patient. In the VA, the drug error rate is .003 percent. Paulson shows me how VistA helps eliminate mistakes. "Let's say you picked up the wrong drug from the cart," she says. Paulson scans the bar code on a bottle she picked at random, and the computer screen flashes in bright red letters the word "error." "If the nurse had picked up the wrong drug, she gets an error message," says Paulson. "She also gets one if she didn't scan both doses of it." Another message will flash on the screen if a doctor prescribes a drug that interacts badly with one the patient is already taking. "We may see errors when the doctor orders the wrong drug, and I'll look at it and say, 'Did you really mean to order this?'" says Paulson. "We don't see errors in drug administration."

VistA has also helped the VHA keep down drug costs. The agency employs pharmacists who are trained to analyze patient data, as well as the results of clinical trials published in medical journals. These researchers weigh the value of different drugs to create an evidence-based formulary, the list of approved drugs the VA keeps in stock. VHA doctors are encouraged to use the drugs on the formulary first, before prescribing a less-effective or more-expensive drug. This cuts down on both costs and patients being given unnecessary medicines. Research has shown, for example, that cheap diuretics are as effective as brand-name high-blood-pressure medicines for most patients, and they often have fewer side effects. Physicians often don't act on this evidence, either because they are unaware of it or because drug company representatives aren't pushing diuretics and don't give out free samples of them. But at the VHA, doctors are urged to try diuretics first. The pharmacists track whether doctors and nurses are prescribing a drug properly, and they look at patient outcomes to see if discouraging the use of a particular drug has inadvertently led to more sickness and more hospitalizations.

The VHA's evidence-based formulary often offers the added benefit of reducing the chances that vets will be prescribed drugs that later turn out to be dangerous or ineffective, or both. In the case of Vioxx, VHA pharmacists knew it was no better for most patients than older painkillers, and they advised against prescribing it for patients who were at low risk of gastrointestinal bleeds.

The computer system also allows the nurses and doctors to monitor their own performance. The rate of hospital-acquired infection, the scourge of surgical wards and ICUs, is lower at VHA hospitals than almost anywhere else in the country. Bringing infection rates down is as simple as getting nurses and doctors to wash their hands between patients and instituting strict rules for inserting central lines and catheters. By tracking infection rates within wards and entire hospitals, nurses and doctors at the VHA are inspired to work together to bring their rates below those at other hospitals in the system.

There are many lessons to be learned from the VHA, the most obvious being that hospitals need electronic medical records, but it would be a mistake to think that VistA alone is responsible for the success of the VHA, or that implementing IT in the rest of the health care system will somehow magically fix its many problems. VistA was a tool, which Kenneth Kizer and the VHA used to measure performance, coordinate care, and reduce error. All those improvements were entirely possible without VistA, but having a computerized system allowed Kizer and his managers to implement change more quickly than they might otherwise have been able to do. Other health care systems, notably Kaiser and the Mayo Clinic, have achieved similar levels of quality while they were still using paper records.

How did they do it? Remember back to chapter 2, where Elliott Fisher showed that hospitals with a high ratio of specialists to primary care physicians did more procedures and tests on his three groups of patients suffering from colon cancer, heart attacks, and hip fractures. And in chapter 4, dying patients who landed in hospitals in Los Angeles that invested in more specialists than primary care physicians, bought more CT scanners and MRI machines, and had more ICU beds, were no better off for all the unnecessary time spent in the hospital and all the extra specialists they saw. What health systems like the Mayo Clinic and Kaiser, as well as Intermountain Healthcare, in Utah and Idaho, have figured out is that they can care for patients by not overinvesting in unnecessary technology and ICU beds. And they do it with a higher ratio of primary care doctors to specialists. The VHA modeled its hospitals and satellite clinics on these highly efficient, successful systems. Having VistA simply made it easier to bring about these changes. By providing rapid feedback to managers, VistA allowed them to test whether or not the changes they made ultimately improved care and helped patients.

That's because every individual patient record goes into a database, which allows the VHA to monitor not only what happens to patients, whether treatments such as flu shots are being delivered, and how long they spend on average in an ICU bed, but also how these factors affect their health. Here's an example. In 2003, in a paper in the *New England Journal of Medicine,* VA quality control officers reported on the effect of Kizer's effort to cut the number of hospital beds between 1997 and 1999. The quality officers found that the number of days patients spent in a hospital bed went down by half. The net effect of this change? Mortality went down among a sampling of three hundred thousand veterans suffering from four out of seven different diagnoses. Mortality was unchanged in the other three. The database showed that the system could cut hospitalizations and at the same time improve survival.

Kizer left the government in 1999, but the VHA's metamorphosis has continued without him. The twelve regions still monitor the performance of their hospitals and the outcomes of their patients. They are constantly trying to improve methods for helping diabetics and cut down on the percentage of patients with chronic heart failure who are repeatedly hospitalized because their disease is not being controlled. Within a region, managers also keep close tabs on patient satisfaction, rates of error, and how long patients wait for their appointments. They push their doctors to do a better job through competition with other hospitals and other regions, and through a combination of exhortation and shame.

The VA also uses its database to ensure it doesn't fail to provide enough care. In 2003, outside auditors were asked to evaluate the quality of the VHA's cardiac care. The auditors looked at records for patients who were admitted to the hospital for any reason involving heart disease, including heart attacks. They then compared the patients' mortality rates to those of similar patients in Medicare. The auditors found that from 1997 to 1999, the VHA had higher mortality rates, in part because it was failing to provide adequate access to invasive procedures, like angiography for patients in the midst of a heart attack. (You'll recall that heart attack patients are the most likely to benefit from these procedures.) Veterans also had to travel twice as far to get cardiac treatment. The VHA immediately developed a plan to improve cardiac care and set goals for its hospitals. It also began a review to determine which facilities needed to upgrade cardiology equipment and hire more cardiologists.

CARE

How can the rest of the U.S. health care system hope to mimic the extraordinary achievements that have come about at the Veterans Health Administration, including its commitment to constant improvement? The necessary steps are pretty obvious: Implement electronic medical records. Reduce the excess capacity in hospitals, the unnecessary beds and extra specialists, that drives a great deal of unnecessary care. Make sure that everybody has access to primary care physicians, and that they aren't overwhelmed trying to handle too many patients. Give them the time to practice preventive medicine. (VHA primary care doctors are responsible for about fifteen hundred patients, at least five hundred fewer than the average internist or family physician.) Use information technology to improve coordination among doctors. Make hospitals and doctors accountable by measuring their performance and the outcomes of their patients. And finally, gather evidence for what works and what doesn't. We could call this strategy CARE, for coordination, accountability, electronic medical records, and evidence.

While the tasks are clear, implementing CARE around the country won't be simple. In order to do it, we have to rethink the way we pay doctors and hospitals. The first step is for Medicare to address the way it overpays for certain procedures, like radiology and bypass surgery, and underpays for less-intensive care. The current system encourages hospitals to invest in expensive doctors and beds and technology that aren't necessarily what patients need. But there are other ways the payment system makes it hard for doctors to coordinate their care and leads to unnecessary hospitalizations. Take the example of caring for diabetics. More than thirty million Americans have diabetes, the product of our ever-increasing girth and sedentary lifestyle. Over 60 percent of Medicare spending goes toward patients with chronic conditions like diabetes and heart disease, and the majority of the money is spent on hospitalizations for complications that could have been prevented with proper care. But keeping diabetics out of the hospital requires constant monitoring. Diabetics who fail to control their blood sugar are more likely to go blind, suffer heart attacks, or have a leg amputated because of a wound that won't heal. Preventing those complications isn't rocket science; it just takes constant work. Patients need to learn to eat better and exercise. They need to monitor their blood sugar and take their insulin or other drugs. They need to see an ophthalmologist regularly to check for damage to the retina and a podiatrist to ensure they are caring for their feet. And their doctors need to check their hemoglobin on a routine basis to make sure they are controlling their blood sugar at home.

How often does all of this coordinated care actually happen? Outside of a few systems, like the VHA, Group Health, and Kaiser, rarely at best. Let's look at just one piece of this puzzle, monitoring hemoglobin. If you have diabetes, your chances are about one in four that a doctor will actually perform that test, let alone teach you to check your own blood sugar level on a regular basis. According to a recent RAND Corporation study, failing to get their blood sugar checked leads an estimated twenty-six hundred diabetics to go blind every year and another twenty-nine thousand to experience kidney failure.

Doctors and hospitals don't neglect to treat diabetics properly because they are lazy or incompetent or don't care about their patients. They fail to do it in part because the payment system punishes them financially when they do. About seven years ago, a group of idealistic doctors in Bellingham, Washington, a bucolic coastal town about an hour north of Seattle, created Pursuing Perfection, a program to help participating medical practitioners prevent diabetes and chronic heart failure and to better care for patients who already have the conditions. The program centers on multidisciplinary teams employing the best practices for counseling patients, helping them to navigate the health care system and control their diseases. It also calls for preventive measures, providing access to nutritionists and nurses to help patients learn to eat better and exercise more in order to avoid getting the conditions in the first place. The doctors have implemented information technology to allow everyone involved in a patient's care to share medical records and support disease management.

Pursuing Perfection has already improved the health of many patients. Rebecca Bryson suffers from both diabetes and congestive heart failure. Before enrolling in the program she was seeing fourteen different doctors and taking forty-two medications. When her lungs would fill with fluid from her congestive heart failure, she would call a doctor's office and tell the nurse what was happening. Sometimes she would get a call back in an hour, sometimes not for a day. She landed in the emergency room routinely. Under the new plan, she has access to a nurse, called a clinical specialist, who knows her case intimately, helps her adjust her medications, and gets her in to see the doctor when she needs it. Bryson also has access to her own electronic medical record, where she can note reactions to a new medication. With the help of her clinical specialist, Bryson has learned how to avoid going to the doctor by doing things like checking on the salt in her diet if her blood pressure goes up. These simple steps have had measurable results for patients across the board, reducing blood sugar levels in diabetics and preventing crises in heart failure patients. Pursuing Perfection has not only improved the lives of patients like Rebecca Bryson, it is saving both Medicare and private insurers thousands of dollars per patient and could cut deaths from diabetes by half.

But Pursuing Perfection is killing the local hospital. Between 2001 and 2008, the initiative will have cost Peace Health's St. Joseph Hospital, in Bellingham, $7.7 million in lost revenue because patients aren't being admitted as often. The county's specialists stand to lose $1.6 million from lost procedures and office visits, and from having to spend time with patients without being compensated. Insurers won't pay for a nutritionist to teach diabetics how to eat properly. They pay podiatrists well to perform procedures, but not to help a diabetic learn to inspect his own feet. One group of sixty doctors, at the Madrona Medical Group, who took part in planning the initiative, have withdrawn from the program because participating will cost them too much money. This is the sorry state of American health care. Doing what's best for patients is bad for business.

The problem here is not that there's no money; it's that the money flows through the system in the wrong way. Hospitals are paid for each episode of care, each hospitalization, and doctors are paid for each office visit, each procedure. They aren't paid to coordinate the care of diabetics or heart failure patients, to hire nurses to track a patient's weight or make sure his lungs aren't filling up with fluid, or a nutritionist to help a diabetic understand what she can and cannot eat. In order for programs like Pursuing Perfection to succeed, hospitals must work with all local doctors, not just those who are willing to lose money in order to help their patients. The way to do that is to pay them as if they were a single, integrated group, hospitals and doctors working together. But that's not how we do it. Instead, our insurers pay the hospital one fee and the individual contractors who work in it—the doctors—another.

Medicare officials are well aware that their own payment system is working against the health of patients, and they have proposed a solution to the problem of poor quality called "pay for performance," or "P4P." In phase one, hospitals receive a small bonus for monitoring their own performance on seventeen measures of quality. Most hospitals are now checking such things as what percentage of diabetics receive an eye exam once a year and how often heart attack patients are given instructions to take aspirin or a prescription for beta-blockers. More performance measures will be added to the list as the plan progresses. In phase two, hospitals will be paid another small bonus for actually improving their scores on each measure. Hospitals that are below average will eventually be fined.

Medicare is also test-driving a similar plan to measure the performance of individual physicians. Doctors fear that they will be measured on things they can't always control. Say a physician has a group of diabetics, for instance, and she's taking great care of them, monitoring their blood sugar regularly and helping them stay out of the hospital. But one of her patients simply won't do what's necessary to keep himself healthy. He refuses to measure his blood sugar. He doesn't take his insulin. And he eats anything he wants, no matter how his doctor exhorts him to change his ways. When Medicare then measures that doctor's performance, she may look bad because of one recalcitrant patient. It's also difficult to measure an individual doctor's performance because patients move between doctors so often, and they see multiple specialists, making it difficult to assign responsibility for an individual patient to a single primary care physician.

But the larger reason we shouldn't be measuring individual doctors is that it doesn't foster cooperation among them. Medicare's P4P plan for hospitals won't either, because it focuses too narrowly on individual aspects of a web of events that must happen in order for a hospital to care properly for a patient. Focusing on a few discrete measures is like saying you are going to make a building earthquake-proof by bolting the furniture to the floor, or reform Social Security by switching to a cheaper brand of ink for writing the checks.

The question is, how can we move the five thousand hospitals and eight hundred thousand physicians in this country to organize themselves into cooperative groups? One way to do it would be to allow the VHA to take over failing hospitals. My colleague Phillip Longman, in his book *Best Care*

Anywhere, outlines a plan for a demonstration project in Massachusetts, where Republican governor Mitt Romney recently struck a grand bargain with the state's Democratic legislature to pass a bill mandating health insurance for all citizens. People in Massachusetts are now required to have health insurance. Those who aren't covered by their employers can purchase individual plans for a reasonable cost, and the state will fund an insurance pool for those who cannot afford it.

Longman's plan, which he calls VistA Health, proposes allowing Boston-area residents to enroll in a system that is run by the VHA, which would assume administrative duties for hospitals in the city that are losing money. The VHA would require these hospitals to implement the VistA electronic medical-record system, which is open source, meaning it's free to anyone who wants to download the code. The VHA would also set the same standards it demands of its own doctors and hospitals and encourage the doctors in the Boston hospitals to practice more integrated care. Doctors would be put on the hospital's payroll, like doctors at the VHA, or they could work under contract to VistA Health. As patients and payers realized that VistA Health offered superior care, they would either put pressure on other hospitals to improve or flock to the VistA system.

Medicare could push for a similar transformation in hospitals around the country by measuring their performance not along the lines of the P4P plan but on the basis of their efficiency. "Efficiency" is a term that we all think we understand, but it has a special meaning in medicine. It doesn't mean the hospital that runs the most patients through in the least amount of time, or the surgeon who can do the most hip replacements in a day. Efficiency in medicine involves delivering the highest-quality care for the lowest cost over the entire course of an illness. For patients with chronic conditions that have no cure, the course of illness is progressive and will eventually end in death. These patients must be cared for over months or years, and efficiency of their care must be measured over the rest of the patients' life. That means quality is more than whether or not your heart attack patients were given prescriptions for beta-blockers on discharge, or any of the other discrete measures in Medicare's P4P plan. It's not just the mortality rate of your heart attack patients, the number of errors committed while treating them, it's also whether the care they received from various specialists and a primary care physician was coordinated over the long haul. High-quality hospitals use an integrated approach to treating chronic conditions, monitoring a heart failure patient's weight once they leave the hospital, for instance, responding quickly if they call to say they're coughing a lot, and adjusting their medication if their weight goes up, which indicates their lungs are filling with fluid. High-quality hospitals do all of this and avoid giving patients unnecessary procedures and tests.

By this yardstick, there are many inefficient hospitals in America. Think back to chapter 4 and the hospitals in Los Angeles where elderly, chronically ill Medicare patients in their last two years of life are subjected to excess, often unpleasant care and endless hospitalizations. At Garfield Medical Center, for instance, Medicare spent $106,254 on the average elderly recipient over the course of his last two years. The Mayo Clinic, by contrast, spent only $34,876. Both hospitals were taking care of patients with multiple conditions, but those who lived near Garfield spent more time in the ICU, saw more doctors, and had many more procedures and tests done to them. Why? Because Garfield has overinvested in physicians and technology and beds in relation to the number of chronically ill patients who use the hospital. With 106 beds per 1,000 Medicare recipients in its patient population, Garfield has nearly twice the number of beds per capita as are found at an efficient hospital like the Mayo Clinic's main teaching hospital in Rochester, Minnesota. Garfield also has 45 ICU beds per 1,000 Medicare recipients and employs 57 physicians. Compare that with the Mayo Clinic's 14.5 ICU beds, less than a third the number at Garfield, and only 20 physicians per 1,000 Medicare recipients.

By every measure, the Mayo Clinic is a more-efficient hospital. It provides superb care—it does much better than Garfield on Medicare's seventeen P4P measures—using fewer resources and spending less money, all without compromising patient satisfaction. Wasteful hospitals like Garfield will say their patients are sicker, and that's why they are giving them more intensive care. But we know from research at RAND and Dartmouth that this isn't the case. We also know that patients who get more intensive care don't live any longer, and the extra care they get actually puts them at greater risk of dying. They certainly aren't enjoying a better quality of life. Think back to Mr. S., the man who was dying of lung cancer and tied down in four-point restraints so the hospital could force-feed him.

Most hospitals, writes Jack Wennberg, are the "Achilles' heel of health care reform: disorganized, dysfunctional systems that are neither aware of the problem [n]or capable of implementing strategies for fixing [it]." Getting hospitals like Garfield to act more like the Mayo Clinic will probably require a combination of rewards and punishment. Jack Wennberg proposes using the Mayo Clinic and other efficient hospital systems, like Intermountain Healthcare and the VHA, as benchmarks, models that other hospitals will be encouraged to emulate with economic carrots and sticks. The first step is to go after the outliers, the most expensive and wasteful hospitals in the country. Wennberg has ranked the nation's hospitals according to how much they overuse acute hospital care on Medicare patients per capita in their last two years of life. If Medicare told the worst offenders—the 3 percent of hospitals at the top of the overuse scale—that it would pay them only as much as it paid the hospitals in the next highest payment category, the federal government would save about $150 million in 2001 dollars. Such a policy would affect 80 hospitals, nearly all of them in Los Angeles, Miami, parts of New Jersey, and downstate New York, regions of the country where hospitals are known to be the most wasteful and to provide the highest rates of unnecessary care. The hospitals affected by this plan would include such prestigious academic medical centers as New York University, as well as small community hospitals. By slowly increasing the percentage of hospitals targeted over a period of years, from the top 3 percent to the top 4 percent and then the top 6 percent, Medicare would save half a billion dollars annually by years seven and eight.

This restriction on payments to the nation's most wasteful hospitals, though not terribly punishing for any individual institution, would nevertheless reverberate through the hospital financing system. South Shore Hospital and Medical Center, in Miami Beach, for instance, would lose on the order of $1.9 million a year, out of its multi-million-dollar annual revenue. But even a small penalty would have an effect on the bond market, says Wennberg. Hospitals go to the bond market when they want to expand or renovate. But if Medicare started levying penalties on wasteful hospitals, it would signal to the market that the government was no longer prepared to subsidize poorly coordinated and unnecessary care, making lenders less inclined to issue bonds for the expansion of inefficient hospitals.

The second step is to promote the growth of organized care throughout the United States. In an increasingly complex medical world, no physician or hospital can stand as an island: The major task facing U.S. medicine is how to move from today's mostly disorganized, chaotic nonsystems to a better model. The Dartmouth researchers and others argue that the key is coordinated care such as that provided in the VHA system, such group practices as Group Health Cooperative or the Mayo Clinic, and organized hospital systems like Intermountain Healthcare. They propose that Medicare should extend P4P to reward providers who don't just follow a few rules of good care, but who also organize their practices to help chronically ill patients over the course of their illness, and develop plans that integrate all sectors of the system—ambulatory care, nursing homes, home health, as well as hospitals. Payment would be based on objective measures of efficiency: resources used, costs incurred, and services provided, as well as selected quality measures. The measures would focus on how well the system performs on the population it serves—not on the performance of individual physicians.

Wennberg proposes a ten-year pathway to reach the goal of giving Americans organized care. The key is a shared savings plan, which would motivate providers to organize themselves and reduce overuse of care, particularly acute care at hospitals. In Wennberg's vision, hospitals or physician groups that began to restructure themselves to look more like the Mayo Clinic, Intermountain Healthcare, and the VHA and that saved money for Medicare, would get to share some of the savings. They would be required to use the money to implement electronic medical records and further improve the coordination of care. Anything that was left over could help defray the costs of downsizing their medical staff, retraining office workers and orderlies, and buying out physician contracts. Medicare would use its share of the savings to help doctors invest in electronic medical records and other infrastructure needed for managing chronic illness that is not now paid for

under traditional Medicare. At the end of a ten-year phase-in, providers that
were not participating in an organized, accountable P4P plan would no
longer receive reimbursement for caring for chronically ill Medicare patients. They would be paid for emergency services only.

Fewer than 10 percent of hospitals in the country have instituted electronic medical records, and the health care industry as a whole spends less
than 3 percent of its revenue on information technology, far less than the
10 percent that other information-intensive industries, like the airlines,
spend. Some hospitals have put in systems only to pull the plug when
doctors rebelled. Cedars-Sinai Medical Center, in Los Angeles, installed a
thirty-four-million-dollar computerized physician ordering system to
streamline drug prescriptions and reduce error rates. The hospital scrapped
it in 2003, after complaints swelled into a full-blown rebellion among
physicians, at least one of whom was caught making routine drug errors
and perhaps didn't appreciate being exposed. Other doctors simply didn't
want to make the change from pen and paper to keyboard, and at least six
other hospitals have shut down computerized drug-dispensing systems.
Kaiser Permanente, in California, is currently struggling to get all the bugs
out of its new four-billion-dollar electronic medical-records system. Such
horror stories have helped to discourage hospitals from investing in IT, but
the main reason so few have installed electronic medical records is that
there's no business case to be made for purchasing a computer system that
won't contribute to the hospital's bottom line. Electronic records can improve care, but hospitals currently don't get rewarded for providing better
care, so they have a hard time justifying the investment. With an incentive
from Medicare to organize care, and their share of the savings, they would
have a reason to do it.

One of the problems facing hospitals that do want to install electronic
medical records is ensuring their system will be compatible with the IT that
doctors in the surrounding community install. There are at least twenty-five
different proprietary electronic medical-records systems in various stages of
development, but no standard exists to ensure they can talk to one another.
One solution to this problem would be for Medicare to simply decree that
all systems must be compatible with VistA. Hospitals and doctors could get

VistA for free, since it can be downloaded from a government site and then adapted to a particular hospital's needs. The high-tech industry wants to sell completely new systems, but they need to be able to talk to one another, and making VistA the common language would allow more rapid adoption of IT.

Working together

Once hospitals have begun to rightsize their staffs and their capital investments in beds and technology, Medicare will want to encourage physicians to start working in cooperative groups. The majority of doctors still practice alone or with at most one or two other physicians. Such small practices have a hard time purchasing IT, but they also are less likely than larger, multispecialty practices to use evidence-based medicine. Getting them to integrate the care of the chronically ill, the way the doctors in Bellingham, Washington, have learned to do would mean restructuring the way they are paid. What we really want doctors to do is start behaving less like independent businesses and more like physicians in integrated health care plans like the VHA, Group Health, and the Mayo Clinic.

The solution to this problem lies in the mountain of data collected over the last decade by Wennberg's group. They now have the tools to define populations of patients who are cared for by a particular hospital, which is crucial to Wennberg's plan for getting hospitals to reorganize. They can also define the set of doctors who either refer the majority of their patients to a hospital, or who do most of their work there. In a recent journal article, Elliott Fisher and several colleagues at Dartmouth proposed a new way to measure the performance of hospitals and the doctors in private practice in the surrounding communities who are affiliated with them. Called the "extended hospital medical staff," their plan would look at how well a hospital and all the doctors affiliated with it care for the entire population of patients who regularly come to that hospital—much the way the VHA monitors the performance of its hospitals. Most doctors who care for hospitalized patients—surgeons, for instance, and cardiologists—tend to be affiliated with no more than two hospitals. Even then, they generally do most of their work almost exclusively in one location. Patients, too, tend to be loyal to a single hospital, usually the one closest to where they live, in part because that's where their doctors refer them. Sure, people sometimes travel to get specialized care—cancer patients go to Sloan-Kettering, in Manhattan, and people fly to a hospital in Vail, Colorado, for orthopedic surgery. But the vast majority of patients, especially Medicare recipients with chronic diseases, who account for 60 percent of Medicare payments, stick to hospitals that are close to home.

That means that Medicare could set performance measures for hospitals and the doctors who work in them, much as the VHA has done, by measuring the population of patients they care for and how well they coordinate care. Medicare would then reward the hospital and its affiliated doctors for excellent performance as a group. This would get rid of the problem that individual doctors have under the current pay-for-performance plan of being penalized for not being able to control what happens to their patients when they go to other doctors. Now all the doctors affiliated with a hospital would have a stake in making sure they were working together to improve care.

It would also further encourage hospitals to begin restructuring the way they deliver care. Hospitals that recruited numerous specialists, built new catheterization labs, or bought the latest CT scanner to increase their volume of reimbursements for radiological tests would soon discover they had overinvested in things that didn't contribute to the outcomes of their patients. Hospitals would be rewarded for recruiting more primary care physicians, on the other hand, and encouraging integrated, coordinated care among their doctors and pushing them to follow established guidelines for appropriate treatment.

Eventually, Medicare should completely transform the way it pays physicians and hospitals. Instead of paying doctors and hospitals separately and reimbursing them for how much care they deliver, it will want to begin paying them as a group on a per capita basis, depending upon the number of patients they care for. (Because outcomes of their patients will be monitored and eventually made public, these integrated systems will not want to attract more patients than they can handle simply to boost their incomes.)

This shift toward a capitated system can be done gradually on a voluntary basis. Hospitals and doctors that decide to switch to the new payment plan will be rewarded with a small bonus, and they can continue sharing savings under Wennberg's proposal. Hospitals and physicians that don't want to play can continue being paid under the old system. But as information accumulates showing that the doctors and hospitals that form integrated groups provide better, more-efficient care, patients will eventually start to shift their allegiance to providers that will serve them best. Private insurers should also encourage their patients to go to the most efficient hospitals and the doctors who provide the highest-quality care.

There are three ways for doctors and hospitals to structure an integrated model of care. One is the physician-led, multispecialty group practice that also owns one or more hospitals. The Mayo Clinic is one example. The Lahey Clinic, in Boston, and the Cleveland Clinic are two more. All the evidence suggests that these groups are more likely than doctors in solo practice or small groups to use evidence-based medicine and employ information technology to deliver more-effective care. Another model is the hospital chain that employs physicians. Intermountain Healthcare owns twenty-one hospitals and clinics and employs twenty-one thousand people, including its doctors. If every hospital in America achieved the same level of efficiency in caring for the chronically ill as Intermountain, Medicare would save more than ten billion dollars a year. The third model is physician-hospital organizations, agreements between groups of doctors and hospitals that allow them to get around some of the legal barriers to cooperating. It doesn't much matter which way a hospital and its affiliated physicians want to organize themselves, as long as they begin working as a cooperative group that uses valid evidence-based medicine.

It's possible to imagine that one day, integrated physician-hospital systems will compete with one another for patients on the basis of the quality of care they deliver and their efficiency. The VHA, if it expanded eligibility to all veterans, would be one place among many that veterans could choose. If VistA Health gets off the ground, as Longman envisions, competing hospitals and doctors will be forced to step up to the plate and show they can care for patients just as well as the VHA-administered hospitals. As the benchmarks for effective and efficient care improve, all hospitals will be pushed to higher and higher standards.

There are, of course, legal and practical barriers to such a plan. Antitrust laws currently make it difficult for hospitals and doctors to share savings. Another impediment is the so-called Stark rules, which currently restrict, but don't eliminate, a doctor's ability to self-refer, or send patients to facilities the doctor owns an interest in or for tests from which the doctor will profit. But if these laws can be made, they can be revoked or amended in order to allow Medicare to bring down costs and improve medical practice. During the phase-in period, Medicare should reform its distorted payment system, first eliminating the excess profitability of many procedures, so that hospitals won't be tempted, as they are now, to focus on certain departments at the expense of others. The next step will be an entirely new reimbursement system that capitates payments to a hospital and the doctors affiliated with it. Medicare will in effect be creating a series of health maintenance organizations, based on multispecialty group practices, which can compete with each other on the basis of quality. How each of these new groups achieves a higher level of quality is up to them, but they now have several model systems to emulate.

Naturally, there's going to be resistance to all of this from many quarters, if only because nobody likes to be forced to change. Hospitals are unaccustomed to being held responsible for the welfare of their patients. Older physicians who don't want to type won't like electronic medical records. Specialists won't like seeing their incomes restrained. Many of them in cities like Los Angeles will find there are fewer positions available. Other doctors will simply resist the idea that the hospital and Medicare can look over their shoulders. An increasingly vocal segment of the American public worries that electronic medical records are not secure enough to prevent employers from getting information that employees would rather keep private, like being diagnosed with a psychiatric condition. But if we can trust banks to protect our money, it seems reasonable to think we can devise a system to protect our medical information.

There are going to be plenty of doctors who will object to such a plan on other grounds. You'll hear them say that Medicare has no business coming between a physician and his patient and that doctors at places like the VHA and Kaiser practice inferior, "cookbook" medicine. This attitude is as understandable as it is wrong. For as long as there have been medical schools, doctors have been taught to think of themselves as small-business owners, as independent entrepreneurs. They don't learn how to cooperate with other doctors or monitor the outcomes of their patients in a systematic fashion. They are required to take a statistics course, but they don't actually learn how to interpret medical evidence. This system worked perfectly well when most people died of acute injury or short-term illness. Today, however, most of us live long enough to develop one or more chronic conditions, which we often suffer from for many years. Treating diabetes and heart disease requires a very different strategy from nursing an elderly patient through a bout of pneumonia. Yet, our entire system is still structured around the outmoded model of acute care.

As more and more physicians grow dissatisfied with medicine, many of them are coming around to the idea that being in a salaried group practice might not be so bad. Doctors who work for the VHA and the Mayo Clinic and staff-model HMOs like Kaiser are a self-selected bunch of idealists. They tend to be more interested in practicing good medicine than in making a lot of money. Salaries for specialists in such systems tend to be slightly lower, on average, than those of doctors in private practice, while primary care physicians enjoy comparable incomes but without the crushing demands of running an office and caring for huge numbers of patients in order to make ends meet. They also express higher levels of satisfaction than the average doctor, and word is beginning to get around. Dr. Lawrence Deyton, chief public health and environmental hazards officer at the Veterans Health Administration, says he has been hearing more and more from doctors who want to come work for the VHA: "Not a day goes by that somebody doesn't call me up asking for a job."

Evidence

This plan can work only if we increase the evidence for effective care. Does every patient who undergoes major surgery need a vena cava filter, the tiny, spiderlike metal device that traps blood clots before they can get to the lungs and cause an embolism? Doctors still disagree. Is lithotripsy, using ultrasound to blast kidney stones into tiny bits, better than surgery? It might not be as safe as doctors and patients think it is. Does everybody with slightly elevated cholesterol really need to take high doses of cholesterol-lowering drugs? These questions represent a microscopic fraction of the mysteries that remain in medicine. The Institute of Medicine estimates that only 4 percent of treatments and tests are backed up by strong scientific evidence; more than half have very weak evidence or none. We can't improve the quality of health care or control costs without better evidence for what works and what doesn't, and we can't expect private industry, which currently funds a majority of clinical trials, to underwrite the research that's necessary to give us that evidence. Getting medicine that's based on reality, rather than potential return on investment, requires a new source of funding. We collectively, as taxpayers and patients, have to find ways to fill the gaping holes in the science of medicine if we want better health care at the best price.

The FDA might seem like the obvious place to turn. But the agency is not set up to fund research, only to regulate the marketing of drugs and devices. The National Institutes of Health, with its thirty-billion-dollar annual budget, might seem like another good choice. The NIH has certainly funded some of the best clinical trials around. The eighty-million-dollar ALLHAT trial, for instance, which compared the effectiveness of different types of high-blood-pressure medications, was paid for by the National Heart, Lung, and Blood Institute. But the NIH isn't actually set up to examine the medical practices of today; its primary mission is to perform basic research that will lead to the cures of tomorrow, and the institutes currently spend only a tiny fraction of their budgets on studies like the ALLHAT trial, research that could change current practice. There's a sense at the NIH that such research, which would compare different drugs, for example, or test existing treatments, is somehow beneath the lofty goals of the agency. As NIH director Elias Zerhouni recently put it, "We don't do Coke versus Pepsi."

We need an institution that is dedicated to providing independent, reputable medical research that can lead directly to improving clinical practice.

One of its first jobs would be assessing the current evidence available for drugs. For instance, the ALLHAT trial has already shown that diuretics, which cost pennies a day, should be the first line of defense against high blood pressure. Armed with such data, insurance companies could adopt a system of "reference pricing," which has been used successfully in Germany to curb drug spending. Insurers reimburse patients fully only for the relatively low-cost, effective drugs, while requiring those who want a higher-priced but no more effective alternative to pay the difference. This would encourage patients to ask their doctors to be more conscious of the available evidence.

But drug research is only the first step. We also need information about devices, and about the wide array of medical practices that have never been put to any kind of real test. Believe it or not, we already have a federal agency that is supposed to produce precisely the sorts of studies we need. When it was created by Congress in 1985, the Agency for Health Care Policy and Research was given three tasks: to fund studies on the effectiveness of medical interventions; to create evidence-based clinical-practice guidelines for physicians; and to make recommendations to Medicare and Medicaid about what drugs, devices, and medical procedures to cover. But most Americans and many doctors have probably never heard of the AHCPR, partly because its name has been changed but also because the agency suffered a near-death experience shortly after the Republican takeover of Congress in 1994.

The AHCPR's troubles began the year before, when it commissioned a panel of twenty-three experts to create a clinical guideline for the treatment of acute lower-back pain. Among the panelists was an expert on back pain from the University of Washington, who had recently published an analysis of existing research on spinal fusion, the surgery that is commonly used for lower-back pain, though there's little credible evidence to suggest that spinal fusion is more effective than nonsurgical treatments. When the AHCPR's expert panel recommended nonsurgical remedies for most lower-back pain, back surgeons went wild. Sensing a threat to their livelihoods, because the AHCPR's guidelines could alter Medicare and Medicaid reimbursement decisions, the surgeons bombarded Congress with letters contending that the agency's panel was biased.

One surgeon, Neil Kahanovitz, founded the Center for Patient Advocacy, a nonprofit group that orchestrated a sustained lobbying campaign not just against the AHCPR's back-pain guidelines but against the entire agency. Kahanovitz found sympathetic ears in the new, antigovernment Republican Congress, led by Newt Gingrich. The agency's name appeared on a House Budget Committee's "hit list" of 140 federal programs targeted for elimination. The surgeons were joined in their efforts to kill the AHCPR by Sofamor Danek, a manufacturer of pedicle screws, devices consisting of plates or rods that are used during spinal fusion surgery—typically adding thousands of dollars to the cost. Sofamor Danek unsuccessfully sought a court injunction to prevent the agency from publishing its guidelines on back pain. Despite support for the AHCPR from the American College of Physicians, the American Medical Association, and the American Hospital Association, the House of Representatives zeroed out its budget. The agency survived thanks to the Senate, but only just barely, with a 25 percent budget cut. The AHCPR was given a new name, the Agency for Healthcare Research and Quality, and stripped of its authority to recommend payment decisions to Medicare and Medicaid.

When the agency's guidelines on treating acute back pain were finally published, they had little impact on medical practice. The number of spinal fusions has continued to rise dramatically over the past decade, going up 127 percent between 1997 and 2004. We spend more than $16 billion each year on spinal fusions, even though there still has never been a rigorous, government-funded clinical trial showing that the surgery is superior to other methods of relieving back pain. We spend an additional $2.5 billion on fusion hardware like pedicle screws, which can add $16,000 to the price of a surgery. Yet there's practically no evidence to show that all those screws and plates improve outcomes either.

Today, the device and drug industries, along with many physicians, remain wary of any form of technology assessment. Companies worry that profit margins will fall when the true value of their products is known and can be compared with alternative treatments. Drug companies enjoy margins that hover in the mid to high teens, a far cry from the 7 percent profit seen on average by companies in the Fortune 500. In 2002, Pfizer, the world's biggest drug company, reported a 28.4 percent return on sales. That was two and a half times better than the 10.7 percent return of General Electric, which is ranked as America's best-managed company. It was nearly nine times better than the 3.3 percent return of Wal-Mart, America's most efficient retailer. Device makers do even better: About 30 percent of the thirty billion dollars we pay for such implantable medical devices as vena cava filters, cardiac defibrillators, artificial hips, and cardiovascular stents is profit. Drug and device makers say they need high profit margins in order to fund their research and development; anything that threatens their margins, they argue, could stifle innovation, and they routinely lobby Congress whenever it looks as if legislation in favor of technology assessment might pass. They argue that technology assessment will lead to lower profits, and lower profits will kill the golden goose of future medical innovation.

That's hard to believe, given that other industries like high tech manage to maintain high levels of innovation on far lower margins. The more likely result of technology assessment is that it will bring about a real market, where only the most effective technologies command the high prices that are now paid for the majority of new devices and drugs, regardless of their real worth. These high prices are sustained in large measure by aggressive marketing, much of it through third parties like academic thought leaders, a tactic that can work only in the absence of reliable, independent, comparative data on effectiveness and safety. Nobody will pay Mercedes-Benz prices for a Hyundai when they can turn to Consumer Reports to comparison shop. But in health care, there's so little comparative information that we pay Mercedes-Benz prices for most devices and new drugs, and for many procedures. The AHRQ, the agency that rose from the ashes of the AHCPR, could provide the kind of information that payers, doctors, and patients need.

In order for the AHRQ to do that, Congress must be persuaded to beef up funding substantially from its current pitiful annual budget of three hundred and eighteen million dollars. Congress would also have to create fire walls to protect the agency from self-interested parties like back surgeons and pedicle screw manufacturers, as well as shifting political winds. The

AHRQ needs the kind of political insulation afforded the Federal Reserve Board, which is able to set sound fiscal policy in part because it is largely immune from congressional pressure. One way to do that would be to create an advisory board of three to six members whose presidential appointments lasted six years and ended in a staggered fashion, so no individual president could clean house. No more than a third of board members should come from industry. This board would help the AHRQ set priorities for appraising existing data and funding clinical trials.

How much would a new AHRQ cost? The U.S. drug industry spends forty billion dollars a year on research. That kind of money probably isn't going to come out of the federal budget any time soon. But we may not need that much, considering that much of the research drug companies now underwrite goes toward "experimercials," clinical trials aimed at increasing market share rather than increasing medical knowledge. If federal and private health insurance programs set aside .005 percent of the two trillion dollars we now spend on health care, the AHRQ would have a ten-billion-dollar endowment. The agency would fund three kinds of studies: comparative technology assessments using existing research; new clinical trials to provide the data needed to evaluate the effectiveness of different treatments; and research to define the most effective clinical pathways for caring for chronically ill patients. The AHRQ would serve as a clearinghouse for all clinical data and its research findings would be made available and accessible to the public.

If the AHRQ became the definitive source for reliable medical information, it could go far in improving the quality of health care. Patients routinely go to Web sites to diagnose themselves, or simply to learn more about a disease, a drug, or a scheduled procedure. But today's medical Web sites vary widely in the quality of information they provide, and even the most reputable sites must rely on what's published in the medical literature, which we've learned is often of dubious value. By going to the AHRQ (which would probably need to be renamed something easier to remember, like the Institute for Clinical Effectiveness, or ICE), both patients and doctors could feel they were making the right clinical choices. Publicizing comparative data could also go far in bringing down prices. It might not be so easy for drug reps to get doctors to prescribe Celebrex when their patients know the drug is more dangerous than over-the-counter ibuprofen and no more effective. It ought to be even harder to get insurers to pay a dollar a pill.

Learning what patients want

Of course, even with a large research budget, it will be many years before the AHRQ can put medicine on firmer scientific footing. Even then, much of what doctors do will remain uncertain. For instance, it may never be possible to conduct a clinical trial to test whether mammography really brings down death rates because too many women and their doctors are already convinced of its merits and will never be willing to enter a trial that might randomly assign them not to be screened for breast cancer. In cases where the benefits of a procedure, drug, or test are uncertain, patients need to be given clear, unbiased information about what's at stake.

Strengthening the patient's role in choosing a particular treatment or test is an important aspect of moving toward more efficient care. Much of the geographic variation in elective procedures arises in large part because of poor communication between physician and patient. Patients don't always understand the competing risks and benefits, and doctors don't always recognize how different patients can be in what they value most when it comes to medical treatment. In the case of the PSA test, for example, one man might fear the possibility of having even a relatively harmless cancer more than he fears the decline in his quality of life that is likely to result from prostate surgery. Over the past two decades, researchers have come up with a variety of aids to help patients come to good decisions. These aids range from short videos to brochures to interactive computer programs, all of which are intended to walk patients through what's known and unknown about a particular treatment or test and what's at stake for them. The aids provide an evidence-based, balanced description of all appropriate treatment options and questionnaires that measure whether the patient was fully informed and the treatment she chose reflected her values.

Decision aids are particularly important for the large number of medical interventions whose merits remain uncertain or whose benefits and risks may be viewed differently by different patients. When physicians discuss such procedures with their patients, they tend to be poor judges of what individual patients really want. One person might find a side-effect intolerable while another is willing to risk it, even if the benefits of the treatment are uncertain. For their part, patients often walk away from discussions with their physicians with unrealistic expectations of both benefits and harms. The net result is overuse of treatments and tests that patients would reject if they had better information. Studies have found that when patients have access to decision aids that present clear, balanced, evidence-based information about a treatment, they are often more wary of the risks of medicine than their physicians are.

More than fifty clinical trials evaluating patient decision aids have shown that they help patients make choices that are more in line with their own values. For example, women with early breast cancer can choose either mastectomy or lumpectomy with radiation. Women who are more concerned about local recurrence of their tumor—and therefore the need for ongoing surveillance—are able to sort out their feelings more easily with the help of decision aids, and they often choose mastectomy; women who are very concerned about losing a breast are more likely to choose lumpectomy. Clinical trials consistently show that decision aids result in better knowledge about options, and in decisions that are more in line with the patient's preferences.

The good news for payers is that informing patients better will very likely decrease overutilization rates: Most clinical trials show that the use of decision aids leads to a decline in demand for surgery—about 25 percent overall. A reduction in surgery rates of this magnitude would result in savings of about four billion dollars a year for Medicare's eleven most common surgical procedures.

Getting decision aids into widespread use will require changes in the legal standards of medical practice. In most states the standard of practice is informed consent, which is based on the idea that the physician is the decision maker who determines medical necessity and informs the patient, who then consents to the doctor's recommendation. Promoting decision aids would require a new standard of practice based not on informed consent, but on informed patient choice. Without this change in the laws doctors who practice shared decision making would be vulnerable to lawsuits. This was evident in a case in Virginia in which a suit was brought against a doctor who used shared decision making with a patient who was considering undergoing the PSA test. The doctor and his patient discussed the test at length, weighing its risks and benefits together, and the patient chose not to undergo the test. When he was later diagnosed with prostate cancer he sued his physician for malpractice for not insisting that he take the test, and won. Malpractice law needs an overhaul for many reasons, not the least of which is its failure to punish and weed out bad doctors, and to compensate patients who are harmed by medical error. But most discussions of malpractice reform have yet to consider patients' need for more balanced and evidence-based information.

Things are beginning to change. The state of Washington recently passed a bill that recognizes the legal status of informed patient choice. The legislature found that high-quality decision aids, which detail the benefits, harms, and uncertainty of available treatment options, improve communication between doctor and patient. The bill will promote effective decision aids and reform the state's laws on informed consent.

The current payment system is another major barrier to informed patient choice. Medicare, like most insurers, pays for utilization, not for shared decision making. Hospitals that implement it will lose money because utilization of their services will go down. Recently, Wennberg and his team recommended that Medicare should expand its P4P agenda to reward hospitals that establish a certified shared decision-making process for ten conditions that often result in elective surgery, such as chest pain due to angina; hip and knee arthritis; silent gallstones; prostate conditions; and breast cancer. The ten conditions account for about 40 percent of Medicare spending for surgery. Hospitals and surgery centers that provided high-quality patient decision aids would receive a small bonus. At the end of an eight-year transition period, Medicare would only reimburse for the ten surgeries if the hospital or surgery center had a certified system in place for supporting informed patient choice.

Medical schools

In the new world of health care, medical schools will have a central role to play, not only in teaching future doctors how to evaluate scientific evidence but also in setting an example of how to organize an efficient hospital system. While some academic medical centers—Oregon Health and Science University and the University of Wisconsin, for example—are models of relative efficiency, the quality of care at many other academic hospitals, even those with superb reputations, is below average. As Medicare begins to measure efficiency and outcomes, it's possible to imagine that academic medical centers will want to lead the way toward higher quality. Instead of hanging banners outside their doors advertising their ranking by U.S. News & World Report, hospitals will want to be known for being rated highly by Medicare.

Medical schools must also begin to redress the state of primary care. The American Medical Association is now calling for fifteen new medical schools in order to train more doctors by 2015. As the baby boomers age, the AMA argues, and doctors retire, we will need to train many more physicians in the coming years. There's considerable disagreement over this, but the most worrisome aspect of the AMA's argument is that those new doctors should be specialists. Why? Because specialists are the doctors that many Americans want to see.

Maybe that's so, but health care economists aren't sure that we should assume the financial burden of those who want to go to specialists. Especially when it's now clear that more specialists in the system will exacerbate the poor quality, high rate of errors, and delivery of unnecessary care. If everybody paid out of pocket for all of their medical care, your desire to go to a specialist wouldn't be anybody else's problem, it would be your right to be seen by the doctors of your choice. But we pay for medicine collectively, and health care is a shared resource. We pay into the system when we are relatively healthy so that the system will be there for us when we fall ill and need expensive care.

What's absolutely certain now is that we don't need more specialists, but we do need more generalists. Many people are already having difficulty finding a primary care physician, and as more and more of them quit practicing or go back into residencies to train to be higher-paid specialists, the shortage of primary care physicians will only get worse. Medicare needs to fix the payment system that overpays for procedures and underpays for the care that's necessary to manage chronic disease and to prevent it. To do a good job at this, primary care doctors need to see fewer patients on average per day. That means we need to pay them more per visit under the current reimbursement system. Eventually, when Medicare pays hospitals and their extended medical staffs a capitated rate, primary care physicians should receive salaries that are closer to what some specialists now make. And part of the money Medicare saves in the early phases of improving hospital efficiency should go toward supporting primary care.

Some of the care that patients need doesn't require a doctor. Dr. Arnold Milstein, a psychiatrist who now works for the Pacific Business Group on Health, a consortium of companies looking for ways to improve health care and bring down costs, envisions a system that employs "health coaches," people who help patients learn to make changes in their lifestyles that can improve their health and prevent disease. You don't need a doctor to learn to monitor your blood sugar or to learn to eat properly. Some insurers have figured this out and now employ battalions of nurses, who spend their time on the phone checking up on patients with chronic conditions. Franklin Health, a company based in Upper Saddle River, New Jersey, manages so-called complex cases for private insurers. Complex cases are the sickest of the sick, patients with multiple or terminal illnesses, who are also the most costly to treat. They typically make up only 1 or 2 percent of the average patient population while accounting for 30 percent of the costs. Franklin's nurses make home visits and spend hours on the phone, sometimes every day, to help patients control pain and other symptoms and stay out of the hospital. For this low-tech but intensive service, the company charges insurers an average of six thousand to eight thousand dollars per patient—but it saves them fourteen thousand to eighteen thousand dollars per patient in medical bills.

Losers and winners

The repercussions from putting medicine on firmer scientific footing and making hospitals more efficient at delivering care will be huge. Many hospital workers and some specialists will find themselves out of a job. Device- and drugmakers will see lower sales for some products and lower profits for many. Investors who hold stock in those companies will see lower returns. Fewer ICU beds means fewer ICU nurses and pulmonologists, the doctors who are often in charge of patients in an ICU. Fewer CT scanners and more judicious use of them could mean fewer radiologists and radiology technicians, and lower sales for GE.

But it's not as if the money that is saved by moving toward a more efficient, effective health care system evaporates. It is made available to do other things in the economy. Companies that are staggering under the weight of their health care obligations, like General Motors, will find themselves able to pay their workers more, to innovate and invest in new product lines. New jobs will be created to support IT systems in hospitals, and medical researchers will be needed to conduct the studies that evaluate the effectiveness of medical treatments. There's no denying that shrinking our health care system will cause dislocation among workers and lower profits for some sectors of the medical industry. But America's industries are undergoing constant change, and in any other arena of our economy we would never tolerate the degree of waste and inefficiency and lack of accountability that's rife in health care.

As we move toward a more efficient, effective system, patients will be the biggest winners of all. As hospitals begin to focus on integrating care, patients will be less likely to fall through the cracks and be deprived of care that they need. They will suffer fewer medical errors, and they will be subjected to less unnecessary, invasive, and potentially dangerous care.

Everybody will begin to save money. Medicare will see the savings first, but as hospitals are pushed toward efficiency, those savings will spill over to private insurance. That means employers and states will pay less for health care. Primary care physicians will find their services once again in demand. Disease-management companies, which help hospitals figure out the best practices to care for their chronically ill patients will have plenty of business.

To reach this point, we have to begin trusting our doctors again. The past two decades have created a sort of schizophrenic attitude about medicine and health care. On the one hand, we want to believe that medicine can cure every disease, if only we could afford the right doctors. We hold on to the fantasy that medicine has become all powerful, that we don't need to exercise any discipline in our lives, because there's a pill to fix the results of smoking and eating to excess. We think we shouldn't have to suffer pain for any reason, or put up with the infirmities of old age.

At the same time, we think our doctors are either incompetent or out to deprive us of the wonderful treatments and medicines that the media tell us will keep us healthy. We go to the Internet to diagnose ourselves and march into our doctors' offices with our sheets of printouts in hand. We demand to be given prescriptions for the drugs we see advertised on TV, and we want to have an MRI for every sprained wrist and swollen knee.

Doctors, too, have come to view us patients with increasing distrust. They worry we will sue them for malpractice, or that we will complain to our insurers if they don't provide the care we demand. Doctors' chat rooms on the Internet are filled with dispirited and angry postings. Emergency physicians especially feel unappreciated by patients who come in for trivial complaints and then grow angry when the doctor suggests they go home and wait until morning. One doctor recounts the story of a couple that came to the emergency room demanding that the woman be given a pregnancy test. When the doctor suggested she could purchase an over-the-counter test, the couple accused him of simply trying to save money.

If you go to a VA hospital, you'll see a very different kind of interaction between providers and patients. Many doctors and nurses who work for the VA are veterans themselves or have family members in the service. Shirley Paulson, the chief nurse in the ICU in Palo Alto, has a son in Iraq. This gives VA workers a sense of pride when they care for the men and women who share that experience, and it shows in the tenderness they display to their patients and their commitment to improving the quality of care they deliver. The patients, too, seem more grateful for the care they receive than patients you see in other hospitals and clinics. Part of that comes from the fact that VA primary care doctors have time to spend with their patients. They can listen to a veteran's list of worries and address each one without having to hustle him out the door in order to see the next patient. But many veterans also know that the care they get is demonstrably superior to what they would see almost anywhere else. The rest of us could enjoy the same quality of care and the same sense of being cared for by our doctors. Getting there is going to mean giving up some of our most cherished notions about the nature of medicine and the economics of our health care. Chief among these is the belief that more medical care is always better.

ACKNOWLEDGMENTS

In any work of nonfiction, the author's name may go on the cover, but the pages that follow would never have been filled without the help of countless others. I'm indebted to so many people I scarcely know where to begin. Every patient, researcher, nurse, and doctor I mention by name in this book gave generously of his or her time and thoughts, and I'm grateful to all of them. But for each person who appears on the page, there are a dozen others standing silently in the wings.

Several institutions provided access to experts who helped me understand the paradox of the hospital business. Chief among them is Johns Hopkins Medicine, where Joann Rodgers helped open doors to administrators who spent many hours walking me through the ins and outs of hospital finances. Johns Hopkins physicians helped me understand the tension between margin and mission at academic medical centers. I owe a debt of gratitude to Diane Meier's palliative care team at Mount Sinai; the doctors and nurses at the Veterans Health Administration Hospital in Palo Alto; to Matt Kestenbaum and the Hospice of Washington Center; Virginia Mason Hospital and Medical Center; and Stanford Hospital & Clinics.

Numerous doctors were more than generous with their time, and their insights inform this book throughout. I spent a day following an extraordinary physician, Harry Rinehart, who runs the rural clinic in Wheeler, Oregon. Cornelius Olcott, of Stanford, provided me the thrill of seeing surgery for the first time. Jonathan Altschuler invited me into the catheterization lab. I leaned heavily on David Elpern, a true hoaloha, and Michael McComb, the kind of doctor we all wish we had. Discussions with Marcia Angell, Robert Berenson, Donald Berwick, Howard Brody, Richard Deyo, Lawrence Deyton, Mark Ebell, Michael Fine, Tonia Fox, Nortin Hadler, Greg Henry, Jerome Hoffman, Chuck Hyman, Jerome Kassirer, Barnett Kramer, Kenneth Kwon, Robert Lindemann, Joanne Lynn, Arnold Milstein, Cyndra Mogayzel, Joe Moser, Shanker Nesathurai, Shawn Newlands, George Sledge, Graham Walker, and Michael Wilkes proved invaluable, and I'm grateful to Roy Poses and the doctors on the Health Care Renewal list for opening my eyes to the struggles of primary care physicians.

For all information economic or historic I turned to Victor Fuchs, Paul Ginsburg, Otha Linton, Mark Miller, Len Nichols, Lawrence O'Brien, Steve Pearson, Chas Rhodes, Sean Tunis, and Gordon Trapnell. A special note of thanks goes to Jack Wennberg and Elliott Fisher. Other Dartmouth researchers, including David Goodman, Megan McAndrew, Lisa Schwartz, Jonathan Skinner, Therese Stukel, James Weinstein, H. Gilbert Welch, and Steven Woloshin gave unsparingly of their time and I took a lot of it, often with the help of Martha Smith.

This book might never have come about without the backing of the New America Foundation, its wonderful staff, and my colleagues there. Sherle Schwenninger, especially, has been an unfailing source of intellectual support. My agent Jay Mandel of William Morris saw a book in me before I did, and gently pushed until I saw it too. I couldn't ask for a better editor than Gillian Blake and a better publisher than the team at Bloomsbury USA.

Numerous friends, family members, and colleagues offered enthusiastic and helpful criticism of various chapters, including Dr. Bernard Carroll, Dr. Diego Escobosa, Gabrielle Gallegos, Kate Glasner, Fruzsina Harsanyi, Barry Lynn, Phillip Longman, Anne MacLeod, Mary MacLeod, Lisa Margonelli, Anne Peticolas, Nancy Smith, Sheri Strite, Dr. Michael Stuart, Alexandra Trower, and Peter Trower. Peter Haugen saved a chapter from terminal muddiness with a few deft strokes of the keys. Donna Jackson Nakazawa provided a keen editor's eye. Jeanne Lenzer, my most faithful and unselfish reader, kept me from making errors of medical fact. Any mistakes that remain are mine alone.

When authors thank their friends, what they don't let on is that after leaning on their friends so heavily for so long for everything from picking up children to taking the dog for a walk, it's a wonder they have any friends left. Carole Feld was a font of brilliant marketing ideas and David Levy produced a wealth of photos. Mary Lynn Bobbitt, Cathy Coney, Jaymie Krens, Selma Manizade, Deacon Ritterbush, and Susan and Lou Wan were always there when I needed them, but George and Mary Pat Peabody did yeoman's duty. I can't thank them enough. Finally, I could never have written this book without the loving support and forbearance of my wonderful husband and son, Greg and Cole Garcia.

NOTES

Introduction

1 Why can't the United States: Malcolm Gladwell, "The Moral Hazard Myth," *NewYorker*, August 29, 2005.

1 Deamonte Driver: Mary Otto, "Boy Dies After Bacteria from Tooth Spreads to Brain," *Washington Post*, March 3, 2007.

2 Instead, we've decided to put up: Cathy Schoen et al., "U.S. Health System Performance: A National Scorecard," *Health Affairs*, September 20, 2006, Web exclusive, http://www.healthaffairs.org.

3 "I look at the U.S. health care system": Henry J. Aaron, "The Costs of Health Care Administration in the United States and Canada—Questionable Answers to a Questionable Question," *New England Journal of Medicine* 349, no. 8 (2003): 801–3.

4 Some policy analysts: Gerard F. Anderson et al., "It's the Prices Stupid: Why the United States Is so Different from Other Countries," *Health Affairs* 22, no. 3 (2003): 89–105.

6 In surveys conducted: Minah Kim, Robert J. Blendon, and Robert M. Berenson, "How Interested Are Americans in New Medical Technologies? A Multicountry Comparison," *Health Affairs* 20, no. 5 (2001): 194–201.

Chapter 1: Too Much Medicine

15 The heroic surgery: Paul Starr, *The Social Transformation of American Medicine* (New York: Basic Books, 1982).

15 Newsmagazines ran weekly reports: Anonymous, "A Healthy Outlook," *Newsweek* 1965.

16 And yet, patients still died: This case was written up in John E. Wennberg et al., "Renal Toxicity of Oral Cholecystographic Media. Bumamiodyl Sodium and

Iopanoic Acid," *Journal of the American Medical Association* 186 (1963): 461–67. The story can also be found in Morton Mintz, *The Therapeutic Nightmare* (Boston: Houghton Mifflin, 1965).

19 The most pressing reason: Starr, *Social Transformation of American Medicine*, 240–60.

19 "My own experience": Ibid, 256–57.

19 The AMA was in effect a labor union: Michael L Millenson, " 'Miracle and Wonder': The AMA Embraces Quality Measures," *Health Affairs* 16, no. 3 (1997): 183–94. The AMA and state medical societies argued at various points against compulsory smallpox and diphtheria vaccination; mandatory reporting of tuberculosis; publicly funded venereal disease clinics; even Red Cross blood banks, on the grounds that public health departments should not be in the business of treating patients—that was the doctor's job. In Chicago, a venereal disease clinic organized in 1919 by some of the city's leading philanthropists provided treatment for $185 a year, a bargain compared with the average of $525 charged by private physicians. Even though the patients were overwhelmingly poor, "the Chicago Medical Society denounced the clinic as unethical, accusing it of unfair competition, and expelled its staff physicians [from the society's ranks]." Clashes with public health clinics and vaccination programs were mild in comparison with the AMA's vitriolic opposition to universal health insurance and prepaid group practices, the earliest HMOs. For more information, see Starr, *Social Transformation of American Medicine*.

19 But the AMA's efforts: Richard Harris, "Annals of Legislation," Part 1–4, *New Yorker*, July 2, 9, 16, and 22, 1966.

23 In 1967, Jack Wennberg left: In the Regional Medical Program, also known as the Program to Conquer Heart Disease, Cancer and Stroke, academic medical centers were to become responsible for care throughout different regions in the United States, and to design systems of care. It was also intended to help technology developed in academic medical centers diffuse outward to community hospitals.

25 Other physicians did not share: John E. Wennberg and Alan Gittelsohn, "Small Area Variations in Health Care Delivery," *Science* 182, no. 117 (1973):1102–8.

30 While Wennberg continued gathering: For a more-recent look at physician workforce estimates, see "The Nation's Physician Workforce: Options for Balancing Supply and Requirements," Institute of Medicine, 1996, at http://darwin .nap.edu/books/0309054311/html/24.html.

30 In passing the legislation: George D. Lundberg, *Severed Trust: Why American Medicine Hasn't Been Fixed* (New York: Basic Books, 2000).

32 Before Medicare: Phillip Longman, personal communication, 2005.

33 inflationary spiral: Gordon Trapnell, pres. Actuarial Research Corp., personal communication, 2005; Lundberg, *Severed Trust*.

33 The government's payment: For a discussion of usual, customary, and reasonable, see Howard Wolinsky and Tom Brune, *The Serpent and the Staff: The Unhealthy Politics of the American Medical Association* (New York: Tarcher/Putnam, 1994), 47–48.

33 Primary care doctors did not play: George D. Lundberg, quoted in Maggie Mahar, *Money-Driven Medicine: The Real Reason Health Care Costs So Much* (New York: HarperCollins, 2006), 15.

33 A cardiac surgeon: Benson R. Roe, "The UCR Boondoggle: A Death Knell for Private Practice?," *New England Journal of Medicine* 305 (1981): 41–45.

33 Between 1950 and 1978: "The Nation's Physician Workforce: Options for Balancing Supply and Requirements," Institute of Medicine.

34 What they found was: *Spine Surgery: A Report by the Dartmouth Atlas of Health Care*, 2006, http://www.dartmouthatlas.com/atlases/Spine_Surgery_2006.pdf; see also Lucian Leape, "Unnecessary Surgery," *Annual Review of Public Health* 13 (1992): 363–83; see also John E. Wennberg et al., "Are Hospital Services Rationed in New Haven or Over-utilized in Boston?," *Lancet* 1, no. 8543 (1987): 1185–89.

34 By 1995, Medicare's bills had hit: *Medicare Chart Book*, 3rd ed., Kaiser Family Foundation, Summer 2005, http://www.kff.org/medicare/upload/Medicare-Chart-Book-3rd-Edition-Summer-2005-Section-6.pdf; see also http://www.publicagenda.org/issues/factfiles_detail.cfm?issue_type—edicare&list=12.

35 Not all parts: For more information about Wennberg's work, see www.dartmouthatlas.com.

35 The differences in cost: John E. Wennberg, Elliott Fisher, and Jonathan Skinner, "Geography and the Debate over Medicare Reform," *Health Affairs*, February 2002, Web exclusive, http://www.healthaffairs.org.

36 In 2000: Estimate of deaths from overtreatment is from Elliott Fisher, personal communication, January 2006.

37 Beyond the excess deaths: Wennberg, Fisher, and Skinner, "Geography and the Debate over Medicare Reform."

41 If you move from Tampa: John Wennberg, from a speech delivered December 2005, in Orlando, Florida.

Chapter 2: The Most Dangerous Place

43 On a chilly Tuesday: The story of Josie King's death is based on interviews with her mother, Sorrel King; see also Erika Niedowski, "How Medical Error Took a Little Girl's Life," *Baltimore Sun*, December 14, 2003, and "From Tragedy a Quest for Safer Care," *Baltimore Sun*, December 15, 2003.

46 Although nobody likes to think: Steven J. Spear and John Kenagy, "Deaconess-Glover Hospital," case study from Harvard Business School, August 25, 2005.

48 In 2003, the *Annals*: Elliott S. Fisher et al., "The Implications of Regional Variations in Medicare Spending," parts 1 and 2, *Annals of Internal Medicine* 138, no. 4
(2003): 273–298.

50 But it was the outcomes: For an in-depth analysis of Fisher's papers, see the
four editorials that accompanied them in the *Annals of Internal Medicine*. Critics argue that there is an alternative explanation for the slightly higher death rate in
the hospitals that are delivering the most care. It's possible that Fisher's team
failed to adequately measure the health of the patients in their study, and that
by some statistical fluke, thousands and thousands of patients who were in the
worst shape landed for the most part in the high-spending hospitals. The patients who were being treated in those hospitals that delivered more care really were sicker—and more likely to die—than those treated in hospitals that
delivered less care. That's why the high-spending hospitals did more for them,
because their condition was worse. That would mean the critics were right;
hospitals that provide more care do so because their patients are sicker and
consequently need more treatment.

This is unlikely. Fisher and his team bent over backward to ensure that
their cohorts of patients were, in fact, equally sick. They looked at several
dozen potential "confounding factors," medical conditions and socioeconomic factors that might skew their results. They tried to ensure, for example,
that the patients in each cohort had similar "comorbidities," additional ailments like diabetes and high blood pressure that could affect their overall
health. There was no consistent difference between the patients who went to
different hospitals.

51 A medical student: Interview with the physician, March 2006.

51 Betsy Lehman: Richard Knox, "Doctor's Orders Killed Cancer Patient," *Boston
Globe*, March 23, 1995.

52 In 1999, the prestigious Institute: Some researchers have taken issue with the
manner in which the Institute of Medicine gathered evidence and categorized
errors, saying it inflated the death rate by including falls as avoidable error.
Other critics argue just the opposite, that most errors go unreported, which
would mean the true number of medical mistakes is even higher. Institute of
Medicine, *To Err Is Human: Building a Safer Health System*, November 1999.

52 Drug errors: D. W. Bates et al., "Incidence of Adverse Drug Events and Potential
Adverse Drug Events. Implications for Prevention. ADE Prevention Study
Group," *Journal of the American Medical Association* 274, no. 1 (1995): 29–34.

52 Why are so many errors: Examples come from Atul Gawande, *Complications:
A Surgeon's Notes on an Imperfect Science* (New York: Picador, 2002).

54 In his book: James Reason, *Human Error* (Cambridge, U.K.: Cambridge University Press, 1990).

55 The chances that multiple errors: Interview with former physician's assistant Jeanne Lenzer; historical death rate from Centers for Disease Control and Prevention, http://www.disastercenter.com/cdc/aacutcar.html.

57 Even aspirin: E. M. Antman et al., "A Comparison of Results of Meta-analyses of Randomized Control Trials and Recommendations of Clinical Experts: Treatments for Myocardial Infarction," *Journal of the American Medical Association* 268, no. 2 (1992): 240–48.

58 This unhappy fact: Stephen Grund, personal communication, May 2006.

61 A telling little study: Elliott Fisher, unpublished data.

62 What Fisher is saying: John E. Wennberg et al., "Evaluating the Efficiency of California Providers in Caring for Patients with Chronic Illnesses," *Health Affairs*, November 16, 2005, Web exclusive, http://www.healthaffairs.org.

64 All of which points: For example, see Regina E. Herzlinger, *Consumer-Driven Health Care: Implications for Providers, Payers, and Policy-Makers.* (New York: Jossey-Bass 2004).

64 In his slim: Donald M. Berwick, *Escape Fire: Lessons for the Future of Health Care* (New York: The Commonwealth Fund, 2002).

66 This astonishing finding: Elizabeth A. McGlynn et al., "The Quality of Healthcare Delivered to Adults in the United States," *New England Journal of Medicine* 348, no. 26 (2003): 2635–45; see also Mark A. Schuster, Elizabeth A. McGlynn, and Robert Brook, "How Good Is the Quality of HealthCare in the United States?," *Millbank Quarterly* 83, no. 4 (2005): 843–95.

67 What is known: See, for example, David C. Goodman et al., "End of Life Care at Academic Medical Centers: Implications for Future Workforce Requirements," *Health Affairs* 25, no. 2 (2006): 521–531; R. L. Ferrer, S. J. Hambidge, and R. C. Maly, "The Essential Role of Generalists in Health Care Systems," *Annals of Internal Medicine* 142, no. 8 (2005): 691–99; Barbara Starfield et al., "The Effects of Specialist Supply on Populations' Health: Assessing the Evidence," *Health Affairs*, March 15, 2005, Web exclusive, http://www.healthaffairs.org.

68 What all of this says: Jeanne Lenzer, personal communication, May 2006; Jeanne Lenzer, "Benefits of Gatekeeping," *Journal of Family Practice* 46, no. 3 (1998): 257–58.

70 This hazard declines: *Morbidity and Mortality Weekly Report*, Centers for Disease Control and Prevention, October 14, 2005, http://www.cdc.gov/mmwr/preview/mmwrhtml/mm5440a2.htm.

Chapter 3: Your Local Hospital

72 Dr. Patrick Campbell: The story of Redding Medical Center and Campbell's role is based on extensive interviews with Campbell as well as newspaper sources and court documents.

73 he graduated in 1972: Kurt Eichenwald, "Operating Profits: Mining Medicare; How One Hospital Benefited from Questionable Surgery," *New York Times*, August 12, 2003.

74 When Moon arrived: Ibid.

74 Primary care physicians: Dorsey Griffith, "Paving the Way: Small Town MDs Grateful to Redding Duo," *Sacramento Bee*, January 12, 2003.

74 Moon sometimes performed: Andrew Pollack "California Patients Talk of Needless Heart Surgery," *New York Times*, November 4, 2002.

74 Between June 2001 and 2002: Eichenwald, "Operating Profits."

75 With the enormous volume of procedures: David Streitfeld, "Tenet Under Closer Exam; Chae Hyun Moon Had His Patients' Respect, if not Love. Now Many Wonder About Him," *Los Angeles Times*, November 11, 2002.

75 In a letter to the editor: Dorsey Griffith, "Beleaguered Doctors Are Heroes to Many: Redding Residents Say Two Heart Specialists Have Saved—and Enriched—Many Lives," *Sacramento Bee*, December 1, 2002.

75 In the summer of 1993: Patrick Campbell, personal communication.

77 Medical records seized: Eichenwald, "Operating Profits."

77 In the opinion of the outside specialists: Maline Hazle, "RMC Duo Called a 'Threat': Board Asks Judge to Suspend Cardiologists' Medical Licenses," *Redding Record Searchlight*, November 9, 2002.

77 In May 2006: Ryan Sabalow, "State Accuses Cardiac Surgeon: Medical Board Wants to Take Realyvasquez's License," *Redding Record Searchlight*, May 17, 2006.

77 By then Redding Medical's: "Tenet Healthcare Corporation to Pay U.S. More than $900 Million to Resolve False Claims Acts Allegations," *U.S. Newswire*, June 29, 2006.

78 Today, hospitals still need: Jack Hadley and John Holahan, "How Much Medical Care Do the Uninsured Use, and Who Pays for It?," *Health Affairs*, February 12, 2003, Web exclusive, http://www.healthaffairs.org. Hadley and Holahan say that 75 percent of uncompensated care is actually reimbursed, either by the government or by private insurance.

79 In their search: Sandra G. Boodman, "Hospitals Go Deluxe," *Washington Post*, September 15, 1998.

79 Billboard ads: See Wikipedia, "Johns Hopkins," http://en.wikipedia.org/wiki/Johns_Hopkins.

82 In other words: Glenn A. Melnick et al., "Emergency Department Capacity and Access in California, 1990–2001: An Economic Analysis," *Health Affairs*, March 24, 2004, Web exclusive, http://www.healthaffairs.org; Susan Headden, "Guns, Money and Medicine," *U.S. News & World Report*, July 1, 1996.

82 Much of the disparity: Rick Mayes, "Causal Chains and Cost Shifting: How

Medicare's Rescue Inadvertently Triggered the Managed-Care Revolution," *Journal of Policy History* 16, no. 2 (2004): 144–74.

83 It was a payment plan: Gregg Easterbrook, "The Revolution in Medicine," *Newsweek*, January 26, 1987.

84 The following year: Len Nichols, New America Foundation, personal communication.

84 But the DRG system: Paul B. Ginsburg and Joy M. Grossman, "When the Price Isn't Right: How Inadvertent Payment Incentives Drive Medical Care," *Health Affairs*, August 9, 2005, Web exclusive, http://www.healthaffairs.org.

84 In 2002, Medicare paid $24,000: *Report to the Congress*, Medicare Payment Advisory Commission, March 2005, 21.

85 more than one hospital: Robert Berenson, Urban Institute, personal communication.

85 From private payers: *Report to the Congress: Physician Owned Specialty Hospitals*, Medicare Payment Advisory Commission, March 2005, Table 10; Liz Kowalczyk, "Small Hospitals Battle for Right to Do Angioplasties," *Boston Globe*, February 13, 2005; Richard A. Lange and L. David Hillis, "Use and Overuse of Angiography and Revascularization for Acute Coronary Syndromes," *New England Journal of Medicine* 338, no. 25 (1998): 1838–39.

85 Dell earns: Alex L. Goldfayn, "TV's Past Meets Its Future as PC Firms Enter Market," *Chicago Tribune*, February 28, 2004.

85 Yet, when hospitals focus: Dr. Joanne Lynn, Centers for Medicare & Medicaid Services, personal communication. See also Ralph Snyderman and R. Sanders Williams, "The new prevention," *Modern Healthcare* 33, no. 19 (2003); "Congestive Heart Failure: Comprehensive Heart Failure Teams Reduce Health Care Costs," *Health & Medicine Week* (2000) http://www.newsrx.com/article.php?articleID=40811; Ian Urbina, "In the Treatment of Diabetes, Success Often Does Not Pay," *New York Times*, January 11, 2006; *Improving Health Care: A Dose of Competition*, the Federal Trade Commission and the Department of Justice, July 24, 2004, http://www.ftc.gov/reports/healthcare/040723health carerpt.pdf.

87 "We were beyond full": Eichenwald, "Operating Profits."

87 "Hospitals need to understand": Quoted in Maggie Mahar, *Money-Driven Medicine: The Real Reason Health Care Costs So Much* (New York: HarperCollins, 2006).

87 With so much riding: Eichenwald, "Operating Profits."

88 By 1999, Campbell had stopped: *United States Court of Appeals for the Ninth Circuit Patrick Campbell, M.D., USA and State of Calif ex rel; Plaintiff and Appellant USA Intervenor and Appellee v. Redding Medical Center, and Tenet Healthcare Corporation, Defendants.*

89 Two weeks later: Melissa Davis, "Insider Sales Cloud the Tenet Tale," TheStreet.com, November 14, 2002.

89 The Justice Department's: Dr. Vincent Yap, chief of cardiology for the Richmond-based Permanente Medical Group and flight surgeon at Travis Air Force Base, reviewed patient records for the California State Medical Board, which filed a temporary restraining order against Moon and Realyvasquez in 2002. See Hazle, "RMC Duo Called a 'Threat' "; Hazle, "Doctor, Hospital Feuded; Mercy Attempted to Monitor Moon's Operating Procedures," Redding Record Searchlight, January 5, 2003; and Ryan Sabalow, "State Accuses Cardiac Surgeon."

90 Other patients: Mahar, Money-Driven Medicine.

90 On August 4: United States Court of Appeals for the Ninth Circuit.

91 There are many lessons: Lawrence O'Brien, Bad Medicine: How the American Medical Establishment Is Ruining Our Healthcare System (Amherst, NY: Prometheus Books, 1999), 150–154.

91 In Los Angeles, for instance: John E. Wennberg, unpublished data.

91 Meanwhile, more than a hundred: See work by Alan Sager, Boston University School of Public Health, http://www.rwjf.org/reports/grr/028054.htm; see also Matt Leingang, "Flu Cases Strain Hospital Capacity," Cincinnati Enquirer, March 1, 2005.

93 In June 2003: Kelly St. John and Mark Martin, "Heart Patient's Many Lives: Redding Whistle-blower Went from Riches to Rags to Robes," San Francisco Chronicle, November 10, 2002.

94 It would take more than two years: Maline Hazle, "RMC 'Whistleblower' Pipes Up," Redding Record Searchlight, September 13, 2003; Hazle, "RMC Whistleblowers Will Share $8.1 Million Reward," Redding Record Searchlight, January 8, 2004.

94 Neither Moon nor Realyvasquez: Streitfeld, "Tenet Under Closer Exam."

94 He wept: Ibid.

Chapter 4: Broken Hearts

101 Only recently have cardiologists: Gina Kolata, "New Studies Question Value of Opening Arteries," New York Times, March 21, 2004.

102 Dr. Nortin Hadler: Nortin M. Hadler, The Last Well Person: How to Stay Well Despite the Health-Care System (Montreal: McGill-Queen's University Press, 2004), 210–12. The studies were all conducted in the 1980s, and cardiologists now say techniques have improved so much that the results of the studies are obsolete. Hadler argues that if that's so, cardiothoracic surgeons and cardiologists should do new studies to find out if they are right that the five hundred thousand bypass surgeries and more than a million stents and angioplasties that are being performed annually are as worthwhile as their supporters contend. See also A. M. Khan and S. Jacobs, "Trash Feet After Coronary Angiography," Heart 89, no. 17 (2003): e17.

102 "An alarming number never": Guy M. McKhann et al., "Cognitive Outcome after Coronary Artery Bypass: A One-year Prospective Study," *Annals of Thoracic Surgery* 63, no. 2 (1997): 510–15; John Carey, "Is Heart Surgery Worth It?," *BusinessWeek*, July 18, 2005; personal communication with David Brown of SUNY Stony Brook, June 15, 2006.

103 "He would ask her": G. Vingerhoets et al., "Short-term and Long-term Neuropsychological Consequences of Cardiac Surgery with Extracorporeal Circulation," *European Journal of Cardiothoracic Surgery* 3, no. 3 (1997): 424–31.

103 In 2001, a group of researchers: Eric C. Schneider et al., "Racial Differences in Cardiac Revascularization Rates: Does 'Overuse' Explain High Rates in White Patients?," *Annals of Internal Medicine* 135, no. 5 (2001): 328–37.

104 More than a billion dollars: The average DRG payment for bypass surgery is twenty-four thousand dollars, according to the MedPAC's March 2005 *Report to the Congress*, "Physician-Owned Specialty Hospitals," http://www.medpac.gov/search/searchframes.cfm. There are four hundred thousand CABG procedures a year.

105 Many doctors are happy to: Roy Poses et al., "Physicians' Judgments of Survival After Medical Management and Mortality Risk Reduction Due to Revascularization Procedures for Patients with Coronary Artery Disease," *Chest* 122, no. 9 (2002): 122–33; Richard A. Lange and L. David Hillis, "Use and Overuse of Angiography and Revascularization for Acute Coronary Syndromes," *New England Journal of Medicine* 338, no. 25 (1998): 1838–39.

106 "The procedure can be done quickly": MGMA Physician Compensation and Production Survey 2003, http://www.scai.org/PDF/SalarySurvey.pdf; American Medical Group Association Compensation and Financial Survey, 2004, http://www.scai.org/PDF/SalarySurvey.pdf.

106 The doctor makes another $800: 2006 Medicare Payment Changes for Physicians and Hospital Outpatient Services, http://www.guidant.com/reimbursement/vi_codes/md_op2006.shtml.

107 Nonetheless, doctors in the south central states: Louise Pilote et al., "Regional Variation Across the United States in the Management of Acute Myocardial Infarction," *New England Journal of Medicine* 333, no. 9 (1995): 562–572.

109 In other words, these doctors have: Therese A. Stukel et al., "Long Term Outcomes of Regional Variations in Intensity of Invasive vs Medical Management of Medicare Patients with Acute Myocardial Infarction," *Journal of the American Medical Association* 293, no. 11 (2005): 1329–37.

111 Yet patients in Boston: John E. Wennberg et al., "Are Hospital Services Rationed in New Haven or Over-utilized in Boston?," *Lancet* 1, no. 8543 (1987): 1185–89.

113 Other researchers have confirmed: M. J. Strauss et al., "Rationing of Intensive

Care Unit Services. An Everyday Occurrence," *Journal of the American Medical Association* 255, no. 9 (1986): 1143–46.

114 This pattern of supply-driven: David C. Goodman et al., "The Relation Between the Availability of Neonatal Care and Neonatal Mortality," *New England Journal of Medicine* 346, no. 20 (2002): 1538–44.

115 He was documenting the fact: The link between specialist supply and utilization has been documented by other researchers. For instance, see Victor Fuchs, "The Supply of Surgeons and the Demand for Operations," *Journal of Human Resources* 13 (1978): supplement 35–56.

116 With sixty-one beds: John E. Wennberg et al., "Evaluating the Efficiency of California Providers in Caring for Patients with Chronic Illnesses," *Health Affairs*, November 16, 2005, Web exclusive, http://www.healthaffairs.org.

Chapter 5: The Desperate Cure

This chapter is based on extensive interviews conducted between 1999 and 2001 with the following sources: Dr. Werner Bezwoda, University of Witwatersrand, South Africa; Paul Goldberg, the *Cancer Letter*; Dr. I. Craig Henderson, University of California, San Francisco; Marilyn MacGregor, Breast Cancer Action; Dr. William P. Peters, Adherex Technologies; Alice C. Philipson, Berkeley, California; Dr. Hope S. Rugo, University of California, San Francisco; Dr. Raymond B. Weiss, National Cancer Institute.

134 We now know that bloodletting: Kevin Patterson, "What Doctors Don't Know (Almost Everything)," *New York Times Magazine*, May 5, 2002.

135 Spinal fusion for low-back pain: Jerome Groopman, *How Doctors Think* (Boston: Houghton Mifflin, 2007).

137 But the first well-designed: James N. Weinstein et al., "Surgical vs Nonoperative Treatment for Lumbar Disk Herniation," *Journal of the American Medical Association* 296, no. 20 (2006): 2451–59.

137 The best that can be said: Richard Deyo and Donald Patrick, *Hope or Hype: The Obsession with Medical Advances and the High Cost of False Promises* (New York: Amacom, 2005).

138 Back surgeons can easily make: Douglas Dammrose, medical director, Blue Cross of Idaho, personal communication, December 2006.

138 Dr. Michael Stuart: Michael Stuart and Sheri Ann Strite, personal communication, January 2007.

140 Over the course of that time: Michelle M. Mello and Troyen A. Brennan, "The Controversy of High-dose Chemotherapy with Autologous Bone Marrow Transplant for Breast Cancer," *Health Affairs* 20, no. 5 (2001): 101–17.

Chapter 6: The Limits of Seeing

142 Socratic master class: Lawrence K. Altman, "Socratic Dialog Gives Way to PowerPoint," *New York Times*, December 1 2, 2006.

147 *Time Magazine* noted: Joshua Cooper Ramos, "Doc in a Box: Computers and
Other Wondrous Machines Have Already Conquered the World of Business.
They Are Now Transforming Medicine and Helping Save Patients' Lives—as
Well as Time and Money," *Time Magazine* Special Medical Issue, Fall 1996, 55.

147 *Newsweek* hailed: Jerry Adler and Deborah Witherspoon, "New Looks Inside the
Body," *Newsweek*, August 1 6, 1 982.

149 In a *JAMA* editorial: George D. Lundberg, "Low-Tech Autopsies in the Era of
High-Tech Medicine: Continued Value for Quality Assurance and Patient
Safety," *Journal of the American Medical Association* 280, no. 1 4 (1998): 1273–74.

149 All of this research: Kaveh G. Shojania et al., "Changes in Autopsy-Detected Diagnostic Error over Time," *Journal of the American Medical Association* 289, no. 2 1
(2003): 2849–56; Shojania et al., "Overestimation of Clinical Diagnostic Performance Caused by Low Necropsy Rates," *Quality and Safety in Health Care* 1 4, no.
6 (2005): 408–13.

150 In a brilliant essay: Malcolm Gladwell, "Mammography, Air Power, and the
Limits of Looking," *New Yorker*, December 1 3, 2004.

152 In 2001, a surgeon: David R. Flum et al., "Misdiagnosis and the Use of Diagnostic Imaging," *Journal of the American College of Surgeons* 201, no. 6 (2004):
933–39; Flum et al., "Has Misdiagnosis Rate of Appendicitis Decreased over
Time?," *Journal of the American Medical Association* 286, no. 1 4 (2001): 1748–53.

153 In 2005, the *Journal*: David M. Studdert et al., "Defensive Medicine Among
High-Risk Specialist Physicians in a Volatile Malpractice Environment," *Journal
of the American Medical Association* 293, no.2 1 (2005): 2609–17.

155 But many breast tumors: Frank D. Gililand et al., "Biological Characteristics of
Interval and Screen-Detected Breast Cancers," *Journal of the National Cancer Institute*
92, no. 9 (2000): 743–49.

157 The Spragues successfully sued: Michael Amon, "$5 Million Awarded in Med-
ical Malpractice Suit," *Washington Post*, February 1 5, 2004.

157 It's easier to acquiesce: Dr. Kathleen Jones, an ER physician in Palo Alto, California, who works at both Kaiser and the Veterans Health Administration Hospital, recently performed a small test of how well ER doctors and nurses
follow the rules for when to do an X-ray on an ankle injury. She found that ER
personnel at Kaiser were less likely to follow the rules and more likely to do
unnecessary X-rays than their peers at the VHA. The reason, she surmises, is
that Kaiser patients are generally more demanding: "Patients expect an X-ray,
and if they don't get one—even after explanations regarding soft tissue injury,
etc.—the patient feels they have received substandard care."

159 One set of rules: Jerome R. Hoffman et al., "Validity of a Set of Criteria to Rule Out Injury to the Cervical Spine in Patients with Blunt Trauma," *New England Journal of Medicine* 343, no. 2 (2000): 94–100.

163 They went on a buying spree: Kelly J. Devers, Linda R. Brewster, and Lawrence P. Casalino, "Changes in Hospital Strategy: A New Medical Arms Race?," *Health Services Research* 38 (2003): 447–469.

164 Doctors in private practice: David C. Levin and Vijay M. Rao, "The Wars in Radiology: Overutilization of Imaging Resulting from Self-referral," *Journal of the American College of Radiology* 1, no. 5 (2004): 317–21; Congressional testimony of Mark E. Miller, executive director of MedPAC, "MedPAC recommendations on imaging services," March 17, 2005, www.medpac.gov/publications/congres sional_testimony/031705_TestimonyImaging-Hou.pdf.

166 One study of twelve hundred whole-body: Claudia D. Furtado et al., "Whole-Body Screening: Spectrum of Findings and Recommendations in 1192 Patients," *Radiology* 237 (2005): 385–94.

168 The average head CT involves: "Radiation Exposure from Medical Diagnostic Imaging Procedures," Health Physics Society, at http://hps.org/documents/meddiagimaging.pdf.

168 In big hospitals: A. F. Mettler et al., "CT Scanning: Patterns of Use and Dose," *Journal of Radiological Protection* 20, no. 4 (2000): 353–59.

168 According to another estimate: Board on Radiation Effects Research, *Health Risks from Exposure to Low Levels of Ionizing Radiation: BEIR VII Phase 2* (Washington, D.C.: National Academies Press, 2006).

170 "This has been huge": Michael LaCombe, cardiologist, personal communication.

170 Meanwhile, the scientific evidence: Phillip Greenland, "Who Is a Candidate for Noninvasive Coronary Angiography?," *Annals of Internal Medicine* 145, no. 6 (2006): 466–67; Gina Kolata "Heart Scanner Stirs New Hope and a Debate," *New York Times*, November 17, 2004.

171 Besides, new devices and drugs: In a seminal paper published in 2001, Mark McClellan, the former head of Medicare and Medicaid Services under the second Bush administration, and his colleague David M. Cutler, a health care economist at Harvard, performed a cost-benefit analysis of several medical innovations. They showed that for every dollar spent on angioplasty and stents, society gained seven dollars in terms of lives saved from heart attacks (a life was estimated to be worth one hundred thousand dollars per year). Extrapolating from this analysis, and that of other new medical technologies, McClellan and Cutler argued that we should be willing to pay for the costs of new technology because it improves the quality of medicine and saves lives. See David M. Cutler and Mark McClellan, "Is Technological Change Worth It?,"

Health Affairs 20, no. 5 (2001): 11–29. In 2006, however, Jonathan Skinner and his colleagues at Dartmouth performed a similar analysis to find that since 1996, when Cutler and McClellan's study ended, the survival rate from heart attacks has stagnated, while spending on stents and angioplasty has continued to rise. See Jonathan S. Skinner, Douglas O. Staiger, and Elliott S. Fisher, "Is Technological Change in Medicine Always Worth It? The Case of Acute Myocardial Infarction," *Health Affairs*, February 7, 2006, Web exclusive, http://www.healthaffairs.org.

171 A study performed: Glenn M. Hackbarth, chairman of the Medicare Payment Advisory Commission, testimony before the U.S. House of Representatives, Committee on Energy and Commerce, Subcommittee on Health, http://www.medpac.gov/publications/congressional_testimony/20050512_Testimony SpecHospEC.pdf.

173 Yet the National Committee: Ibid.

Chapter 7: The Persuaders

177 "Dear Doctor" letter: http://www.yourlawyer.com/topics/overview/effexor.

177 A more-recent FDA study: David Gunnell, Julia Saperia, and Deborah Ashby, "Selective Serotonin Reuptake Inhibitors (SSRIs) and Suicide in Adults: Meta-analysis of Drug Company Data from Placebo Controlled, Randomised Controlled Trials Submitted to the MHRA's Safety Review," *British Medical Journal* 330, no. 7488 (2005): 26–30.

179 In 2002, doctors wrote: Gianna Rigoni, testimony at the meeting of the Psychopharmacologic Drugs Advisory Committee, February 2, 2004, http://www.fda.gov/ohrms/dockets/AC/04/transcripts/4006T1.doc.

179 Rates of pediatric prescriptions: Julie M. Zito et al., "Trends in the Prescribing of Psychotropic Medications to Preschoolers," *Journal of the American Medical Association* 283, no. 8 (2001): 1025–30.

180 More than 90 percent: Kenneth E. Towbin, "Gaining: Pediatric Patients and Use of Atypical Antipsychotics," *American Journal of Psychiatry* 163, no. 12 (2006): 2034–36.

180 Among boys ages six to twelve: Thomas J. Moore, senior scientist and health policy analyst at the George Washington University Medical Center, http://drugsafetyresearch.com/downloads/med_use_antidep.pdf.

180 In 2005, according to an analysis: Gardiner Harris, "Proof Is Scant on Psychiatric Drug Mix for the Young," *New York Times*, November 23, 2006.

180 When you look at Americans: David M. Walker, "New Spending Estimates Underscore Need for Reform," U.S. General Accounting Office, testimony at http://www.gao.gov/new.items/d01101ot.pdf.

181 We spend as much: Patricia M. Danzon and M. F. Furukawa, "Price and

Availability of Pharmaceuticals: Evidence From Nine Countries," *Health Affairs*, October 29, 2003, Web exclusive, http://www.healthaffairs.org.

182 For example, the redefinition: A. Baumgaertel et al., "Comparison of Diagnostic-criteria for Attention-deficit Disorders in a German Elementary-school Sample," *Journal of the American Academy of Child and Adolescent Psychiatry* 34, no. 5 (1995): 629–38; see also Tracy L. Skaer and Linda M. Robinson, findings presented May 2004 at American Psychiatric Association meeting, http://www.news-medical.net/print_article.asp?id=1300.

182 For instance, the criteria: National Cholesterol Education Program guidelines, http://www.nhlbi.nih.gov/new/press/01-05-15.htm.

183 The beginning: This section of the history of drug advertising is drawn largely from two sources: Greg Critser, *Generation Rx: How Prescription Drugs Are Altering American Lives, Minds, and Bodies* (New York: Houghton Mifflin, 2005): 32–35; J. Erlen and J. F. Spillane, *Federal Drug Control: The Evolution of Policy and Practice* (New York: Pharmaceutical Products Press, 2004), http://haworthpressinc.com/store/SampleText/5012.pdf.

185 Network executives: Anonymous, "Drug Companies Go Directly to Consumers in Quest for Doctors' Prescriptions," *Adweek*, January 4, 1988; Carla Lazzareschi, "Drug Ads: Prescription for Controversy: Pharmaceutical Firms Bypass Doctors to Aim Pitch Directly at Consumers," *Los Angeles Times*, May 1, 1988.

186 Pfizer ran an ad: Barbara Mintzes, "Direct to Consumer Advertising Is Medicalizing Normal Human Experience," *British Medical Journal* 324, no. 7342 (2002): 908–11.

187 Every dollar: Anonymous, "Prescription Drugs and Mass Media Advertising," National Institute for Health Care Management, September 2000, www.nihcm.org/DTCbrief.pdf.

187 That's a better return: Pierre DeLegge Consulting, "2004 Advertising to Sales Ratios for the 200 Largest Ad Spending Industries," *Marketing Today*, http://marketingtoday.com/tools/ad_to_sales_2004.htm.

187 Nearly one in three adults: Richard Frank et al., "Trends in Direct to Consumer Advertising of Prescription Drugs," Kaiser Family Foundation Report, http://www.kff.org/rxdrugs/loader.cfm?url=/commonspot/security/getfile.cfm&PageID=14881.

189 Reporters, she says: Trudy Lieberman, "Bitter Pill," *Columbia Journalism Review* 4 (July/August 2005).

189 Dedicated to: Mike Snider, "Sleepy Days Caused by Restless Nights," *USA Today*, June 20, 1991.

191 Australian journalist Ray Moynihan: Ray Moynihan and Alan Cassels, *Selling Sickness: How the World's Pharmaceutical Companies Are Turning Us All into Patients* (New York: Nation Books, 2005).

192 In 1998, SmithKline: Brendan I. Koerner, "Disorders Made to Order," *Mother Jones* 27, no 4 (2002): 58.

194 That year, New York's: "Settlement Sets New Standard for Release of Drug Information," New York State Department of Law press release, August 26, 2004, http://www.oag.state.ny.us/press/2004/aug/aug26a_04.html. The press release says: "GSK conducted at least five studies on the use of Paxil in children and adolescents but only released one of these studies, which showed mixed results on efficacy. The lawsuit alleged that the company suppressed the negative results of the other studies, which failed to demonstrate that Paxil is effective and which suggested a possible increased risk of suicidal thinking and acts in certain individuals."

195 Where drug manufacturing was once: Vince Parry, "The Art of Condition Branding," *Medical Marketing & Media*, May 2003, 42–49.

196 Take Viagra: Ibid.

196 In *Better than Well*: Carl Elliott, *Better than Well: American Medicine Meets the American Dream* (New York: W. W. Norton & Company, 2003).

198 It was his dream: Centers for Medicare and Medicaid Services, http://www.cms.hhs.gov/charts/healthcaresystem/chapter1.pdf.

199 It's hard to imagine: J. Coe, "The Lifestyle Drugs Outlook to 2008: Unlocking New Value in Well-being," Datamonitor, *Reuters Business Insight*, Healthcare, PLC, 2003, pp. 42–3. Quoted in Moynihan and Cassels, *Selling Sickness*, xii and 179.

199 Now there are triple-wide: Deborah Baldwin, "Medicine Cabinets: Walk Right In," *New York Times*, March 18, 2004.

200 On the surface: Barnett Kramer, National Cancer Institute, personal communication, 1999, 2004; Shannon Brownlee, "Perils of Prevention," *New York Times Magazine*, March 16, 2003; Shannon Brownlee, "Unkind Cuts," *The New Republic*, March 12, 1999.

203 But there's not a single: John Abramson, *Overdo$ed America: The Broken Promise of American Medicine* (New York: HarperCollins, 2004): 210–20.

204 For whatever reason: Peter Rothwell, neurologist, Radcliffe Infirmary, Oxford, U.K., personal communication, January 2003; Jean-Louis Mas et al., "Endarterectomy Versus Stenting in Patients with Severe Symptomatic Carotid Stenosis," *New England Journal of Medicine* 355, no. 16 (2006): 1660–71.

205 James Goodwin: James S. Goodwin, "Geriatrics and the Limits of Modern Medicine," *New England Journal of Medicine* 340, no. 16 (1999): 1283–85.

207 A former geriatrician: R. Sean Morrison, Diane E. Meier, and Christine K. Cassel, "When Too Much Is Too Little," *New England Journal of Medicine* 335, no. 23 (1996): 1755–59.

Chapter 8: Money, Drugs, and Lies

210 The company had recently published: Claire Bombardier et al., "Comparison of Upper Gastrointestinal Toxicity of Rofecoxib and Naproxen in Patients with Rheumatoid Arthritis," *New England Journal of Medicine* 343, no. 21 (2000): 1520–28.

210 In parallel campaigns: "Offensive Position for Vioxx," July 28, 2000; "Bulletin for Vioxx: New Obstacle Response," May 1, 2000; "Bulletin for Vioxx," April 20, 2001; Representative Henry A. Waxman "Memorandum to Democratic Members of the Government Reform Committee," May 5, 2005, http://over sight.house.gov/documents/20050505114932-41272.pdf.

211 By the time new data: Bruce M. Psaty and Curt D. Furberg, "COX-2 Inhibitors—Lessons in Drug Safety," *New England Journal of Medicine* 352, no. 11 (2005): 1133–35.

211 Food and Drug Administration safety: David J. Graham et al., "Risk of Acute Myocardial Infarction and Sudden Cardiac Death in Patients Treated with Cyclooxygenase 2 Selective and Non-selective Non-steroidal Anti-inflammatory Drugs: Nested Case-control Study." *Lancet* 365, no. 9458 (2005): 475–81; Jeanne Lenzer, "FDA is Incapable of Protecting US 'Against Another Vioxx,'" *British Medical Journal* 329, no. 7477 (2004): 1253; see also David J. Graham, testimony before Senate Finance Committee, November 18, 2004, http://www.senate .gov/~finance/hearings/testimony/2004test/111804dgtest.pdf.

212 The pharmaceutical industry itself: Marcia Angell, *The Truth About the Drug Companies: How They Decieve Us and What to Do About It* (New York: Random House, 2004).

212 In his essay: Malcolm Gladwell, "High Prices: How to Think About Prescription Drugs," *New Yorker*, October 25, 2004.

214 As a soldier in Pfizer's army: See, for example, Daniel Morelli and Marlon R. Koenigsberg, "Sample Medication Dispensing in a Residency Practice," *Journal of Family Practice* 34, no. 1 (1992): 42–48.

215 In an alarming yet funny: Carl Elliott, "The Drug Pushers," *Atlantic Monthly*, April 2006.

216 But the research says otherwise: See, for example, Howard Brody, "The Company We Keep: Why Physicians Should Refuse to See Pharmaceutical Representatives," *Annals of Family Medicine* 3 (2005): 82–85; J. P. Orlowski and L. Wateska, "The Effects of Pharmaceutical Firm Enticements on Physician Prescribing Patterns. There's No Such Thing as a Free Lunch," *Chest* 102 (1992): 270–273; Ashley Wazana, "Physicians and the Pharmaceutical Industry: Is a Gift Ever Just a Gift?," *Journal of the American Medical Association* 283, no. 3 (2000): 373–380; Jerry Avorn et al., "Scientific Versus Commercial Sources of Influence on the Prescribing Behavior of Physicians," *American Journal of Medicine* 73 (1982): 4–8.

217 In an essay: D. Katz, A. L. Caplan, and J. F. Merz, "All Gifts Large and Small: Toward an Understanding of the Ethics of Pharmaceutical Industry Gift-giving," *American Journal of Bioethics* 3, no. 3 (2003): 39–46.

217 In the same way: Michael Oldani, "Thick Prescriptions: Toward an Interpretation of Pharmaceutical Sales Practices," unpublished manuscript.

218 In 1992, under pressure: Melody Petersen, "Doctor Explains Why He Blew the Whistle," *New York Times*, March 11, 2003.

221 Thought leaders are also: Maggie Mahar, *Money-Driven Medicine: The Real Reason Health Care Costs So Much* (New York: HarperCollins, 2006).

222 Today, a third of academic clinicians: Jennifer Washburn, *University Inc: The Corporate Corruption of Higher Education* (New York: Perseus Books 2005).

224 So how did Wyeth manage: Carl Elliott, "Pharma Goes to the Laundry: Public Relations and the Business of Medical Education," *Hastings Center Report* 34, no. 5 (2004): 18–23; Matthew Kaufman and Andrew Julien, "Scientists Helped Industry to Push Diet Drug," *Hartford Courant*, April 10, 2000; Alicia Mundy, *Dispensing with the Truth: The Victims, the Drug Companies, and the Dramatic Story Behind the Battle Over Fen-Phen* (New York: St. Martin's/Griffin, 2002) 81, 121–25.

225 In a subsequent editorial: Marcia Angell and Jerome Kassirer, "Editorials and Conflicts of Interest," *New England Journal of Medicine* 335, no. 14 (1996): 1055–56.

225 Later, Manson and Faich: JoAnn Manson and Gerald Faich, "Conflict of Interest: Editorialists Respond," *New England Journal of Medicine* 335, no. 14 (1996): 1064–65.

226 The article discussed: Garret A. Fitzgerald and Carlo Patrono, "The Coxibs, Selective Inhibitors of Cyclooxygenase-2," *New England Journal of Medicine* 345, no. 6 (2001): 433–42; John Abramson, *Overdo$ed America: The Broken Promise of American Medicine* (New York: HarperCollins, 2004).

227 The discrepancies that Abramson: Gladwell, "High Prices: How to Think About Prescription Drugs."

228 This situation has only: Drummond Rennie, "Thyroid Storm," *Journal of the American Medical Association* 277, no. 15 (1997): 1238–43; Thomas Bodenheimer, "Uneasy Alliance—Clinical Investigators and the Pharmaceutical Industry," *New England Journal of Medicine* 342, no. 20 (2000): 1539–44; J. E. Bekelman, Y. Li, and C. P. Gross, "Scope and Impact of Financial Conflicts of Interest in Biomedical Research: A Systematic Review," *Journal of the American Medical Association* 289, no. 4 (2003): 454–65; H. T. Stelfox, G. Chua, K. O'Rourke, and A. S. Detsky, "Conflict of Interest in the Debate over Calcium-channel Antagonists," *New England Journal of Medicine* 338, no. 2 (1998): 101–6.

228 In the view of Richard Horton: Richard Horton, "The Dawn of McScience," *New York Review of Books*, March 11, 2004; Washburn, *University Inc.*

228 In a hilarious spoof: David L. Sackett and Andrew D. Oxman "HARLOT plc: An Amalgamation of the World's Two Oldest Professions," *British Medical Journal* 327, no. 7429 (2003): 1442–45.

229 What's not so funny: S. Heres et al., "Why Olanzapine Beats Risperidone, Risperidone Beats Quetiapine, and Quetiapine Beats Olanzapine," *American Journal of Psychiatry* 163, no. 9 (2006): 185–94.

230 All of this might be laughable: PharmaReports, "Novel Antipsychotics Driving Market Evolution," http://www.leaddiscovery.co.uk/reports/Antipsychotics%20-%20Novel%20Antipsychotics%20Driving%20Market%20Evolution.html.

230 But in 2006, a study: "NIMH Study to Guide Treatment Choice for Schizophrenia," press release from the National Institute of Mental Health, September 19, 2005.

230 This pattern repeats: Carol Tamminga, "Practical Treatment Information for Schizophrenia," *American Journal of Psychiatry* 163, no. 4 (2006): 563–65.

231 "Although M.D.'s like objective": Alex Berenson, "Eli Lilly Said to Play Down Risk of Top Pill," *New York Times*, December 17, 2006.

231 As of January 15: Tom Zeller, "Documents Borne by Winds of Free Speech," *New York Times*, January 15, 2007.

233 Only when all the pieces: Elliott, "Pharma Goes to the Laundry," 18–23.

236 The second problem is that: Mahar, *Money-Driven Medicine*, 285–324.

Chapter 9: The Doctor Isn't In

238 Gordon Peabody: This chapter is based on extensive interviews with several primary care physicians, including Gordon Peabody (not his real name). Also interviewed: Paul B. Ginzburg, Center for Health Systems Change; Dr. Fitzhugh Mullen, editor, *Health Affairs*.

240 Embraced by employers: For an excellent primer on managed care, see Paul Starr, *The Social Transformation of American Medicine* (New York: Basic Books, 1982); Cara S. Lesser, Paul B. Ginsburg, and Kelly J. Devers, "The End of an Era: What Became of the 'Managed Care Revolution' in 2001?," *Health Services Research* 38, no. 1 (2003): 337–55.

242 By 1980, there were nearly: Derek R Smart, *Physician Characteristics and Distribution in the US*, 2007 Edition, (Chicago: American Medical Association, 2007), 326.

243 At staff-model HMOs: Frances C. Cunningham and John W. Williamson, "How Does the Quality of Health Care in HMOs Compare to That in Other Settings? An Analytical Review: 1958–1979," *Group Health Journal* 1, no.1 (1980): 4–25.

243 Yet traditional HMOs had: Richard Harris, "Annals of Legislation," Part 1–4, *New Yorker*, July 2, 9, 16, and 22, 1966.

243 By 1970, there were only: Michael Millenson, *Demanding Medical Excellence: Doctors and Accountability in the Information Age* (Chicago: University of Chicago Press, 1999).

243 A little more than a decade: Mimi Swartz, "Not What the Doctor Ordered," *Texas Monthly*, March 1995.

245 Over the course of a decade: Pamela Moore, "Dividing Overhead and Keeping the Peace" *Physician's Practice*, September/October 2002.

245 Doctors, notes Guy Clifton: Guy L. Clifton, "No Health Care Reform Without Cost Containment," unpublished manuscript.

247 In 1985: Alvin R. Tarlov, "HMO Enrollment Growth and Physicians: The Third Compartment" *Health Affairs* 5, no. 1 (1986): 23–35; Millenson, *Demanding Medical Excellence*, 301–309.

247 Capitation worked best: Millenson, "Growing Pains Afflict HMOs," *Chicago Tribune*, June 16, 1987.

248 Wall Street only added: For a history of the commercialization of medicine, see Donald L. Barlett and James B. Steele's excellent *Critical Condition: How Health Care in America Became Big Business and Bad Medicine* (New York: Doubleday, 2004).

250 In 1995, average income: Thomas Bodenheimer, Robert A. Berenson, Paul Rudolf, "The Primary Care–Specialty Income Gap: Why It Matters," *Annals of Internal Medicine* 146, no. 4 (2007): 301–6.

250 Eventually the press: Millenson, *Demanding Medical Excellence*; Millenson, "Health-Care Debate Rages; Cost-Paring: Good Business or Bad Medicine?" *Chicago Tribune*, June 14, 1987; Millenson, "Growing Pains Afflict HMOs."

256 Doctors had other ways: Hoangmai H. Pham et al., "Financial Pressures Spur Physician Entrepreneurialism," *Health Affairs* 23, no. 2 (2004): 70–81.

258 "Doctors never bought": Robert J. Blendon, personal communication; see also Robert J. Blendon et al., "Understanding the Managed Care Backlash," *Health Affairs* 17, no. 4 (1998): 80–94.

259 In a recent report: American College of Physicians, "State of the Nation's HealthCare: A Report from the American College of Physicians," January 30, 2006; see also "Creating a New National Workforce for Internal Medicine: Recommendations of the American College of Physicians," April 2006, http://news.acponline.org/college/pressroom/as06/workforce_paper.pdf.

259 In 1949, 59 percent: New York Chapter, American College of Physicians, "The Future of Primary Care: A Report on Primary Care Medicine in New York State," November 2006, http://www.acponline.org/chapters/ny/future_primary.pdf.

259 Ten years later, 21 percent: Bodenheimer et al., "The Primary Care–Specialty Income Gap"; see also Bodenheimer, "Primary Care—Will it Survive?," *New England Journal of Medicine* 355, no. 9 (2006): 861–63.

260 Americans will usually pay: Lisa Sanders, "The End of Primary Care," *New York Times Magazine*, April 18, 2004; see also Abigail Zuger, "For a Retainer, Lavish Care by 'Boutique Doctors,' " *New York Times Magazine*, October 30, 2005.

261 Two ingredients are necessary: Kerr White, "The Ecology of Medical Care: Origins and Implications for Population-based Healthcare," *Health Services Research* 32, no. 1 (1997): 11–21.

261 The second ingredient: See Jerome Groopman, *How Doctors Think* (Boston: Houghton Mifflin, 2007), for an excellent overview of how doctors make diagnoses, and a description of Roter and Hall's work on pages 13–16.

262 Cyndra Mogayzel: Cyndra Mogayzel, personal communication, May and November, 2006.

264 While the family practitioner's status: See, for example, Barbara Starfield, Leiyu Shi, and James Macinko, "Contribution of Primary Care to Health Systems and Health," *Milbank Quarterly* 83, no. 3 (2005): 457–502.

264 In one recent *Consumer Reports*: Buzz McClain, "Tell Me Where it Hurts: Poll: Doctors and Patients Often Let Each Other Down," *Washington Post*, February 6, 2007.

Chapter 10: Less Is More

267 This thought experiment: Norman Daniels, *Just Health Care* (Cambridge, U.K.: Cambridge University Press, 1985).

269 The VHA's prescription accuracy: Catherine Arnst, "The Best Medical Care in the U.S.: How Veterans Affairs Transformed Itself—and What It Means for the Rest of Us," *BusinessWeek*, July 17, 2006; see also D. J. Ringold, J. P. Santell, and P. J. Schneider, "ASHP National Survey of Pharmacy Practice in Acute Care Settings: Dispensing and Administration—1999," *American Journal of Health-System Pharmacy* 57, no. 19 (2000): 1759–75.

269 According to a RAND Corporation study: Steven M. Asch et al., "Comparison of Quality of Care for Patients in the Veterans Health Administration and Patients in a National Sample," *Annals of Internal Medicine* 141, no. 12 (2004): 938–45; see also Elizabeth A. McGlynn et al., "The Quality of Healthcare Delivered to Adults in the United States," *New England Journal of Medicine* 348, no. 26 (2003): 2635–45.

270 Raymond B. Roemer: Arnst, "The Best Medical Care in the U.S."

270 The VHA manages: Phillip Longman, "The Best Care Anywhere," *Washington Monthly*, January 1, 2005; see also Veterans Administration statistics at http://www.va.gov/vetdata/ProgramStatics/stat_app99/table_11.xls; http://www.va.gov/vetdata/ProgramStatics/stat_app02/Table%2010%20(02).xls; http://www.cms.hhs.gov/NationalHealthExpendData/downloads/tables.pdf.

271 At the same time: William Safire, "Most Sacred Cow," *New York Times*, January 12, 1995.

271 President Bill Clinton signed: The Library of Congress Veterans' Health Care Eligibility Reform Act of 1996, http://www.presidency.ucsb.edu/ws/index.php?pid=52074.

276 That's because every individual: Carol. M. Ashton et al., "Hospital Use and Survival among Veterans Affairs Beneficiaries," *New England Journal of Medicine* 349, no. 17 (2003): 1637–46.

276 In 2003, in a paper: Ashish K. Jha et al., "Effect of the Transformation of the

Veterans Affairs Health Care System on the Quality of Care," *New England Journal of Medicine* 348, no. 22 (2003): 2218–27.

278 How often does all: The First National Report Card on Quality of Health Care in America, http://www.rand.org/pubs/research_briefs/RB9053-2/; see also Jane E. B. Reusch, "Diabetes, Microvascular Complications, and Cardiovascular Complications: What Is It about Glucose?," *Journal of Clinical Investigation* 112 (2003): 986–88.

279 Doctors and hospitals don't neglect: Gina Kolata, "Health Plan That Cuts Costs Raises Doctors' Ire," *New York Times*, August 11, 2004; Carolyn Nielson, "Helping Chronically Ill Manage Care Improves Lives, Cuts Costs: 'Pursuing Perfection' Program Is so Simple, It's Brilliant," *Bellingham Herald*, July 14, 2003; and Pursuing Perfection in Whatcom County (WWPP), http://www.hinet.org/chic/PursuingPerfectionWeb/.

280 But Pursuing Perfection is killing: Jack Homer et al., "Models for Collaboration: How System Dynamics Helped a Community Organize Cost-effective Care for Chronic Illness," *Systems Dynamics Review* 20, no. 3 (2004) 199–222 ; see also Kolata, "Health Plan That Cuts Costs Raises Doctors' Ire."

280 Medicare officials are: Performance measures and P4P pitfalls described at http://www.delfini.org/page_Publication_PerformanceMeasures.htm.

281 Medicare is also test-driving: Hoangmai H. Pham, Center for Studying Health System Change, personal communication.

283 At Garfield Medical Center: John E. Wennberg, unpublished manuscript; see also Wennberg et al., "California Hospitals," *Health Affairs*, November 16, 2005, Web exclusive, http://www.healthaffairs.org.

286 Fewer than 10 percent of hospitals: Ceci Connolly, "Cedars-Sinai Doctors Cling to Pen and Paper," *Washington Post*, March 21, 2005.

287 The solution to this problem: Elliott S. Fisher et al., "Creating Accountable Care Organizations: The Extended Hospital Medical Staff," *Health Affairs*, December 5, 2006, Web exclusive, http://www.healthaffairs.org.

289 There are three ways: Denis Cortese and Robert Smoldt, "Taking Steps Toward Integration," *Health Affairs*, December 5, 2006, Web exclusive, http://www.healthaffairs.org.

289 If every hospital in America: Megan McAndrew and Kristen Bronner, "The Care of Patients with Severe Chronic Illness: An Online Report on the Medicare Program," The Dartmouth Atlas of Health Care, 2006.

292 The Institute of Medicine estimates: Marilyn J. Field and Kathleen N. Lohr, eds., *Guidelines for Clinical Practice: From Development to Use* (Washington: National Academies Press, 1992).

293 The AHCPR's troubles: Richard A. Deyo and Donald L. Patrick, *Hope or Hype: The Obsession with Medical Advances and the High Cost of False Promises* (New York: Amacom, 2005).

294 The number of spinal fusions: AHRQ Web site HCUPnet tool used to calculate the percentage increase, based on hospital discharge data in 1997 and 2004, http://hcupnet.ahrq.gov/HCUPnet.jsp?Id=238CB6D4E63F3E88&Form=SelALL LISTED&JS=Y&Action=%3E%3ENext%3E%3E&_ALLLISTED=No.

294 Drug companies enjoy margins: Maggie Mahar, *Money-Driven Medicine: The Real Reason Health Care Costs So Much* (New York: HarperCollins, 2006), 285–293; For- tune 500, April 17, 2006, http://money.cnn.com/magazines/fortune/fortune 500/performers/industries/return_on_revenues/index.html; Kaiser Family Foundation, "Profitability among Pharmaceutical Manufacturers Compared to Other Industries, 1995–2004," http://www.kff.org/insurance/7031/ti 2004-1-21.cfm.

295 In order for the AHRQ: AHRQ Web site, "Budget Estimates for Appropria- tions Committees, Fiscal Year 2008," http://www.ahrq.gov/about/cj2008/ cjweb08.htm, see page 9.

297 Strengthening the patient's role: Annette M. O'Connor et al., "Towards the Tip- ping Point: Accelerating the Diffusion of Decision Aids that Help Patients to Weigh Benefits Versus Risks," unpublished manuscript; see also O'Connor et al., "Decision Aids for People Facing Health Treatment or Screening Deci- sions," Cochrane Review, in *The Cochrane Library*, Issue 4 (Chichester, U.K.: John Wiley and Sons Ltd. 2006), http://cochrane.org/reviews/en/ab001431.html.

298 Getting decision aids: Jaime Staples King and Benjamin W. Moutlon, "Rethink- ing Informed Consent: The Case for Shared Medical Decision-Making," *Ameri- can Journal of Law and Medicine* 32 (2006): 429–501.

299 This was evident: For an excellent discussion of all cancer screening tests, see H. Gilbert Welch, *Should I Be Tested for Cancer? Maybe Not and Here's Why* (Berkeley: University of California Press 2006).

299 But most discussions of malpractice: Decision aids are available from such commercial sources as Health Dialog; at several medical centers including Dartmouth-Hitchcock Medical Center and the Mayo Clinic; and clearing- houses located at the National Cancer Institute and U.S. Centers for Disease Control and Prevention. For an inventory of decision aids and a review by the Cochrane Collaboration, see Ottawa Health Research Institute, "A–Z Inventory of Decision Aids," decisionaid.ohri.ca/AZinvent.php.

INDEX

note: page references followed by n refer to footnotes.

A NOTE ON THE AUTHOR

Shannon Brownlee is an award-winning journalist whose stories and essays about medicine, health care, and biotechnology have appeared in such publications as the *Atlantic Monthly*, the *New York Times Magazine*, the *New Republic*, and *Time*. Her work has been featured in *The Real State of the Union*, a collection of the best policy analyses from the *Atlantic*'s "Real State of the Union" series, and in *The New Science Journalists*, a collection of the best science writing. Born and raised in Honolulu, Hawaii, she holds a master's degree in biology from the University of California, Santa Cruz. She is a Schwartz Senior Fellow at the New America Foundation, in Washington, D.C. Brownlee lives in Annapolis, Maryland, with her husband and son.